SIMONA MORINI'S ENCYCLOPEDIA OF HEALTH AND BEAUTY

By the same author:
BODY SCULPTURE

SIMONA
MORINI'S

THE BOBBS-MERRILL COMPANY, INC.

ENCYCLOPEDIA OF HEALTH AND BEAUTY

BY SIMONA MORINI

ILLUSTRATIONS BY CAROL DONNER

INDIANAPOLIS/NEW YORK

Published by the Bobbs-Merrill Company, Inc.
Indianapolis   New York

Designed by Jacques Chazaud
Manufactured in the United States of America

First printing

LIBRARY OF CONGRESS CATALOGING IN PUBLICATION DATA

Morini, Simona, 1932–
   Simona Morini's Encyclopedia of health and beauty.

   Includes index.
   1. Beauty, Personal—Dictionaries.   2. Women—
Health and hygiene—Dictionaries.   I. Title.
II. Title: Encyclopedia of health and beauty.
RA778.M766   646.7′2′024042   75–6403
ISBN 0–672–51913–5

With special thanks to:

Dr. John McCredie, general surgeon,
Department of Surgery, Victoria Hospital, London, Ontario;

Dr. Ann C. Hill, dermatologist,
Cornell University Medical School-New York Hospital;

Alfred F. Zobel, director of communications,
Hoffmann-La Roche, Inc., Nutley, New Jersey;

for reviewing and checking the manuscript for accuracy.

ABORTION

On January 22, 1973, the United States Supreme Court overturned the superconservative attitude of most states toward abortion. The court stated that no longer can a state interfere with a woman's right to have an abortion within the first three months of pregnancy. During the second and third trimesters, the states can interfere only to see that procedures conform to safe medical practice. Only in the final trimester of pregnancy do the states have the authority to prohibit abortion altogether, and then only when there is no threat to the mother's life or health, including mental health.

This doesn't mean that the controversy over abortion has been settled once and for all. There are many countries where abortion laws have not yet been liberalized, and even in the United States powerful groups opposing abortion are still actively trying to reverse legislation. What makes the matter even more confused is the fact that birth control methods which work *after* conception have blurred the traditional legal distinction between abortion and contraception.

Laws against abortion are the product of an age that could not foresee the more recent contraceptive chemicals and techniques. These laws are no longer answerable to the ambiguities created by medical progress because they do not deal with scientific reality. Most abortion laws are based on the postulate that pregnancy begins at the time of conception, while the scientific opinion is that pregnancy begins after nidation, the implantation of the fertilized OVUM in the uterus. The introduction of the INTRAUTERINE DEVICE and the MORNING-AFTER PILL, however, blurred the distinction between contraception and abortion, for both allow conception but prevent nidation. And should PROSTAGLANDINS become used widely as a MENSTRUATION-inducing contraceptive, the distinction will become even more vague.

Ideally, an abortion should be performed by a gynecologist, because, for one, some of the preferred techniques are blind surgical procedures; that is, the surgeon does not actually see the uterus, a structure with which few physicians have much experience.

The choice of ANAESTHESIA depends on the patient's health, on whether she suffers, for instance, from diabetes, an ALLERGY, HYPERTENSION, or has had a Caesarian section. It also depends on her psychological stability. A *local* anaesthetic is often enough for a resolute, healthy woman; however, some doctors prefer *general* anaesthesia on principle. In the opinion of Dr. Albert Altchek, associate professor of obstetrics and gynecology at Mount Sinai School of Medicine in New York, "General anaesthesia puts all the guilt on the operator," while a frightened, remorseful woman under a local anaesthetic "may feel a partner to the 'crime.' "

There are four abortion techniques: dilatation and curettage (commonly referred to as D&C); suction (or vacuum aspiration); saline injection (or salting-out); and prostaglandins.

The first two procedures are called "early" abortions because they are performed within the first twelve weeks of gestation—twelve weeks from the first day of the last menstruation. The third and fourth are "late" abortions. At present the saline injection is the best choice for women who are at least sixteen weeks pregnant; prostaglandin injections are still experimental.

An early abortion is undoubtedly the easier and the safer of the two to perform; the risk rate of a late abortion is at least four times higher. However, many women are not able, for a variety of reasons, to have an early abortion. Thus, once the twelve-week limit has passed, the doctor has to decide whether to advise the patient to wait through the so-called interim period (between the thirteenth and the fifteenth week) or whether it is still safe to perform one of the early abortions. Many gynecologists prefer to wait.

Dilatation and Curettage—A procedure used by gynecologists not only to induce abortion but also to treat miscarriage and for diagnostic purposes in nonpregnant women. The physician carefully examines the patient to determine the size, contour, and position of the uterus. The opening of the cervix, the neck of the uterus, is gradually stretched until it is wide enough to accept a curette, a rod-shaped instrument with a sort of sharp-edged spoon on the end. The doctor inserts the curette into the uterus and gently scrapes the walls.

Suction—This is the best technique for a woman with a small, rigid uterus, a tight cervix, and a long, narrow VAGINA. Here, too, the cervix is dilated, but less than in the D&C. A slender hollow tube, called a suction hose, is inserted into the uterus. The hose usually is made of clear sterile plastic, with a swivel connection in the hollow handle and a hole that can be opened or closed by a plastic ring to release or transmit suction. The hose is connected to a small vacuum pump, and a gentle suction empties the uterus. This is usually followed by a final cleanup with a small curette.

Both D&C and Suction last about ten minutes.

Saline Injection—With a long hypodermic needle inserted into the uterus through the abdomen, the physician removes most of the fluid from the amniotic sac (in which the fetus is developing) and replaces it with a solution of salt and water. Some time later—the waiting period lasts from five hours to two days—the uterus begins to contract, as in labor. Contractions continue until the uterus expels the fetus. The reason why the saline injection should not be performed before the sixteenth week is that before this time the amniotic sac may not be large enough for the doctor to locate easily.

Prostaglandins—Recently the FDA has approved for late abortions the injection of some of these hormonelike substances—among the most powerful of all biological materials—which occur naturally in the body and which only recently have been synthetized by inexpensive processes. During some early research, prostaglandins were found useful for inducing labor. Later, it was discovered that prostaglandins brought about expulsion of the product of conception at *any stage* of pregnancy.

When it is too late for a D&C and too early for a saline injection, 15 to 25 mg of the prostaglandin PGF_2 can be injected instead into the amniotic cavity, without having first to remove the amniotic fluid.

After a successful abortion, a woman should expect a few cramps and a certain amount of weakness as aftereffects of anaesthesia and psychological reaction. Bleeding should not be heavier than that of a menstrual period.

ABRASION

Abrasion is the scraping or rubbing off of the most superficial layers of cells from an area of the skin or the mucous membrane.

ACEROLA

Acerolas, also called Barbados cherries, are slightly acid berries that grow in shrubs in the West Indies. Acerola is a rich source of VITAMIN C and is sometimes used in "natural" vitamin preparations.

ACNE

Acne is one of the most common, but by no means the least serious, of skin diseases. It is a result of the inflammatory changes on the so-called pilosebaceous unit—any oil gland in the skin that opens into a hair FOLLICLE.

Young people between the age of puberty and their early twenties are most susceptible to acne. Adolescence is the time when the whole body undergoes extraordinary physical changes—when sex HORMONES, for instance, initiate the sebaceous glands' development.

Adults, too, may have acne: cortisone therapy, for instance, used in treating certain illnesses, may cause acnelike eruptions in some patients. Also, in a few women, CONTRACEPTIVE PILLS cause, or aggravate, acne. Still, the fact that castrated people never suffer from acne—unless they receive androgen (male sex hormone) therapy—confirms the theory that acne is related to the activity of hormones, although there is no explanation yet as to why not all adolescents have acne, and why only a portion of those who do have scars, regardless of the severity of the acne. All we know for the moment is that some people are genetically susceptible to acne and/or to scarring.

The function of sebaceous glands is to send up to the surface of the skin a small amount of sebum (oil) to soften and protect the skin. If stimulated by a disproportionate amount of sebum, the fatty acids contained in the sebum collect on the skin and deep within the follicles, causing their walls to thicken and shed particles that mix with the fatty acids. This forms a waxy plug called a comedo which obstructs the normal passage of sebum to the surface. Open comedones are usually called blackheads; closed sebum-containing comedones underneath the skin are called whiteheads, or milia.

Often, the pressure of the comedo causes the follicle to break, allowing sebum and some fatty acids to filtrate into the surrounding tissue, which, apparently because of the intensely irritating action of the fatty acids, becomes inflamed. The result is a papule or pimple. Sometimes pus forms as part of the body's defense mechanism against infection, and the papule turns into a pustule. The following stage is an accumulation of pustules, some of which—especially the milia—may turn into CYSTS.

Acne with comedones and pustules is called acne vulgaris; when deep cysts are involved, it is called acne conglobata. People with acne usually have only one type or the other, but sometimes both are present.

Scars appear when the inflammation is allowed to spread to the skin's deeper layer, the dermis, which does not regenerate as does the epidermis, the superficial layer. Once the follicle is broken, the original tissue will be replaced by scar tissue.

There are no *cures*, but excellent treatments for acne are available. Basically, acne therapy consists of drying and "peeling" the skin so that the comedones will loosen, allowing sebum to move to the surface, and of preventing inflammation from developing and deepening. However, acne therapy depends, more than most other treatments, on the patient's unique hormonal and immunological response, on his cooperation, and on the doctor's understanding of his specific problems.

There is a wide choice of methods available for treating acne, and a dermatologist may use several of them in proper sequence. First, he may apply SOAPS and CLEANSERS with added sulfur or abrasives, such as pumice or aluminum oxide particles, which are designed to loosen comedones, to remove the film of oil that spreads over the skin surface, and to reduce bacteria. Deeper comedones are removed with an extractor. Milia must be punctured, after first being covered with an antibiotic cream. Cysts can be treated with injections of cortisone, or with ANTIBIOTICS such as tetracycline—500 to 1000 mg a day, depending on the severity of the acne, and a reduced prescription of 250 mg a day as soon as the acne improves, continuing until it disappears. Improvement may take some time, because antibiotics affect *developing* rather than *existing* lesions. Antibiotics seem to work independently of their ability to suppress bacteria: they have the ability here to diminish the concentration of fatty acids in the sebum. Occasionally women taking these drugs develop vaginitis, which should be treated immediately.

The use of ultraviolet rays from a quartz lamp is a popular treatment. The dose must be high enough to produce a slight reddening of the skin, but the eyes should be shielded, and exposure timed carefully and increased gradually to allow the skin to become used to the rays.

Estrogen and progesterone have been used, alone or in combination, to counteract the hormonal mechanism probably responsible for the development of acne. Some doctors simply prescribe contraceptive pills to treat women with acne. Estrogen does indeed reduce sebum flow, but some feel that the dose needed is too high for the drug to be effective for men; in women, estrogen has been known to produce a number of side effects.

Recently cryotherapy (use of extremely cold temperature) has been quite successful in the treatment of superficial pustules and cysts. The pustules are daubed with a cotton applicator soaked in liquid nitrogen, which freezes them for three to five seconds. The skin reddens and small blisters form; these usually last for a few days. More recently, a liquid nitrogen spray has been successfully tested.

Vitamin-A acid (or tretinoin), produced by oxidizing VITAMIN A, is excellent for the local treatment of acne because it accelerates the natural turnover of the epidermis, increases the skin's permeability, and is not toxic, even if inadvertently ingested. It is usually applied daily, one hour before bedtime. (Application in the morning would be futile, as ultraviolet rays inactivate vitamin-A acid.) With increased permeability, the skin becomes extremely though temporarily sensitive to other substances such as COSMETICS, PERFUMES and aftershave lotions, which may irritate and chap the skin for a few days. The acne begins to clear up about four or five weeks later, after a brief flare-up.

In at least one study, three out of two thousand dark-skinned patients noticed a gradual (and reversible) lightening of the skin after vitamin-A acid treatment. Another study, completed in 1969 by Dr. Albert M. Kligman of the University of Pennsylvania School of Medicine, is now a classic. It investigated the effects of chocolate on acne vulgaris. Dr. Kligman and his team discovered that chocolate—to this day emphatically forbidden to acne patients, and high on the list of such blacklisted delicacies as nuts, candy, shellfish, cheese and malted milk—has no influence on the composition or output of sebum. In fact, the study suggested that sebaceous glands are quite autonomous and that skin functions are hardly influenced by such things as the environment or, in this case, diets.

ACTINOTHERAPY

Actinotherapy means treatment of disease by rays of light, especially ultraviolet (actinic) light.

ACNE, for instance, often improves with exposure to ultraviolet rays, either from sunlight or from a sunlamp, because the light kills bacteria in the skin. Ultraviolet rays also have a drying and peeling effect on the skin's outer layer, thus opening an exit to plugged glands.

ACUPUNCTURE

Acupuncture is a method of therapy that has been used in China for centuries to treat disorders of the internal organs through stimulation by very fine, sharp, pliable needles inserted into the body at specific points called *loci*.

For more than three thousand years the therapeutic value of acupuncture has been recognized in the Orient, but it has become popular in this country only recently. And in spite of recent spectacular successes, modern Chinese physicians tend to avoid expressing any fanciful theories concerning acupuncture; they prefer to base their techniques on the empirical results of hundreds of years of research and observation.

Indeed, the underlying mechanism of acupuncture is still not

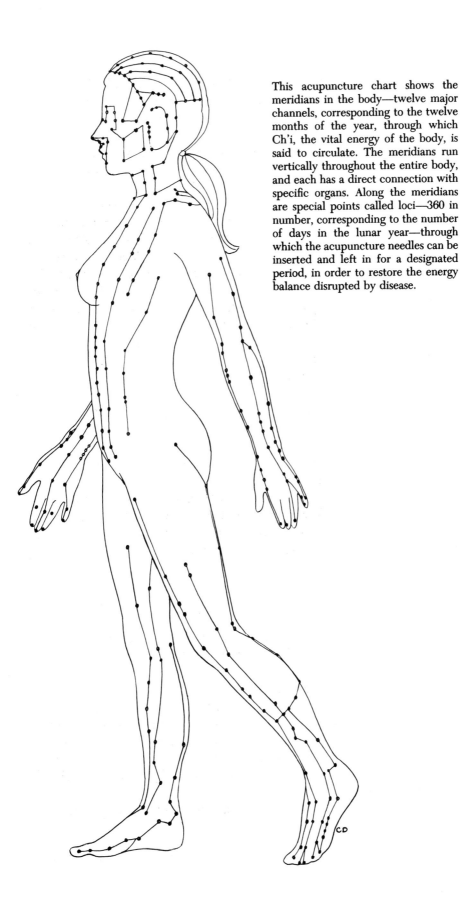

This acupuncture chart shows the meridians in the body—twelve major channels, corresponding to the twelve months of the year, through which Ch'i, the vital energy of the body, is said to circulate. The meridians run vertically throughout the entire body, and each has a direct connection with specific organs. Along the meridians are special points called loci—360 in number, corresponding to the number of days in the lunar year—through which the acupuncture needles can be inserted and left in for a designated period, in order to restore the energy balance disrupted by disease.

7

understood. The treatment does not restore destroyed tissue, eroded bones, or dislocated joints, but it has shown dramatic results with diseases of the nervous system, such as MIGRAINE and deafness, and with chronic diseases, such as BACKACHE, ARTHRITIS, ASTHMA, diabetes, ulcer, and INSOMNIA.

Acupuncture is based on the ancient Chinese philosophical concept of Ch'i, the vital energy of the body. If the flow of Ch'i is normal, the body is healthy; disease or pain results if the flow of Ch'i is impeded. Acupuncture is used to regulate the flow of Ch'i, and thereby cure disease or diminish pain.

Ch'i is a physical manifestation of the two opposing and complementing principles of Yin and Yang. Yin represents the *negative*—night, cold, dark, female, and the interior of the body. Yang is the *positive*—day, hot, light, male, and the exterior of the body. Yang actuates Yin, and Yin produces Yang; health is dependent on their harmonious balance.

Ch'i circulates through the twelve organs of the body along twelve major channels called *meridians,* which run vertically throughout the body and have a direct connection with every part of the body, thus furnishing the best access to the center of any disturbance. The loci, through which the needles can be inserted, are found along the meridians.

The loci are often far removed from the apparent source of discomfort and were probably first determined empirically. For instance, an ancient Chinese soldier might have been struck in the leg by an arrow, causing the stomach pain he had suffered all his life to disappear miraculously. Today, there are Chinese and American companies which manufacture electric devices that can actually determine where the various loci are. Experts disagree, however, over the number of loci in the body; some say 365, while others identify as many as 642. One of the tasks of the recently founded American Society of Chinese Medicine is to standardize the terminology and to distribute the loci on acupuncture charts.

Acupuncture as a form of ANAESTHESIA—allowing a patient to undergo an operation while completely conscious—was first used in China in 1958. For operations that either are very painful or last too long, acupuncture, used together with some other local anaesthetic and an appropriate painkiller, can reduce the danger or the various difficulties inherent in *general* anaesthesia. In these cases, it is important that the patient experience the so-called Teh Ch'i sensation: a feeling of soreness, swelling, and numbness that accompanies the insertion of the needles and is maintained throughout the operation by twirling the needles, either manually or electrically.

A supplement to acupuncture is moxibustion—the application to specific loci of small, combustible cones of dried leaves of wormwood, which are ignited and burned down to the skin until a blister forms.

Acupuncture has been practiced and taught in France since 1934; in England it has been practiced for at least ten years, and in the Soviet Union it has been taught in medical schools since 1959. In the United States, seminars and courses are being offered throughout the country, and several doctors are enthusiastically studying acupuncture techniques. However, there are many distinguished physicians who oppose acupuncture as "just rubbish." Others resort to it only when conventional treatments have failed. Some think that acupuncture works in China only because of the cultural factor of more than three thousand years of belief, and that a regimented society such as modern China can achieve a uniform behavior in the masses without their conscious cooperation. But in the West, they feel, acupuncture can only work for people who are also susceptible to hypnosis, or suffer from ailments that are psychosomatic in origin. However, it is now accepted that acupuncture does not require cooperation from the patient, for it is not a psychological phenomenon.

American medical authorities, alarmed by acupuncture's sudden popularity, have adopted a very cautious official attitude. They fear, for one, that acupuncture might become a perfect tool for quacks, who could claim they can treat cancer with it. Another concern is the influx of hundreds of foreign-trained acupuncturists—with or without professional degrees—into the United States. Already there have been reports of severe burns and scars following moxibustion, and of inexperienced acupuncturists piercing blood vessels or hollow organs with the needles.

Appropriate legislation to regulate the practice of acupuncture and the licensing of practitioners in this country is already under way. As of 1974, Arizona, California, the District of Columbia, Maine, Massachusetts, New York, Nevada, Oregon, Tennessee and Texas permit the use of acupuncture by a physician or by an acupuncturist under a physician's direct supervision, provided the patient's informed consent has been obtained.

AEROSOL

Aerosol, a generic term used in chemistry, refers to a suspension of microscopic liquid or solid particles in air or gas. The term was first coined in the early 1940s for space insecticides, but the system is now applied to the packaging of various drugs and such cosmetics as HAIR SPRAYS and dyes, DEODORANTS, shaving lather, PERFUMES and breath fresheners.

The principle on which an aerosol dispenser is built is relatively simple: all liquids exert pressure on the walls of any container in which they are placed. When a propellant (liquefied or compressed gas such as nitrogen or fluorocarbons) is sealed in a container together with a liquid, part of the liquid settles at the bottom and part of it vaporizes, rising to the top. The vaporized layer exerts pressure not only against the walls of the container but also on the liquid layer, forcing it through a tube to the opening of the valve. When the valve is released by pressing the button, the liquid is forced out for as long as the valve's orifice remains open and sufficient propellant is left inside the container.

The propellant, whose boiling point is usually far *below* room temperature, vaporizes almost instantly, producing a spray of liquid particles. If the spray is directed toward the hair or the skin, the propellant vaporizes *before* hitting the surface, leaving behind particles of the active ingredient.

For the packaging of two different ingredients, a two-compartment container has recently been devised, with a special dispensing mechanism that allows one substance to rise from its compartment and automatically mix with the other in the right proportions at the moment the valve is opened.

AFTERPAINS

As soon as a baby is born, the mother's uterus begins to shrink. During this reduction—or involution—the uterus undergoes contractions, called afterpains, that feel very much like menstrual cramps.

It usually takes about six weeks for the uterus to reduce gradually from about two pounds to about two ounces. Its muscles keep contracting during this time, as they did during pregnancy.

As the uterus becomes smaller, lochia, which consists of clots of blood and tissue, is eliminated from the body. Lochia gradually subsides, and by the end of the first week it has changed from bright to dark red, similar to menstrual blood.

Women who breastfeed their babies may notice afterpains more, since the sucking of a baby at the breast stimulates the contraction of the uterus.

Afterpains, despite their name, are not painful; at most they are slightly uncomfortable, and they certainly are welcome, as they mean that a woman's figure is returning to normal.

AGE RETARDATION

The mechanism of human aging is still little understood. For centuries man has accepted aging as the inevitable step following birth and growth, as the common fate of plants, animals, and human beings. And yet, prolonging life has been, and still is, man's most passionate dream. Though most of us are living longer than our ancestors—we now survive tuberculosis and pneumonia, childbirth infection and appendicitis, which used to be fatal—we still are within the original LIFESPAN of cavemen. However, for the first time scientists are seriously trying to do something about halting the human aging process.

There are presently two categories of *savants* active in this field: the *rejuvenators* and the *gerontologists*. The first category comprises a heterogeneous group of people (some are downright quacks, others have legitimate medical degrees) who aim to produce the classic elixir of youth. These modern rejuvenators differ from their ancient counterparts only in the ingredients used: HORMONES, ENZYMES, fresh animal cells, glands, VITAMINS, instead of powdered dragon teeth, nightingale tongues, and so forth.

Among the most famous "rejuvenating" centers are:

The clinic La Prairie, in Clarens-Montreux, Switzerland. Created by the late Dr. Paul Niehans, a Geneva physician, the clinic still offers to aging patients its famous injections of fresh cells selected from various organs of unborn lambs (corresponding to the ailing human organ the injection is meant for) and extracted from newly slaughtered pregnant sheep.

Renaissance Revitalization Spa, a combination of rejuvenating center and BEAUTY SPA, in Nassau, Bahamas, headed by Dr. Ivan M. Popov, a Yugoslavian physician. At Renaissance, too, cellular therapy is currently available. The only difference is that the compounds to be injected are prepared at the Medical Faculty of the University of Heidelberg, Germany, and shipped frozen to the Bahamas. Also available are incubated chicken embryos, which are administered either orally or as a rejuvenating facial cream.

The Institute of Geriatrics in Bucharest, Rumania, directed by Professor Ana Aslan, a Rumanian physician who twenty-five years ago discovered that one of the cheapest, mildest, easiest-to-synthetize ANAESTHETICS—procaine (better known by one of its brand names, Novocaine®)—has invigorating effects on humans. Ever since, she has been treating thousands of people suffering from a variety of physiological and psychic disorders usually connected with age but not unknown to youth: ARTHRITIS, HYPERTENSION, ulcers, DANDRUFF, nail problems, etc.

Dr. Aslan's original drug is called Gerovital H_3, a deceptively simple formula (which chemists in various countries have tried in vain to duplicate exactly) of procaine hydrochloride, benzoic acid, potassium metabisulphite and disodium phosphate.

Not that Dr. Aslan has been tried for sorcery, but for years she has been the subject of acrimonious rows in the medical world and even in the political world. But, by now, not only is she a national heroine in Rumania but at the beginning of 1974 she has finally been accepted by the skeptical American medical community. Gerovital may soon be available in America.

The Niehans cellular therapy has not been so lucky. Though both La Prairie and Renaissance seem to be highly successful, judging from their impressive lists of rich and internationally prominent patients, these clinics have no scientific status in the United States.

The gerontologists are in a different league, although they don't dismiss the rejuvenators' work, as the possibility of discovering an elixir of youth is not to be ruled out entirely. Gerontology is a relatively new discipline—about twenty years old—which is not yet and may never become a specialty, for it requires the knowledge and skills of a colossal team of specialists: biologists, biochemists, geneticists, embryologists, immunologists, sociologists, psychologists. Such interdisciplinary cooperation is necessary because there is no single self-evident process which explains or causes the aging of all living creatures. The secret of aging is probably locked inside the cells: any organism's life-span is most likely programmed in the genetic code, determined by the particular set of genes that the organism has inherited. Aging, it appears, is a combination of several phenomena, such as:

1) Accumulation of faultily reproducing, and imperfectly functioning, cells due to wear over a period of time;
2) Accumulation in certain cells of insoluble waste products of metabolism, which slowly poison the organism or interfere with its functions;
3) The organism's progressive inability to withstand the stress of the environment and the gradual disorganization of its organs *at different rates;*
4) The development of autoimmune reactions; i.e., the body's defense mechanism, which is meant to immunize it against invading germs and other antigens, becomes so inefficient with age that the body seems to react against and reject its own tissue.

The goal of gerontology is not so much to extend human life as either to slow down the period of growth or to prolong that of youthful maturity. Already the speed of aging has been slowed down in laboratory mice by reducing their intake of food (and thus of CALORIES), by lowering their body temperature, and by other manipulations of their metabolisms. The next step will be to see whether the same techniques can be used on human beings.

Among the most important centers of gerontological studies in this country are:

1) Duke University Center for the Study of Aging and Human Development;

2) Gerontology Research Center at the Baltimore City Hospitals in Maryland;

3) State University of New York's School of Medicine in Buffalo;

4) Albert Einstein College of Medicine in New York City;

5) Hillside Hospital on Long Island, New York.

ALCOHOL

Alcohol is the major chemical ingredient of wines, beers and distilled beverages. It is a natural substance formed by the reaction of fermenting sugar with yeast spores. Although there are many alcohols, the kind in alcoholic beverages is called ethyl alcohol, a colorless, inflammable liquid which has an intoxicating effect.

Alcohol has no nutritional value but is often classified as a food because it contains CALORIES. It is also classified as a drug, because it affects the central nervous system.

Different sources of sugar are used for the fermentation process for different alcoholic beverages. Wine, for example, is made from grapes or berries; beer from germinated barley; rum from molasses. Hard liquors, such as gin, scotch, vodka and whiskey, result from the further concentration of the alcohol produced by fermentation through a process called distillation.

The rapidity with which alcohol enters the bloodstream and affects the brain and body depends on:

1) *The kind of drink*—Hard liquors are absorbed faster than wine and beer, because the latter contain small amounts of nonalcoholic substances that slow down the absorption process. Diluting an alcoholic drink with WATER also helps to slow down absorption, but carbonated drinks may increase it.

2) *The rate of drinking*—Half an ounce of alcohol can be burned up in the body in about one hour; and if a person sips a drink slowly and doesn't have more than one drink an hour, the alcohol will not build up in the blood. But gulping a drink may well produce immediate intoxication.

3) *The state of the stomach*—Eating before, as well as with, a drink will slow down the absorption rate of alcohol in the blood.

4) *Body weight*—The same amount of alcohol has more effect on a slight than on a heavy person, and, in general, more on a woman than on a man. Alcohol is quickly distributed uniformly within the circulatory system; therefore, the heavy person has a smaller concentration of alcohol in his blood.

5) *The circumstances*—Drinking in a relaxed atmosphere while sitting comfortably will have less impact than drinking while standing.

13

When a person is emotionally upset, tired, or under stress, alcohol may have a stronger effect than normal.

When a person drinks an alcoholic beverage, 20 percent of the alcohol in it is immediately absorbed into the bloodstream through the stomach walls, without having to be digested first. The blood carries it directly to the brain, where it acts by slowing down brain activity. The other 80 percent is processed only slightly slower through the gastrointestinal tract and into the blood.

A low level of alcohol in the blood has a mild tranquilizing effect; however, at first, alcohol may act as a stimulant—a person may talk more freely, become aggressive. Higher alcohol levels in the blood depress brain activity to a point where memory, muscular coordination, and balance may be temporarily impaired. Still higher alcohol levels within a short period of time may produce loss of control and a severe reduction of sensory perception.

Alcoholism is a general term that covers many diseases, all of which have in common excessive drinking. Alcoholism seems to proceed through psychological dependence, progression, loss of control, adaptive metabolism, and, eventually, physical dependence. Chronic alcoholism, especially when combined with malnutrition, may result in cirrhosis, liver failure, heart failure, or permanent mental damage.

Alcoholism would be impossible without alcohol; however, alcohol is not the only cause: alcoholism is a consequence of a complex interaction of biological, psychological, and sociological factors. Scientists are still researching the multiple causes of alcoholism, such as genetic and biochemical abnormalities in the human body, poor nutrition, emotional problems, and environmental conditions.

ALLERGIC RHINITIS (HAY FEVER)

Hay fever is not a fever, and hay is only one of its many causes. A more accurate name for this condition is allergic rhinitis, which refers to an allergic reaction, chiefly involving the lining of the nose, due primarily to the seasonal inhalation of POLLENS.

Hay fever seasons vary in number, length, and time of the year, according to the weather and the kinds of plants found in the area. For instance, one major allergen, RAGWEED pollen, is the primary cause of fall hay fever in the Central states, while the Eastern states produce less ragweed; and there are places in the United States that are completely free of it.

Other allergens, such as dust, MOLDS, feathers, food, and animal DANDER, often combine to aggravate hay fever's symptoms; worse, they may cause symptoms that resemble those of hay fever but which

14

continue year round. This condition is called perennial allergic rhinitis.

Allergic rhinitis is not dangerous and does not cause permanent damage, but some of its complications can be troublesome. Sneezing, stuffed-up and runny nose, itching and swollen eyes, and infection of the sinuses are among hay fever's major symptoms.

The most serious complication of hay fever is bronchial ASTHMA, with such symptoms as spasms of coughing, difficulty in breathing, and wheezing. Asthma *is* serious if not kept under control.

Hay fever varies in kind and intensity from region to region and from person to person; only an allergy specialist can advise the best treatment for a specific case. As is usual with most allergens, avoidance is the best remedy. However, sometimes it is impossible to escape windborne pollens altogether, though of course there are more of these pollens in the country than in the city, and fewer near a large body of water.

The most effective treatment of hay fever consists of administering desensitized injections of the particular pollen's extract, beginning with minute doses which are gradually increased. The injections may be given during or just before the hay fever season, or all year round, depending on the allergist's diagnosis.

Antihistamines give temporary relief to milder cases, though it doesn't work for asthma, for which cortisone preparations seem more effective. Antihistamines, cortisone, and nasal drops and sprays all are powerful drugs and should never be used without a physician's directions.

ALLERGY

Allergy is a condition in which a person is made ill by a substance that is harmless to most others. When the allergic person touches, smells, breathes, eats, or is injected with one of the substances to which he is sensitive (allergens), he develops one or more abnormal reactions: itching, sneezing, wheezing, hives, migraine, asthma. In the worse cases, even shock and sudden collapse occur.

Allergies are perhaps the most elusive phenomenon in the human body: no two allergy patients are quite the same, no two are allergic to the same things, no two have identical symptoms under different circumstances, yet different allergies can have identical symptoms.

The tendency to develop allergies is usually inherited; however, they are not transmitted in a linear way. We still don't know what factors control their genetic transmission. For one, if a person inherited, let's say, the tendency to develop RAGWEED HAY FEVER, he may *never* develop hay fever if he is not exposed to ragweed. Also, the same substance may upset different parts of the body in different members of the same family. Some allergies develop before birth, others appear only late in life; often they spring up seemingly from nowhere, singly or in clusters, sometimes overlapping and reinforcing each other, only to disappear suddenly forever.

The causes of allergy are many, and the almost endless list of allergens is apparently growing—plastics, cosmetics, synthetic fabrics, food additives and preservatives, detergents, drugs, metals, pesticides, household gas, industrial fumes, even sperm . . . in addition to the traditional allergens, such as dust, pollen, mold, insect stings, animal fur, and food.

Allergic reactions don't always affect the same part of the body: the skin, the nose, the lungs, the stomach, the intestines, or the bladder can be disturbed by an allergic process. Even blood vessels can be affected: capillaries may become *dilated* (allowing fluids to leak out into the tissue spaces, causing a rash) and arteries *constricted* (which, inside the skull, for instance, reduces the supply of glucose oxygen to the brain, thus causing painful MIGRAINES).

For reasons that are not yet fully understood, it is the bodily functions normally regulated automatically by the autonomic nervous system that are affected by the allergic reaction: breathing, digesting, urinating, the sweat glands, the heart beat, blood pressure. All these functions can be, and are, so frequently disturbed in allergic diseases that, in the words of Dr. John W. Gerrard, professor of pediatrics at the University of Saskatchewan in Canada, we could almost call allergies "diseases of the autonomic system."

The activities of the autonomic nervous system are regulated (the way a computer or a thermostat is) by the region in the brain called the hypothalamus. We cannot consciously control its activities, yet it is not entirely independent of will and emotions, for the hypothalamus has connections with other areas of the brain concerned with both thought and feeling. Therefore the problems, the worries, the stresses that exist in our minds can have repercussions on the hypothalamus and may in this way precipitate allergic symptoms. However, it is sometimes difficult to decide whether the patient's symptoms are caused by an allergic reaction or by an emotional disturbance. Many laymen, and some physicians, tend to believe the latter: it's easier to substitute a catch-all psychological answer for a complicated, perhaps unsolvable physical explanation. This doesn't mean that psychological disturbances are not associated with allergic reactions; but it is important to keep in mind that there is no conclusive evidence that allergies have a psychogenic origin, and that as far as we know psychological disturbances tend to *compound* rather than *cause* an allergy.

In the development of an allergy there is first a sensitization and then

APPROXIMATE TIME OF APPEARANCE OF MAJOR POLLENS AND MOLDS IN VARIOUS REGIONS OF THE UNITED STATES

REGION	JAN.	FEB.	MARCH	APRIL	MAY	JUNE	JULY	AUG.	SEPT.	OCT.	NOV.	DEC.
Northeast			Ash Maple	Elm Maple	Oak	Grass	Alternaria Hormodendrum	Ragweed Alternaria Hormodendrum	Ragweed Alternaria Hormodendrum	Alternaria Hormodendrum		
Southeast		Elm	Ash Maple	Oak Sycamore	Pecan Oak Bermuda grass	Bermuda grass Hormodendrum	Alternaria Hormodendrum	Ragweed Alternaria Hormodendrum	Ragweed Alternaria Hormodendrum	Ragweed Alternaria Hormodendrum	Hormodendrum	
North Central				Elm Maple	Oak	Grass Hormodendrum	Alternaria Hormodendrum	Ragweed Alternaria Hormodendrum	Ragweed Alternaria Hormodendrum	Alternaria Hormodendrum		
South Central		Elm	Oak Maple Sycamore	Pecan Alternaria	Bermuda grass Alternaria Hormodendrum	Bermuda grass Alternaria Hormodendrum	Alternaria Hormodendrum	Alternaria Hormodendrum	Ragweed Alternaria Hormodendrum	Ragweed Alternaria		
Plains			Maple	Cottonwood		Grass Hormodendrum	Russian thistle Kochia† Hormodendrum	Ragweed Russian thistle Kochia Hormodendrum Alternaria	Ragweed Sagebrush			
Southwest	Alternaria*	Alternaria Cottonwood	Alternaria Ash Mountain cedar	Alternaria Bermuda grass False ragweed	Bermuda grass	Bermuda grass Hormodendrum		Alternaria Russian thistle Kochia	Alternaria Russian thistle Kochia	Alternaria		
Intermountain Basin			Elm	Cottonwood	Sycamore	Grass		Russian thistle Kochia	Sagebrush			
Pacific Coast North			Alder	Maple Oak	Grass	Grass Plantain	Grass					
Pacific Coast South	Alternaria		Oak Walnut	Oak Walnut Olive	Bermuda grass	Bermuda grass	Bermuda grass	Various compositae	Elm Compositae	Elm Compositae Alternaria	Alternaria	Alternaria

* E.g., daisy, dandelion, goldenrod, etc.
† E.g., cypress, spurge, etc.
Source: Reprinted with permission from the American Lung Association, from *Asthma, a Practical Guide for Physicians.*

a reaction. Sensitization causes a change in the body chemistry, leading to an allergic reaction when the person is exposed *again* to the same substance. An allergic reaction takes place when a person has over-stepped his own *level of resistance*, either because he is suddenly exposed to a higher concentration of the allergen or because his resistance has been weakened by illness. After the first allergic reaction has occurred, a person's level of resistance is permanently weakened; in the future, even small amounts of that particular allergen may cause a reaction.

The most common allergens are:

Inhalants—Substances that are breathed in: house dust; pollens from trees, grasses, and weeds; emanations from feathers and animal fur; perfumes; aromas from paints and from food; insecticides; tobacco smoke; gases; smog. These particles are caught up in the nose or penetrate the lungs; they may also be absorbed through the bowel if saliva containing them is swallowed.

Ingestants—Substances that are swallowed: foods; food additives; drugs taken by mouth.

Injectants—Such as antibiotics; or the sting of bees, wasps and hornets.

Contractants—The countless substances the body comes in contact with: silk, wool, soaps, creams, zippers, and jewels containing nickel; poison ivy; and so forth.

Infections—Suffered by people who are actually allergic to whatever germ is causing the infection, though often the infection merely aggravates an underlying allergy.

Physical factors—Such as exposure to cold air and cold water and to heat and sunshine; exercise, which may aggravate asthma, urticaria and eczema.

Although several allergic disorders were known and described in the nineteenth century, this subject was not developed on a scientific basis until the turn of the century. Even more recently the study of allergy has become related to IMMUNOLOGY, the study of the body's defenses against the bacteria and the viruses that try to invade it. These defenses result in various forms of *immunity*, namely, the body's increased resistance or tolerance to the action of germs. Modern allergists have discovered that an allergic organism produces specific ANTIBODIES that react to the substances to which the organism is allergic as if these normally harmless substances were germs. In other words, the study of allergy developed as the study of those unusual reactions which occur when the body becomes *sensitive* rather than *immune* to something that it is exposed to more than once.

The keys to the body's immunological defense are the white blood cells, called lymphocytes, which are provided with antibody-forming proteins called immunoglobulins, which in turn help to destroy germs

18

attacking the body. There are five categories of immunoglobulins—Ig M, Ig G, Ig A, Ig D and Ig E—each with a specific function at different stages of the defense process. Most organisms produce just immunoglobulins M, G and A, with only insignificant amounts of D and E. But allergic organisms may produce large amounts of Ig E, some of which become attached, for unknown reasons, to a special group of cells called mast cells. These cells contain a powerful chemical, histamine; and when the Ig E on their surface comes in contact with an allergen, the mast cells immediately discharge histamine into the surrounding spaces. Histamine in small quantities helps in the battle against germs, but it also makes the bronchial tubes contract, the capillaries dilate, the arteries constrict and the stomach contract—all the various unpleasant reactions that occur when an allergic person comes into contact with whatever it is he is allergic to. Sometimes the release of histamine is so swift, so powerful, that it may lead to death. This violent reaction is called ANAPHYLAXIS and is sometimes observed in people extremely allergic to penicillin or to insect stings.

The first and most important aid in diagnosing an allergy is a thorough history. The patient is asked to think back to times and events associated with allergic episodes, in order to provide the allergist with clues in his search for the specific allergens that are troubling the patient. A physical examination follows, to establish whether the symptoms are indeed allergic. Next, skin tests are made with specially prepared extracts of house dust, pollens, weeds, molds and various foods. These extracts may be placed on the skin and a scratch made at that point, or they may be injected directly. If a patient is allergic to any of these substances, his skin becomes red, itchy and swollen because of the histamine discharged into the tissue, and the test is *positive*. If he is not allergic, no reaction occurs and the test is *negative*. However, such skin tests are not conclusive because, although we know that a positive test indicates that an allergic reaction is taking place, it does not necessarily mean that the same allergic reaction is taking place in the nose, the lungs, the blood vessels, or wherever else it usually occurs in that patient. A person with asthma may have a positive skin test to horse dander, and yet horse dander may not be the cause of his asthma.

What often confuses the patient and the allergist is the fact that an allergic reaction may or may not have any relationship to the manner in which the allergen comes in contact with the body. For instance, *inhalants* may cause digestive problems, while a person may have an asthma attack from something he has eaten. A medication taken orally may produce a skin rash, while something rubbed into the skin may produce hay fever.

The most successful principle of allergy treatment is to remove the allergen. If the allergen is an air pollutant, or worse, the very tools of a person's occupation—hair-tint chemicals for the hairdresser, gasoline for the mechanic, mouse fur for the lab technician—it may be almost impossible to treat it unless the person's life is totally rearranged. But if the allergen is a pet, feather pillows, house dust, food or even pollens or molds, an allergic person can remove it or at least avoid it most of the time. Interestingly, the best way to avoid house dust is to let it lie undisturbed, rather than scattering dust particles around by dusting and vacuum cleaning.

When allergens cannot be removed, allergies have to be controlled with medications:

Antihistamines—These work well with allergies that cause nasal congestion. They do not prevent the formation of histamine; rather, they *displace* histamine so that it cannot act on the mucous glands in the nose and the bronchial tubes. But since histamine is not the only substance released in an allergic reaction, antihistamines are of no help in controlling wheezing, for example.

Epinephrine—This is excellent for relaxing the bronchial tubes and is a quick relief for asthma. Epinephrine is the synthetic counterpart of a natural substance produced by the adrenal glands and normally released in great amounts in times of stress. Epinephrine must be injected in small quantities and subcutaneously, because if taken by mouth it is destroyed by digestive juices.

Ephedrine—Ephedrine is similar to epinephrine, but its action is slower. However, it can be taken by mouth, and it stimulates the heart.

Cortisone—Cortisone, also produced naturally by the adrenal glands, is very useful in treating severe asthma attacks and eczema. However, some people may experience some side effects and, more important, may become dependent on it.

Disodiumcromoglycate—Useless in the treatment of acute attacks of asthma or hay fever, disodiumcromoglycate is excellent in their prevention. Some people find much relief in inhaling it at regular intervals every day.

Desensitization—This entails injecting small quantities of the allergen, which probably stimulates the production of immunoglobulin G, which, unlike Ig E, does not lead to the release of histamine but grasps the allergen when it is still in the bloodstream, before Ig E can catch up with it. But since it may take months before a useful amount of Ig G is built up in the system, and the shots may need to be continued for years, this treatment is justified only when it is very difficult to eliminate allergens from the environment or when symptoms are so severe that they cannot be controlled by medication. The treatment of allergy is obviously not a simple matter; however, there are few allergies that cannot be controlled by a good allergist who has the full and alert cooperation of the patient. We will have to learn to live with allergies until immunology—apparently the key word for allergy—will come up with a solution to this malady once and for all.

AMBLYOPIA (LAZY EYE)

Sometimes called "lazy eye," amblyopia is a major cause of partial loss of vision. It is a condition of reduced or dim vision in an eye which otherwise appears to be normal. If the two eyes do not see objects with the same degree of clarity, the eye with the poorer image is not stimuluted during the formative years to develop or maintain clear vision.

Thousands of people suffer some degree of amblyopia that could have been prevented. Prevention depends upon very early discovery, when a child is three to five years old.

AMNIOCENTESIS

Amniocentesis is a procedure that consists of inserting a hollow needle through the abdomen into the uterus of a pregnant woman and withdrawing a small amount of amniotic fluid—the serumlike liquid in which the developing embryo is suspended.

The fluid is then sent to a laboratory, where the cells grow in a culture and the CHROMOSOMES are examined under the microscope to establish whether the fetus suffers from some chromosomal or metabolic disorder. Often, the fetus's sex can be determined this way.

However, amniocentesis is not a routine procedure; it is a delicate operation that is performed only when there are reasons to suspect that the fetus has, for instance, a serious congenital disease such as mongolism, in which case an ABORTION may be considered. Many gynecologists feel that any woman over thirty-five who becomes pregnant should undergo amniocentesis, as her chances of giving birth to a mongoloid child are considerably greater than those of a younger woman.

Amniocentesis requires a gynecologist's flawless skill and is usually performed during the early weeks of pregnancy. As a rule, the later it is performed, the safer it is for both the mother and the fetus; but if an abortion is advisable, amniocentesis is best done within the first sixteen to eighteen weeks of pregnancy.

AMYL NITRITE (SEX DRUG)

Amyl nitrite is a flammable, clear, volatile, yellowish liquid used mainly (as a second choice after nitroglycerin) for the relief of attacks of angina pectoris. In the last several years, however, it has become extraordinarily popular as a sex drug.

Amyl nitrite is sold in fragile glass vials covered by finely spun cloth, which can be easily crushed with two fingers and inhaled immediately. The only pharmacologically known action of amyl nitrite is relaxation of smooth muscles and dilation of blood vessels, which causes an abrupt lowering of blood pressure, an increase in pulse rate, blushing of the skin and a feeling of giddiness. The most common side effect is a severe though brief and harmless headache. However, the drug's properties of lowering blood pressure and increasing pulse rate may be harmful to people with certain other heart diseases.

Though difficult to prove, this feeling of giddiness is reported to increase the intensity of orgasm of both men and women, and to increase the sensitivity of the skin. Also, dilation of blood vessels may slow down erection in a man. Thus, if the amyl nitrite inhaling is well timed, it could pleasantly delay orgasm and ejaculation.

ANAESTHESIA

Anaesthesia refers to entire or partial loss of feeling or sensation, a state of paralysis of the sensory apparatus. Anaesthetics are the drugs used to obtain a state of painlessness, necessary for almost all kinds of surgery.

Anaesthesia can be general, regional or local.

General anaesthesia—A general anaesthetic produces complete unconsciousness, muscular relaxation and absence of pain sensation. It can be administered as inhaled gas or injected intravenously. A tube has to be put into the trachea in order to control a patient's breathing. Its effects last approximately six or seven hours.

Regional anaesthesia—Regional anaesthesia is obtained by injecting cocaine derivatives to block a large nerve which supplies the area that needs to be anaesthetized.

Local anaesthesia—Local anaesthesia is a loss of sensation confined to a limited part of the body. It may be a locally applied solution of cocaine for nose operations, for instance, or ethyl chloride, used to "freeze" the skin for such procedures as DERMABRASION.

ANALGESICS

Algesia means sensitivity to pain, and analgesic is the generic term for any substance that relieves PAIN—anything from ALCOHOL to ASPIRIN or HYPNOSIS. But the analgesics commonly referred to are chemical compounds, which are classified into two categories: *strong* and *mild*. However, because of the question of addiction and the consequent legal restrictions imposed on certain drugs, analgesics are also classified as *narcotic* and *nonnarcotic*.

Narcotic analgesics include morphine (strong) and codeine (mild)—both of which are opium alkaloids—their semisynthetic derivatives, such as heroin and oxymorphone, and a number of synthetic preparations, such as meperidine and methadone. Narcotic analgesics should be used only for short-term treatment of intense pain, such as pain caused by surgery. Also, different dosages must be used for different types of pain: a high dose of morphine, for instance, can be quite effective in cases of intolerable pain, but may cause difficulty in respiration. As a rule, narcotic analgesics should never be used for mild or moderate pain that can be relieved by nonnarcotic analgesics, as their side effects—drowsiness, nausea, and, most important, dependence—can be quite serious.

Narcotic analgesics relieve pain by acting on the central nervous system. Their euphoric action probably relieves anxiety, and although the patient may still retain a sensation of pain, his pain threshold is raised.

Nonnarcotic analgesics include aspirin, other salicylates, and a group of unrelated synthetic compounds, many of which are excellent for treating rheumatism and inflammations, and are generally referred to as antipyretic, i.e., fever-relieving analgesics.

Nonnarcotic analgesics act on the receptors in the nervous system periphery. It is believed that antipyretics control fever by lowering the temperature center in the hypothalamus elevated by the fever.

Analgesics can be used alone or together with tranquilizers, sedatives or hypnotics, in order to increase the analgesics' effectiveness by promoting rest and sleep. In other instances, a stimulant such as caffeine may be added to reduce mental confusion.

Whether narcotic or nonnarcotic, however, the action of analgesics is no more clearly understood than the nature of PAIN itself.

ANAPHYLAXIS

The term anaphylaxis was originally used only to describe a severe and unusual physiological reaction in laboratory animals produced by the injection of foreign matter, such as horse serum (serum obtained from the blood of horses inoculated with bacteria). Such an injection may render the animal hypersensitive to a subsequent injection; this phenomenon is called *active anaphylaxis*. Anaphylaxis produced in an animal by injecting the blood of a sensitized animal is called *passive anaphylaxis*.

However, anaphylaxis also refers to a rapid, exaggerated allergic reaction of the human organism to a foreign substance which acts as an antigen, i.e., stimulates the formation of specific ANTIBODIES in the organism.

The course of anaphylaxis is extremely varied: it may occur minutes after antigen exposure or hours later; the duration of the reaction is also variable, and so is the severity of the symptoms, although antigens that are *injected,* such as penicillin or INSECT STINGS, often trigger the most severe anaphylactic reactions.

Whether mild or severe, anaphylaxis should be treated immediately: prompt recognition of early symptoms may prevent progression to more serious and even fatal reactions.

ANEMIA

Anemia is a disorder of the blood resulting when the production of red blood cells is reduced, or when the turnover of these cells is faster than their maturation, or when the concentration of hemoglobin—the red pigment of the red blood cells that carries oxygen to the blood—is reduced. If the amount of hemoglobin is below normal or if there are too few red blood cells, not enough oxygen will get to the tissues.

Anemia is not a disease in itself but rather a symptom of a number of disorders, all of which involve difficulty in transporting oxygen throughout the body. Excluding sudden massive loss of blood, all anemias—there are more than one hundred different types—ultimately result from: 1) inadequate blood production; 2) hemolysis, i.e., disintegration of the red blood cells; or 3) a combination of the two.

Anemia's own symptoms—increased heart-beat rate, decreased blood circulation rate, pallor, weakness, dizziness, susceptibility to colds, excessive menstrual blood loss—are often vague and difficult to establish. When anemia develops slowly, the body adjusts to it so perfectly that even very anemic people may have few or none of these warning signs. Only a severe and quickly developing anemia can be clearly recognized; a person with an anemia resulting from chronic loss of blood because of cancer of the stomach, for instance, very likely would not recognize his condition. He may feel weak and tired and look pale, but he may not think he ought to see a doctor.

One of the easiest anemias to identify is the so-called nutritional anemia, caused by a deficiency in IRON, folic acid or VITAMIN B_{12}. But in a high percentage of patients, diagnosis of one or a combination of these deficiencies is not enough: the associated illness must be sought. Poor diet alone may or may not cause anemia—in fact, some people who don't eat properly may have anemia but still not be deficient in iron, folic acid or vitamin B_{12}. Foods rich in iron include liver and parsley. Also quickly recognizable is anemia in pregnancy, a result of increased demands of the body for iron. And, in general, women have a greater tendency to be anemic than men because of loss of blood during MENSTRUATION. In either case, these deficiencies are successfully treated with the administration of the specific missing nutrient.

ANORECTICS (APPETITE SUPPRESSANTS)

Some of the drugs that some doctors prescribe for obesity are anorectics, which are believed to diminish appetite, though scientists are not entirely sure how they work.

Most, though not all, anorectics contain amphetamine, a central nervous system stimulant that has a known potential for dependence.

In 1972, the Food and Drug Administration conducted an investigation of anorectic drugs in order to establish whether these drugs really work in reducing excessive weight and whether they are safe. The FDA concluded that "patients receiving anorectics *will* lose more weight than those who are not treated with them. But patients who take the drugs and diet will lose only a fraction of a pound more a week than those who resort only to dietary restriction. And the rate of weight loss is greater during the early stages of taking the pills." Anorectics, then, have a limited usefulness in the treatment of obesity, not to speak of the fact that anorectic drugs are habit-forming and have been extensively abused in the United States as well as in other countries. Those anorectics containing amphetamine, which have been used as pep pills, have been especially abused. They can create dependence, psychotic behavior and severe withdrawal symptoms.

As a result of the FDA findings, such drugs as Dexedrine®, Biphetamine®, Obotan®, Preludin®, Tepanil® and Pre-Sate® have been put under strict government control, with labels warning physicians to use them with extreme care. However, many doctors still believe that, when used for short periods of time (a few weeks) as an adjunct to DIET and EXERCISE and only for selected patients who are not likely to become addicted to them, anorectic drugs are useful. Others feel that appetite suppressants should be prescribed only to help patients adapt to a diet, and then only to people who are serious about losing weight and whose obesity is not due to mental depression, which would make them more vulnerable to drug dependency.

An appetite suppressant that was quite popular in the 1950s is thyroid extract. Its use was banned in the early 1960s because of its many side effects, the worst of which is damage to the heart.

ANOREXIA NERVOSA

Anorexia nervosa and OBESITY are the two extremes of energy imbalance; the obese person compulsively eats *more* than he can burn in energy; the anorectic person denies himself food so stubbornly and for so long that he literally can starve himself to death.

Anorexia nervosa is a rather uncommon psychological disorder that occurs almost exclusively in young women. Anorectics exaggerate to themselves the size of their bodies, so that they view themselves as enormously fat while they already may be grotesquely thin.

Anorectics not only share with the obese an obsession with their bodies and contempt for their fatness, but experience the same sense of inadequacy, rejection and social isolation—they feel that they must become thinner in case they should be unable to refrain from overeating.

In certain cases, obese adolescents may take too literally the recommendation that reducing will make them slim, beautiful and happy, and become what Dr. Hilde Bruch, professor of psychiatry at the Baylor College of Medicine in Houston, Texas, calls "thin fat." This condition is similar to anorexia nervosa in that "thin fat" girls, though they have succeeded in becoming and staying thin, are emotionally crushed by the effort of starving themselves, for the ugliness of being fat no longer prevents them from putting their unrealistic dreams to the test. However, there are definite differences between "thin fat" people and anorectics, because the latter continue to lose weight down to a level *below* normal and are not only in psychological danger but in physical danger as well.

Anorexia nervosa can be diagnosed according to the following criteria:

1) A tremendous loss of weight due to prolonged avoidance of fattening foods, especially CARBOHYDRATES; and excessive EXERCISE.
2) Cessation of MENSTRUATION at the onset of the illness or even preceding the loss of weight.
3) A morbid fear of becoming fat.

Anorexia nervosa is undoubtedly a psychological disorder, but it also has an endocrine component. Moreover, it is conceivable that anorexia nervosa might be the result of an impairment in the food-regulating center of the hypothalamus, analogous to the disturbances observed in animals with experimental lesions of the hypothalamus. Such animals may either starve themselves or, if the lesion is in a different location, become enormously fat.

Treatment for anorexia nervosa remains, for the moment, essentially empirical. Psychotherapy is seldom effective when used without a program of weight gain. On the other hand, drugs aimed exclusively at stimulating appetite are also not enough. By the time an anorectic asks for medical help, a physician has to move fast—a 50 percent loss of normal weight can be fatal—and cautiously at the same time, because the very nature of the illness makes the patient resist treatment. Often, the presence of a skillful and friendly nurse can make the difference: she can establish a rapport with the patient and gently cajole her into finishing every day the food that is put on her plate.

Despite the lack of any specific treatment, this general method is usually effective: patients gain weight in matters of weeks, and their obsession with thinness diminishes proportionately to their weight gain.

To avoid relapses, doctors recommend periodic check-ups over a period of one to five years.

ANTACIDS

Antacids are substances employed (mostly empirically and self-pre-scribed) to diminish the quantity of hydrochloric acid—a normal constituent of gastric juice needed for good digestion that sometimes is produced in too large quantities—in the stomach.

There are on the market hundreds of different antacids (though only about a dozen brands)—in the form of tablets, liquids, powders, lozenges, gums, granules and pills—competing to soothe a variety of symptoms, loosely called indigestion, resulting from causes as diverse as gastric disorders and depression or anxiety. However, antacids are also fre-quently prescribed by physicians for the treatment of peptic ulcer (ulcers in the stomach or duodenum caused by excessive irritation from gastric acid) and of gastro-esophageal reflux (called heartburn in its mild form), caused by a defective junction of the stomach and the esophagus (the tube leading from the pharynx to the stomach), which allows reflux of acid gastric juice into the esophagus.

Antacids seem to work in four different ways: 1) direct neutralization of the gastric acid; 2) dilution of the acid to a lower concentration; 3) direct absorption of hydrogen from the hydrochloric acid; 4) a combina-tion of dilution, partial neutralization, and absorption of hydrogen. Each has specific advantages and drawbacks; the ideal antacid may not have been found yet.

Most antacids in use today contain one or more of the following ingredients:

Aluminum hydroxide—Dissolves slowly, thus neutralizes gastric acid slowly, but its effect lasts long. Safe for long-term use but may be constipating.

Calcium carbonate—Insoluble, it leaves the stomach relatively slowly. Slow neutralizer, lasting effect. However, it may stimulate an increased amount of stomach acid, which may persist long after the antacid's action has ended. Also, it may be constipating and may raise the calcium level in the blood, and possibly cause the formation of stones in the kidneys. (Tums®; Pepto-Bismol®)

Magnesium hydroxide—More soluble than aluminum hydroxide, it is a faster neutralizer, but may have a laxative effect. Safe for long-term use, although doses must be regulated for patients with kidney disturbances. Since it tends to cause diarrhea, most antacid preparations mix aluminum and magnesium compounds to balance the constipating and the laxative effects.

Magnesium trisilicate—Slow in the onset but lasting in effect. May have laxative effect but safe for long-term use. Dosage must be regulated for patients with kidney disturbances. (Phillips' Milk of Magnesia®)

Sodium bicarbonate—Highly soluble, it reacts rapidly with hydrochloric acid. Short-lived in effect, because it is rapidly emptied from the stomach. Unsuitable for frequent or long-term use, for its alkaline quality may affect body chemistry. It should not be used by patients on low-salt diets, especially in those preparations in which the sodium content of a daily dose is higher than 115 mg. (Brioschi®)

Citric acid—Sometimes added to sodium bicarbonate. The chief end product is sodium citrate, a very effective antacid. However, sodium citrate is metabolized by the body into sodium bicarbonate—with the same disadvantages of this compound.

Some antacid preparations such as Bromo-Seltzer® also contain caffeine, which stimulates acid secretion in the stomach. Others, such as Bufferin® and Alka-Seltzer®, add ASPIRIN, which may irritate the stomach of an ulcer patient without being of any antacid use. Vanquish® combines aspirin, antacid, *and* caffeine. Thus, it would seem that an antacid combining aluminum and magnesium salts would be the best agent for long-term use. Still, as of 1974, few adequate studies comparing efficacy and side effects have been made.

As for peptic ulcer, the efficacy of antacids has not been demonstrated in rigorously controlled studies. Yet antacids do seem to improve this disease, the same way they do "indigestion."

In the reflux symptoms, antacids neutralize the refluxed material, so as to protect the esophagus tissue from thinning and letting the acid reach sensitive nerve endings, thus causing pain.

For the moment, then, there is no *rational* therapy for either indigestion, heartburn or peptic ulcer, but many patients who seem to have these disorders do respond to antacids. It is important, however, that a person who has an ulcer avoid caffeine in tea and in coffee, and also avoid preparations that contain aspirin.

ANTIBIOTICS

Antibiotics are organic compounds formed by living microorganisms—such as bacteria or fungi—that have the capacity, in dilute solutions, to inhibit the growth of or to destroy other bacteria, such as disease germs.

Penicillin, one of the early antibiotics, is one of the greatest medical discoveries of this century. In 1928 Sir Alexander Fleming, a British chemist, first observed that a mold of the germ *Penicillium* produced a substance that inhibited the growth of staphylococci. Penicillin's early purification and use were slowed by technical difficulties; a great part of the present understanding of penicillin came from its use by the American and the British armies between 1942 and 1946.

Basically, doctors now know that these powerful drugs, while efficiently eliminating the bacteria of an infection, also radically modify the normal bacterial content of the human body. These changes are not important in most cases, but in some the presence of new organisms may eventually produce other, more serious infections known as "superinfections." It has also been discovered that any bacteria repeatedly exposed to inadequate doses of an antibiotic will eventually become resistant to it. (This is why hospital-borne infections are often more difficult to treat than infections contracted in the outside world.) Some people may develop sudden, violent allergic reactions (ANAPHYLAXIS) to antibiotics.

Careful physicians never administer antibiotics—even in an emergency—without an accurate diagnosis, which may include the particular patient's history and the exact nature of the infection. There are many other antibiotics, such as sulfonamides, streptomycin, and tetracycline, which act selectively on certain infections. To discover which one will work against a certain type of infection, the doctor removes a specimen of pus and applies it to a plate containing different antibiotics. The antibiotic that prevents growth of the organism should then be administered to the patient.

Antibiotic therapy is most successful when the bacterial growth of an infection is reduced in such a way as to allow the patient's immunological defense mechanism to control the remaining bacteria.

ANTIBODIES

Antibodies are various substances synthetized in the tissues and the blood of an organism for the purpose of fighting the invasion of foreign bodies—such as bacteria or toxins—called antigens.

Each kind of antigen provokes the formation of a specific type of antibody. These tend to keep developing in the body even after the antigens are gone, thus creating immunity to those particular antigens.

ANTICOAGULANT

An anticoagulant is a natural substance or other agent which interferes with, delays or suppresses coagulation of the blood.

ANTIOXIDANTS

Antioxidants are substances—such as VITAMIN E—capable of slowing the rate of oxidation, the decomposition process that occurs naturally in many organic materials.

Both natural and synthetic antioxidants are added to many manufactured or processed products such as FATS, SOAPS, COSMETICS and drugs.

In fats and fatty foods, oxidation means rancidity—a rank taste and smell, destruction of fatty acids and fat-soluble VITAMINS, and possible toxic effects.

Antioxidants are in great demand in the manufacture of pastry, frozen fruits, meats and poultry, potato chips, candies, chewing gum and dehydrated vegetables.

ANTIPERSPIRANTS (DEODORANTS)

Antiperspirants are substances that reduce the flow of PERSPIRATION from the sweat glands to the skin's surface. None of the available products completely stops perspiration, which would be undesirable, as sweating is an important function of the skin, concerning temperature regulation and water metabolism in the body. Antiperspirants are by their very nature also DEODORANTS, because they contain antibacterial ingredients, that is, ingredients which temporarily destroy the microorganisms that decompose the pure liquids of the eccrine glands and the milky secretions of the apocrine glands, thus causing BODY ODOR.

The most common antiperspirant ingredients are aluminum chlorhydroxide and aluminum chloride. (Salts of metals such as aluminum, IRON, mercury or zinc all have astringent properties, but some produce discoloration and others are toxic; salts of aluminum and zinc are those most commonly used in antiperspirants.) These ingredients are themselves antibacterial, but generally are combined with other antibacterial substances that provide additional protection.

Although scientists know a great deal about antiperspirants and their effects, the basic mechanism by which they reduce perspiration is still being investigated. One theory is that an antiperspirant may partially block the sweat ducts, or that it may cause the duct walls to swell, thus reducing their size. Another theory is that antiperspirants may alter the walls of the ducts, allowing less water to reach the surface of the skin.

While most antiperspirants are also deodorants, the reverse is not true. Apparently not everyone is aware of the difference; many people seem concerned primarily with concealing body odor. This explains in part the success, for instance, of feminine hygiene sprays. Doctors—including a few psychiatrists, who feel that the advertisements for the sprays imply that women are *by nature* dirty—advise against them.

Washing with soap and water, they point out, is still the most effective and safest way to eliminate the mildly odorous secretions of glands contained in women's external genitals. Soap and water cannot take care of odors caused by fungal infection, menstrual flow, or by a forgotten tampon or DIAPHRAGM, but neither can chemical sprays. In fact, there have been several reports of irritation and rashes caused by vaginal sprays.

Physicians and the FDA also caution against Mennen E®, an antiperspirant/deodorant which, according to one of its advertisements, represented "a new era in deodorant protection," thanks to the gentle action of VITAMIN E. However, by late 1973 and early 1974, several dermatologists reported cases of contact DERMATITIS rapidly spreading from the underarm to the trunk and arms and probably caused by the vitamin.

The best antiperspirants are the *unscented* ones, since those containing PERFUMES may be allergenic and, from the aesthetic point of view, may compete with a woman's favorite perfume.

Some antiperspirants include the word "unscented" on their labels, though when the product is scented the label doesn't always say so. In any case, as of January 1, 1976, all cosmetic products in this country will have to list the ingredients they contain in order of predominance.

Antiperspirants can be a cream, a roll-on, a liquid (usually in an AEROSOL spray can) or a powder. The powder is more practical when the label specifies "light" or "invisible," for the heavier powder often smudges on dark clothes.

Antiperspirants are most effective when applied on scrupulously clean skin (soap considerably reduces the number of bacteria) but not right after a bath; it is best to wait until the body is cool and at rest. Some antiperspirants claim to be most effective when applied at bedtime, allowed to stay on all night, and washed off in the morning. For the underarm, since hair tends to collect skin debris, bacteria, and stale perspiration, depilation makes it easier for the antiperspirant to reach the skin.

AREOLA
Areola refers to the pink or pigmented circular area around the nipple of the breast.

ARTHRITIS
Arthritis literally means inflammation of a joint; however, the word refers to dozens of different conditions causing aches in the joints and the connective tissue throughout the body, not all necessarily involving

inflammation. Some people call it rheumatism, a vague word used for unexplained pains in joints and muscles. Even arthritis specialists don't agree on a precise definition.

Arthritis is an extremely common disease—almost everyone is susceptible to it, and people who live long enough are almost certain to develop one type or another. The most serious forms of arthritis are accompanied by inflammation. It starts with a tissue injury inside the joint or somewhere else, followed by an inflammatory reaction, which causes more damage, which increases the inflammation, which in turn causes still more damage. The damage that occurs changes the structure of the bones and other tissues of the joints, making them stiff, sometimes

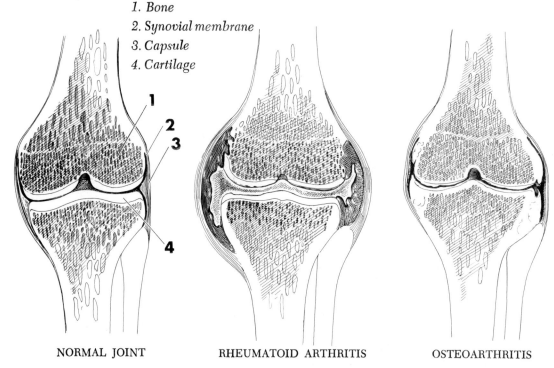

1. Bone
2. Synovial membrane
3. Capsule
4. Cartilage

NORMAL JOINT   RHEUMATOID ARTHRITIS   OSTEOARTHRITIS

Left: Drawing of a normal joint: the space where two bones meet is enclosed in a capsule. The capsule has an inner lining called the synovial membrane. The bone ends are covered by a thick cartilage, and the joint space contains a small amount of synovial fluid.

Middle: Rheumatoid arthritis, i.e., inflammation of a joint. The cause is possibly a dormant virus or reaction to an organism that affects the capsule and causes swelling of the synovial membrane. Many joints are usually involved; inflammatory tissues invade the cartilage surrounding the bone ends and eventually destroy it. Finally, scar tissue may form between the bone ends and may turn into bone, causing the joint to become rigid and painfully distorted as a result of muscle contractures.

Right: Unlike rheumatoid arthritis, which is inflammatory and involves many joints, osteoarthritis usually affects only individual joints and is rarely accompanied by inflammation. The most common characteristic of osteoarthritis is the wearing out of the joint of an aging person.

distorting them, and sometimes making movement impossible. Fractures that involve joints are especially liable to be complicated by the development of degenerative arthritis, the effects of which may not become evident until years later.

The major forms of arthritis are chronic, and whatever damage takes place is permanent and tends to get worse unless proper precautions are taken and treatment continued for long periods of time.

The most common kinds of arthritis are:

Rheumatoid arthritis—The most serious, most painful and most crippling. It can affect the whole body, but it primarily attacks the joints. It tends to subside and flare up unpredictably, causing progressive damage to the tissues. Women are more susceptible than men.

Osteoarthritis—This is essentially a wear-and-tear disease of the joints that comes with age. It is usually mild and not generally inflammatory.

Rheumatic fever—A severe systemic disease that follows a streptococcus infection. It frequently damages the heart and causes a form of arthritis in the joints that subsides quickly and is never crippling.

Gout—A painful, inherited disease that most often attacks the small joints, especially those in the big toe. Men are much more susceptible than women.

The precise cause of rheumatoid arthritis is not yet known. Because the inflammation looks as if it were due to infection, researchers have looked for years for an infectious agent as the source of the disease— without success. Recently, scientists have suggested that arthritis may be due to a latent viruslike organism that lies dormant in the body for years before suddenly becoming active and causing illness.

The area where two bones meet is enclosed in a capsule, containing the so-called synovial fluid. The capsule has an inner skin called the synovial membrane. Inflammation starts there, swelling the membrane and spreading to other parts of the joint system. The enflamed membranes form a mass growing over and under the cartilage surrounding the bone ends, into and around the tendons. Finally, scar tissue can form between the bone ends and sometimes change to bone, so that the joint becomes fused, permanently rigid. While a joint is undergoing this deterioration, muscle contractions can cause distortions. This is most apparent when arthritis attacks the hands.

All this can happen, but proper treatment started before it happens can prevent it in most cases. There are many drugs available for treating rheumatoid arthritis. Because the disease varies so much from person to person and because people vary in the way they react to certain drugs, a physician may have to try different ones until the most effective in a specific case is found.

ARTHRITIS

One of the most frequently prescribed drugs is ASPIRIN, which reduces inflammation and PAIN. But in order to be effective it has to be taken in large doses every day; if a person cannot tolerate aspirin in high dosage, the physician must prescribe some other anti-inflammatory drug. Gold salts, too, have been used for years in treating rheumatoid arthritis. They reduce the severity of the inflammation, but since they are toxic they must be administered in very carefully regulated doses. Cortisone can reduce the pain and the inflammation in a matter of hours; however, it cannot stop the progress of the disease. Worse, it can cause side effects that may be more severe than arthritis itself.

Much of the crippling from rheumatoid arthritis develops because of an arthritic's tendency to keep painful joints in a comfortable position for long periods of time. This causes the joints to stiffen and the muscles around the joints to become weak because of inactivity. Special exercises have been devised to keep arthritic joints mobile and in functioning condition. Hot baths, HEATING PADS and heat lamps are also recommended, because heat is relaxing and helps joints to move better and with less pain.

Having discovered that, when diseased tissue is removed from a joint before much damage has taken place, normal tissue grows back and may remain healthy for a long period of time or even indefinitely, surgeons have developed countless surgical techniques to solve the problem of crippling in rheumatoid arthritis. Among the most distinguished surgeons in this field is Dr. Alfred B. Swanson, chief of orthopedic surgery at the Blodgett Memorial Hospital in Grand Rapids, Michigan. Dr. Swanson has also been conducting research since 1962 to develop flexible SILICONE rubber implants to replace joints of the hand, wrist, elbow, and big toe which are already distorted because of untreated rheumatoid arthritis. Meanwhile, newer materials that have greater toughness than silicone but with the same stability and inertness have been developed, which opens new hopes for people suffering from this disease.

Treatment for osteoarthritis and rheumatic fever is similar to that for rheumatoid arthritis, except that cortisone is not used orally for osteoarthritis but in special situations is injected into the joint to bring temporary relief.

As for gout, treatment is now available to control it effectively, indeed more successfully than any other form of arthritis. The purpose of this treatment is to reduce the level of uric acid, a normal body substance which in this disease is either overproduced or produced faster than the kidneys can eliminate it. There are drugs, such as colchicine, which control acute attacks. Others, such as probenecid and allopurinol, act, respectively, by helping the body discharge more uric acid and by reducing the body's production of it.

34

ARTIFICIAL NAILS

Artificial nails, also called nail elongators, are a synthetic material that is either preshaped or designed to be pasted over natural fingernails for the purpose of hiding stubby nails and giving them a long and attractive appearance.

First, the natural nail surface is slightly filed with an emery board to remove excess oil, smooth rough spots and increase adhesion to the plastic film. Then, if the artificial nails are preshaped, they are glued to the natural nails and filed to the desired shape and length. The other type is manufactured as a fine pink powder which was developed from material used by dentists for filling teeth. Basic ingredients include a vinyl compound, a catalyst, and a plasticizer. The powder is diluted immediately before application into a viscous liquid or thick dough that quickly—in seven to nine minutes—hardens to a tough, nonporous plastic.

A stiff silvered paper or plastic, shaped to follow the contours of the fingertips, is fitted under the tip of the natural nail, and the artificial one is built over this guide.

To prevent plastic deposits on the skin around the nails, a coat of "separator"—an easy-to-remove, water-soluble resin—is applied to the skin.

According to manufacturers, artificial nails remain firm and light on natural fingernails for about four or five weeks, after which a skillful operator can fill in the gap left by the nail's new growth. They are recommended to strengthen soft and injured nails and for nail-biters, as the plastic film is so hard that the teeth slip off rather than bite into it.

However, many dermatologists disapprove of plastic nails. For one thing, local allergic reactions are common. Also, if the artificial nails are left on too long, moisture may accumulate under the impermeable plastic, causing the nail plate to soften and even lift from the nail bed—a condition known as ONYCHOLYSIS.

ASPIRIN (ACETYLSALICYLIC ACID)

Aspirin, or acetylsalicylic acid, is one of the most successful, most widely used synthetic drugs in the entire field of pharmacology. Aspirin does not require a prescription and is used the world over as a favorite antineuralgic, as a mild painkiller, and as a mild sedative.

The mechanism of aspirin's action is one of the many processes not yet fully understood. We know, however, that it has four distinct effects: 1) it acts against PAIN; 2) it lowers fever; 3) it reduces inflammation; 4) it creates a feeling of well-being, perhaps as a result of the first three effects, or perhaps as an independent effect—*without* inducing addiction, sedation, or euphoria, or in any way affecting mental processes. Only recently has it been demonstrated that aspirin works where the pain originates; one theory is that aspirin and aspirinlike drugs block or fill nerve endings so that no pain impulses can get to them. Another theory is that aspirin acts by inhibiting a specific ENZYME or group of enzymes.

Almost without exception, so-called extra-strength medications contain aspirin; and the "ingredient doctors recommend most" mentioned in commercials is nothing but aspirin. Interestingly, researchers have discovered that there is practically no difference, as far as relieving pain is concerned, among plain, buffered, coated, compounded, or seltzer-type aspirin. In fact, plain aspirin is *less* stomach-upsetting than either buffered aspirin or the other ingredients used in a compound. Still, the question of aspirin dosage has not yet been answered. As an ANALGESIC (painkiller), aspirin's potency is *not* increased in proportion with the dose: for most people, two tablets provide all the analgesic power that is needed for at least three or four hours. Some, however, find slightly higher doses more effective; and recent studies have shown that it is safe for arthritic patients to take—under medical supervision—up to twelve aspirins a day without, as it was previously believed, causing kidney damage.

But aspirin in high enough quantities becomes quite toxic and may cause erosion in the gastric mucosa. In general, aspirin should be used only for the kind of ailments described on the label or specified by a physician. It should not be taken by a person who has a kidney disorder, has an ulcer, or is taking ANTICOAGULANTS (blood-thinning drugs), and a person should immediately discontinue using it if, after taking it for a HEADACHE, he has reactions such as nausea, asthma, intestinal disorders and so forth. In these cases, a safe aspirin substitute—not quite so effective or powerful—is a drug called acetaminophen.

The safest way to take aspirin is with a full glass of water or milk, after a meal. However, the fastest way to obtain relief with aspirin is also a rather distasteful one—by taking it with a glass of hot water.

At the beginning of 1974, three University of Georgia scientists reported that they had found a way to make aspirin in a liquid form—with the consistency of maple syrup, flavored with orange or peppermint—that should considerably reduce many of its undesirable side effects, such as lodging and then dissolving only in one area of the stomach, producing irritation or, in severe cases, hemorrhage. And in Italy, a doctor at the hospital of Livorno announced at the end of 1973 that he had developed a water-soluble, injectable aspirin, which could be used much more widely than the oral preparation and with no side effects.

More recently, Dr. John R. J. Sorensen of the University of Cincinnati

Medical Center has proposed a solution for lessening the danger of peptic ulcer for people who depend on aspirin to reduce the inflammation of ARTHRITIS. A peptic ulcer may start when aspirin attracts and binds the organic copper present in stomach tissues, forming a compound that acts on the enflamed tissues. By adding copper to aspirin—copper aspirinate —the necessary copper is provided without removing it from the stomach.

ASTHMA

Asthma is a generic term for a number of symptoms, brought about by different causes, in which the trachea (windpipe) and the bronchi (the two main branches of the trachea leading, respectively, into the right and the left lung) become excessively irritated by various stimuli and therefore narrowed. This causes abrupt, recurrent, suffocating attacks of asthma, which may last from a few hours to days or even weeks and then gradually subside. Because of this constant irritation of their lungs, asthmatic people are more susceptible to lung and bronchial infections.

An asthmatic attack consists of:

1) *Shortness of breath*, due to increased effort required to breathe air through narrowed bronchial tubes, either because of swelling of the membrane lining the tubes or because of contraction of the muscles around them;

2) *Wheezing respiration*, due to excessive air trapped in the lungs that cannot be exhaled through the narrowed tubes;

3) *Cough*, caused by the irritation of the membrane and the secretion of mucus.

In their struggle for breath, the asthmatic lungs become distended, the chest swells, the neck muscles strain, and the veins become engorged.

There are two types of asthma: *allergic* and *nonallergic*.

Allergic asthma, which is often inherited, usually occurs in children and young adults with a previous history of ALLERGY in the form of HAY FEVER, HIVES or eczema. In a particular patient, one or more substances can consistently provoke asthmatic attacks. The most common of these substances are POLLEN, DANDER, dust, MOLDS and the sting of wasps; also, drugs such as ASPIRIN or ANTIBIOTICS, heat, cold or sunlight. Even though virus infections, FATIGUE and anxiety may play roles in an asthmatic attack, it is seldom possible to prove that any of these is the *direct* cause of the attack.

Nonallergic asthma usually occurs in adults with no previous history of allergy. No specific cause can be demonstrated to produce this kind of asthmatic attack.

Not all substances provoking asthmatic symptoms are ALLERGENS.

A person who is hypersensitive to a foreign substance (allergen), such as ragweed, develops marked difficulty in breathing on exposure to the allergen.

The allergen interacts with previously sensitized mast cells, causing the release of a number of chemicals, including histamine, which are responsible for the allergic reactions. In the asthmatic, histamine causes contractions of bronchial muscles, thus restricting the free flow of air into the lung.

1. *Normal bronchus, with plenty of space for air*
2. *Antigen*
3. *Mast cell*
4. *Histamine*
5. *Allergic reaction in a muscle cell*
6. *Contracted muscle*
7. *Blocked bronchus*
8. *Alveoli (air sacs)*

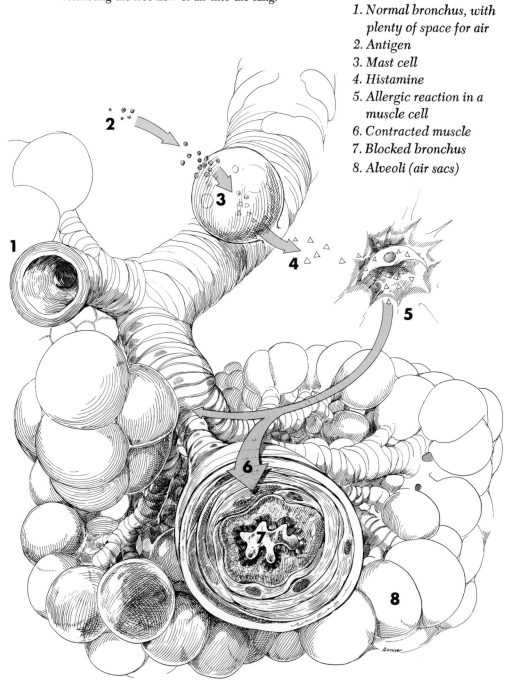

Some are simply nonspecific irritants—sulfur dioxide, for instance, which is found in smog, and which can cause bronchospasms (convulsive contractions of the bronchi) both in asthmatic and in healthy people. Thus, just because a person may have a few occurrences of wheezing does not necessarily mean that he is asthmatic.

Contrary to common belief, asthmatic children rarely outgrow their condition without treatment of the cause. The younger the patient and the sooner the treatment is started, the better are the prospects for recovery.

In order to diagnose asthma and rule out lung infection or other diseases with similar symptoms, the physician may need to perform a number of laboratory examinations, among which are a blood count; X-rays of the chest and nasal sinuses; skin tests, and a lung-capacity test, i.e., how much air the lungs are capable of taking in with each breath.

The same types of treatment are used for both allergic and nonallergic asthmatic attacks. They include:

1) So-called bronchodilator drugs, such as Epinephrine®, Ephedrine®, or Aminophylline®, administered by mouth, injection or with an aerosol sprayer;

2) Expectorants, such as iodide compounds, to dissolve thick mucus and ease the coughing;

3) Cortisone, the synthetic equivalent of the adrenal gland hormone of the same name.

The general health measures that should be taken, too, are the same for both types of asthma: avoid irritants such as tobacco or smog; any drugs—sedatives, VACCINES—without consulting a physician; extremes of heat and cold; physical fatigue and emotional stress.

For allergic asthma, the specific allergens have to be identified, and treatment is similar to that used for other forms of allergy. Allergic asthma attacks, however, can be prevented with cromolyn sodium, a relatively new drug in powder form that is inhaled directly into the lungs from a pocket-size instrument called an insufflator. Cromolyn sodium is thought to prevent certain cells in the lungs from releasing histamine, the powerful chemical that causes the bronchial tubes to contract and the capillaries to dilate—the first step in an asthmatic attack.

B

BACKACHE

Backache is extremely common: every day, seven million Americans are under some form of treatment for this disorder.

Backache is a symptom of some elusive injury to the spinal column—twenty-four adjoining, movable bones called vertebrae (seven cervical; twelve thoracic; five lumbar), which transmit most of the body's weight to the sacrum, which consists of five vertebrae fused together.

The possible causes of backache are almost countless—poor POSTURE, badly fitting shoes, overweight, pregnancy, ARTHRITIS, osteoporosis, too little or too much EXERCISE, a too soft bed, a spinal-cord injury, or cancer. But it can also be caused by anxiety, tension, and sexual problems; these, of course, don't show on an X-ray of the spine, but they can provoke muscle spasms similar to, if not worse than, those resulting from a physical injury. It is therefore most important that a patient with a backache for more than one week see a doctor for an accurate diagnosis. To rely on painkillers or to have one's back manipulated can be dangerous if the underlying disorder is, for instance, cancer.

One of the physician's basic problems when faced with a patient complaining of a "bad back" is to narrow down the diagnosis from the great number of possible causes. He has to question the patient closely about his family, daily activities, sports, moods, and sleeping habits. And even when there seems to be a direct cause—that is, the backache started suddenly after a stumble, after the lifting of a heavy suitcase, after a too vigorous sneezing—the disparity between the insignificance of the trauma and the intensity of the back pain it triggered is a signal of a more serious underlying cause.

Among the more serious backaches is the slipped disc, the well-known though improperly named diagnosis of the rupture of one of the discs, the tough, elastic rings (fibrous on the outside, with a jellylike nucleus) found between each vertebra and acting as shock-absorbers.

When a disc ruptures, the nucleus protrudes, and when it presses on some sensitive nerve ending it causes a sudden, piercing backache.

When the rupture occurs in a disc between two lumbar vertebrae—most often it happens between the fourth and the fifth (the so-called L4-L5 disc)—it sets off a diffuse, severe pain known as lumbago. When it happens at the bottom of the spinal column, where this joins with the sacrum—the L5-S1 disc—it is appropriately known as sciatica, as the sciatic nerve, which originates there, is rubbed and enflamed, with pain radiating through the buttocks, down the thigh and the leg, sometimes as far down as the toes. In some cases, both the L4-L5 and L5-S1 discs rupture, which means that the unfortunate patient suffers from both lumbago *and* sciatica.

For certain cases of severe "slipped disc," a surgical procedure called laminectomy is recommended: the orthopedic surgeon first removes part of a plate of bone behind the vertebra next to the disc and then the protruding disc itself. Sometimes, with the removal of the disc, the vertebrae get so close together that their bony protuberances may hit each other. To avoid this, arthrodesis, better known as spinal fusion, is performed: the vertebrae above and below the removed disc are fused together with grafts of chips from the patient's hip bone.

Once serious underlying causes of backache that would require hospitalization have been ruled out, treatment consists mainly of home remedies: a few days' bed rest on a hard mattress (a too long bed rest would weaken the muscles supporting the lower back); ANALGESICS; MASSAGES followed by mild EXERCISE; HEATING PADS or ice packs—depending on whether a particular doctor believes in *heat* or *cold* to ease the pain by relaxing the tension in the muscles—or some more powerful muscle relaxant, such as ethyl chloride, often used by athletes. Also, especially for an anxious, tense patient, a physician may prescribe an antidepressant medication.

Sometimes, however, backache seems to reject any treatment at all and becomes chronic, as if the body had reached some sort of painful equilibrium—a vicious circle of muscle spasms that cause pain, in turn making a person tense, in turn leading to more spasms.

Because backache is so often unmanageable, many doctors are reluctant to treat it. This leaves the field open to osteopathy and chiropractic, two controversial schools of medical practice based on the theory that most diseases are due chiefly to a loss of structural integrity in the tissues, and that health can be restored through manipulative therapy—in the case of backache, through manipulation of the spine.

More recently, at least in the United States, people have experienced dramatic relief of chronic backache with ACUPUNCTURE, the original Chinese medical practice of puncturing the body with special gold or silver needles.

BACK-COMBING (TEASING)

Back-combing, or teasing, the hair is meant to add body to hair styles. If done properly (and if the hair is healthy), teasing doesn't do any damage. Naturally it should be done gently and not too often, in order to minimize the tangling and the tension, especially if the hair is dry or breaks easily.

One way of teasing hair more effectively and gently is to use a brush rather than a comb. To remove the tangles, one should begin brushing (or combing) at the hair's end, working toward the scalp.

BARBITURATES

Barbiturates are a large family of chemicals with powerful hypnotic effects; that is, they are drugs that act to induce profound sleep.

Barbituric acid, the first barbiturate, was synthetized in 1864 by the famous German chemist Adolf von Baeyer. Since then, hundreds of different hypnotics and dozens of similar compounds, as well as combination drugs, each with a different brand name, have been produced from the original barbituric acid molecule.

One of the ways barbiturates act on the organism is by reducing the brain's utilization of oxygen, which causes the activity of nerves and muscles, including the heart, to slow down. Barbiturates are sometimes classified as *short-acting* (such as Amobarbital® and Thiopental®) and *long-acting* (such as Phenobarbital®). The speed with which a barbiturate induces sleep depends on the time it takes to dissolve in myelin, the fatlike substance forming a sheath around certain nerve fibers and found in the white matter of the brain. The duration of a barbiturate's effect depends on the rate at which it is metabolized by the body, which means that short-acting barbiturates act quickly on and disappear quickly from the organism, while traces of long-lasting ones can still be found in the urine after several days. If taken every night for several months, barbiturates may have a cumulative effect and cause physiological side effects, as well as addiction and intellectual impairment.

Moreover, barbiturates taken together with alcohol or with other drugs such as stimulants or tranquilizers may provoke DRUG INTERACTIONS, which in turn may cause excessive central nervous system depression, including respiratory difficulties. Paradoxically, small doses of certain barbiturates may cause excitement and restlessness. And finally, as barbiturates suppress the dreaming stage of sleep (REM sleep), they may provoke a "dream rebound"—the nightmares that often follow a drug-induced sleep as compensation for suppressed REM sleep—which in turn causes INSOMNIA, thus perpetuating a vicious circle of barbiturate dependency.

All things considered, one may wonder how barbiturates could still be prescribed legitimately. One explanation is that barbiturates are indeed very effective hypnotics and that physicians are often pressured by chronic insomniacs. Also, some general practitioners may not yet be aware of the psychological disturbances sometimes underlying insomnia, of the problems of sudden withdrawal or of the relatively new concept of drug interaction. Often, a doctor may be unable to surmise such interaction should a patient fail to mention that he is already taking large doses of nonprescription drugs, such as anthihistamines, ASPIRIN, or cough medicines, many of which are themselves combinations of drugs.

The conscientious physician, then, will carefully investigate each patient suffering from insomnia to see whether the underlying cause of the sleep disturbance can be eliminated. He will be aware of the influence of the patient's age upon the quality of sleep, and the possibility of drug allergy; and he will recommend barbiturates or other hypnotics only in rare cases, for short periods of time, and, above all, will prescribe the right dosage.

BARIATRIC MEDICINE

Bariatric medicine, a relatively new word in the medical vocabulary, refers to the work of bariatricians, specialists in the treatment, prevention and dissemination of information concerning the complex problem of obesity.

BATH OILS

Bath oils are preparations of mineral or vegetable oils and PERFUMES, available in sprays, liquids, capsules, beads or powder, that are added to baths. There are two kinds of bath oils: *emollient* and *nonemollient.*

Emollient bath oils—These help control dry skin caused by age, excessive bathing, low humidity of winter, and over-heated apartments. In general, mineral bath oils adhere better to the skin than do vegetable oils.

Some bath oils disperse throughout the water, while others float on the surface. The latter are generally preferred, because they leave only a thin film on the body, rather than depositing a heavy coating on towels and all over the tub, making it slippery and difficult to wash off.

However, there are so-called "instant bloom" bath oils that give to the water a rich, milklike appearance and are good moisturizers. They disperse in the water but don't leave a ring around the tub.

Nonemollient bath oils—These are merely fragrant products with no therapeutic claims. A few drops of these bath oils just give a bath a pleasant odor.

BATH SALTS

Bath salts are capsules, pellets, granules, or powders designed to soften and to give fragrance and color to bath water, and to act as a mild cleanser. The oldest and simplest bath salt is rock salt crystals, which, since it is inert, can be scented with practically any perfume, and colored with certified dyes. However, rock salt won't soften the water, doesn't dissolve quickly, and won't cleanse the body.

Sodium chloride, borax, sodium sesquicarbonate and epsom salts are among the most widely used bases for bath salts. The residues formed by the evaporation of spring water—spring water salts—make another excellent base. Sodium phosphates are considered one of the best water softeners.

Substances such as sodium perborate, peroxide and sodium bicarbonate are also used because of their property of releasing oxygen when they come in contact with water; the bubbles rising to the surface of the bath produce a pleasant tingling sensation on the skin. Oxygen bath salts have to be kept completely dry before use to prevent the oxygen from being released prematurely.

Effervescent bath salts are lovely but less popular, as it is difficult to keep them from getting moist.

Some bath salt preparations include herbs such as chamomile, lavender blossoms, dandelion, thyme, sage or spearmint.

BEAUTY MACHINES

The term beauty machine is not in the dictionary, and it was probably first used by a fashion-magazine editor hard-pressed to think of yet another euphemism. But it is a good term to describe the dozens of electrically and manually operated appliances favored by cosmeticians and beauty salons.

Technically, beauty machines include everything from ELECTRIC HAIR STYLERS to ELECTROLYSIS needles and DERMABRASION wire brushes. In practice, people tend to make a distinction between "reasonable" and "fancy" beauty machines. Fancy beauty machines usually are found at expensive beauty salons and have alluring trademarks. To name a few: Spiralator®; Tension-Ease®; Esthetron®; Firmatron®; Carbatom®.

Some of them, naturally, are disapproved of by physicians, as they are often manufactured and operated without sound scientific basis. Think of the various "bust developers," for instance, or Perma-Tweez®, the battery-powered, do-it-yourself electrolysis device. Just as naturally, fancy beauty machines fascinate many women, who see them as an extension of COSMETICS and beauty devices in general.

Other beauty machines are quite harmless—Dermascope®, for instance, simply magnifies the skin, permitting both client and consultant to study particular skin conditions. Vapodyne® flows lukewarm water over the surface of the skin. Judging from the description of its U.S. Government patent, the electric cream dispenser that Marie McGrath, the well-known New York hair colorist, invented in a moment of frustration will be extremely useful to anyone who wants to apply creams, hair colors, medicated lotions, even dog shampoos, without having to immerse the hands in them.

And then there are beauty machines which, one hopes, won't be *too* harmful. Esthetron®, for instance, is a gadget equipped with two types of electric current—a stabilized galvanic current used for deep-skin cleaning, with a so-called disincrustation attachment for deep-skin stimulation; and a modulated and polarized current of low voltage to permit deep penetration of special ionized products.

Firmatron®, imported from France, is a high-powered machine with brush attachments that rotate on the body to increase circulation. Another attachment features rotating wooden balls, which are meant for the same purpose but with a more vigorous effect.

Biotron-Activ® looks like part of a vacuum cleaner, and it acts like one when its metal suction cup is applied on the skin for the purpose of "drawing up excess fat and loosening and breaking down fatty deposits."

Carbatom® is a high-power spray meant to "help stimulate blood circulation, nourish skin cells and increase surface skin acidity for protection against germ penetration."

The list of beauty machines is much longer, and growing. Still, questions such as whether certain beauty machines break tiny blood vessels; whether electrodes are traumatic to the skin; whether blood circulation ought to be stimulated electrically; whether wrinkles should be irrigated, or whether blackheads should be treated with suction instruments may well remain unanswered for a long time.

BEAUTY SPAS

The common term "spa" is derived from the Belgian town of Spa, which, because of the curative value of its mineral springs, was the most fashionable resort of Europe in the eighteenth century. Not all beauty spas, however, are located near mineral springs. The term "spa" can refer to a beauty-and-health resort where people can rest, lose (or gain) weight, exercise, learn good health habits, slow down aging—in a word, give up for a while responsibility for their looks and well-being and entrust them to a staff of well-trained specialists, usually including dieticians, physical instructors, cosmeticians and masseurs, supervised by a physician.

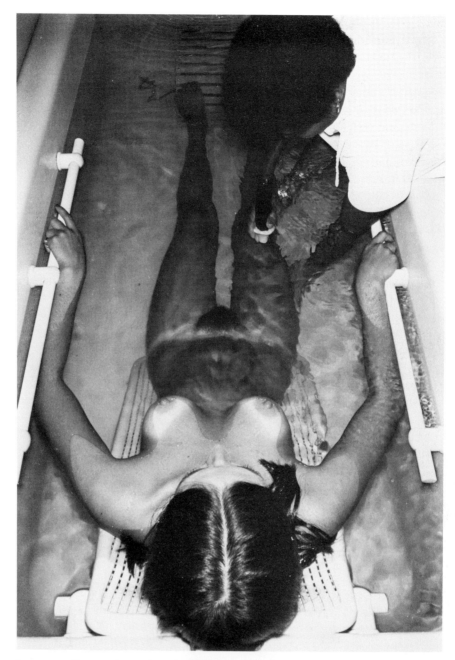

A guest at Renaissance in Nassau, Bahamas, enjoying her daily session of one of the various "thalassotherapies" available at this spa.

The oversize tub is filled with circulating sea water—one of the few still unpolluted sea waters in the world—piped in directly from the nearby shore.

The operator is giving the young woman an underwater massage by moving a jet of heated sea water over her submerged thighs.

GUS ROBERTS

Successful beauty spas in this country—such as La Costa near San Diego, California; The Golden Door, near Escondido, California; Main Chance (owned by Elizabeth Arden) in the Arizona desert; The Greenhouse (run by Charles of the Ritz and Neiman Marcus) at Arlington, Texas—usually offer luxurious quarters, calorie-minded but excellent food, large swimming pools, whirlpool baths, SAUNAS, gyms and dancing and yoga classes. Some of the spas are small and secluded, surrounded by tropical gardens or luscious countrysides. Others are self-contained units in large resorts, with tennis courts, golf courses, riding stables, private beaches. At least one, Murieta Hot Springs in Southern California, is a spa in the literal sense of the word: it has not only mineral springs but also mud baths.

Among well-known beauty spas abroad are the Rancho la Puerta in Mexico and the Renaissance Revitalization Spa in Nassau, Bahamas. More ambitious than the other beauty spas, Renaissance offers specific programs of rejuvenation such as cellular therapy (i.e., injections of cells extracted from various organs of unborn lambs) and oral treatment with incubated chicken embryos. Renaissance, which is located on a lovely, unpolluted beach, also offers hormone therapy, mud and seaweed baths, inhalations of aromatic oils, and the so-called thalassotherapy, which consists of scotch douches (alternating jets of hot and cold water) and whirlpool baths of filtered and heated sea water.

In a way, small, secluded beauty spas are better than large ones that bustle with social activities. For one thing, "temptations" such as rich foods, alcohol, cigarettes and unsupervised sports are less accessible. On the other hand, small beauty spas tend to acquire some of the more negative characteristics of an enclosed community. Persons attending a smaller spa may band together in a fairly cohesive group with a similar aim—to pamper themselves, which can become tedious work if done twenty-four hours a day. Also, as in a small community, conflicts may arise.

The expert beauty-spa administration is aware of all this and often succeeds in providing the right atmosphere, so that the spa's slightly absurd routine not only makes sense but becomes a pleasure—at least for two weeks, the minimum time it takes for any kind of invigoration and beautification to take place.

BIOFEEDBACK

Biofeedback, a term coined in 1969 by a group of physicians subsequently called The Biofeedback Research Society, refers to a number of techniques that use electronic instruments to give a person immediate and continuing signals of changes in bodily functions of which he is normally unaware—such as fluctuations in blood pressure, muscle tension, skin temperature, and brain-wave activity.

Despite the accepted belief that physiological functions regulated by the autonomic nervous system are beyond a person's conscious control, physicians have reported that people undergoing biofeedback experiments quickly learn first to recognize and then to control their physiological "involuntary" functions.

Though biofeedback has still to be explored further, and in any case cannot be seen as a remedy for organic diseases, it already shows extraordinary potential in the understanding and treatment of conditions such as HYPERTENSION, ASTHMA, MIGRAINE, tension HEADACHE and epilepsy.

Biofeedback instruments usually can detect, transmit and amplify precise information about a subject's internal changes, and the information is usually channeled through a computer and presented to the subject as a buzzer (which he hears through earphones), as a light flashed in a soundproof room from a box resembling a traffic light, or as a moving chart. Once a person can "hear" or "see" his own heart beat, blood pressure, or brain waves, he can learn to manipulate them mentally, increasing or decreasing his internal processes' frequency, volume, speed or intensity. At first the desired physiological events occur only by chance, but when they do occur the feedback instrument informs the subject that the feeling he is experiencing is the "right" one. As the process is repeated, the subject learns to distinguish the right feeling more accurately and finally to *produce* the feeling (and the associated physiological processes) at will. Eventually, he is able to do so *without* the use of the instrument. Obviously, the capacity to learn such control is inherent in all human beings, and biofeedback, which could be compared to such classic practices as yoga or meditation, only simplifies and accelerates the learning process.

BIOPSY

A biopsy is the examination, usually under a microscope, of a piece of living tissue removed from the body, usually under local anaesthesia, in order to help formulate an otherwise uncertain diagnosis of infection, benign tumors, and cancer.

There are three basic types of biopsy, depending on the amount of tissue removed:

Open biopsy—In open biopsy, a specimen of tissue is either scraped with a curette, a spoon-shaped knife, if the lesion is superficial, or excised, if it is deep. Sometimes, some normal tissue is also removed to allow the pathologist to make a comparison. The pathologist usually decides what size the specimen should be and whether it should be treated chemically or frozen to avoid distortion of the cells in the air before the specimen reaches the laboratory.

Punch (or aspiration) biopsy—This is used mostly for diagnosis of skin lesions, such as SKIN CANCER, or of breast CYSTS, with a minimum of trauma. It is performed by puncturing the lesion with a hollow needle, which then sucks up part or all of the lesion's tissue for examination. Punch biopsy is preferred when the biopsy tissue has to be removed from so-called cosmetic areas, because it leaves only a minuscule scar.

Surface biopsy—In surface biopsy, cells obtained from the secretions of an organ are specially stained and examined, as in the PAP SMEAR TEST, in order to detect early cancer of the cervix.

BLEACHING CREAM

There is no bleaching cream on the market that is truly safe and effective in lightening uneven, dark spots on the skin such as freckles, birthmarks, age spots, flat moles, and chloasma, also called "mask of pregnancy."

Despite the apparent increased frequency of disorders in the pigment of skin, no practical progress has developed in the cosmetic industry. As for pigmentation studies in medical centers, much theory and a few scientific observations about how different preparations work are all that is available.

The bleaching creams of the early 1970s are not much different from those of the 1940s, except that today the risks of certain concentrations of bleaching ingredients are better understood.

The most effective skin lighteners available today are:

1) Masking makeups containing titanium dioxide. These products do not truly bleach the skin, but just effectively *cover* the blotchy areas.
2) Oxidizing agents such as peroxide, or organic acids such as lemon juice which decolorize melanin, the skin pigment.
3) Specific bleaching substances, of which mercury is the best, that act by preventing the synthesis of tyrosinase, the enzyme that catalyzes various compounds in the body into melanin.

Other bleaching compounds, such as hydroquinone and its derivatives, act by destroying melanocytes (the color-producing cells) or by poisoning some of the steps of the formation of melanin.

However, there are disadvantages to each type of product:

1) Titanium dioxide not only is just a coverup but is opaque, reflecting the light differently from the rest of the skin. Unless the spot is small, these products are aesthetically unsatisfactory.
2) Peroxides and organic acids are frustratingly slow, unpredictable, and often reversible in their action.

3) Mercury compounds may produce a little lightening of the excessive pigment, but they may become toxic and cause allergic reactions.

The best bleaching creams, then, are those containing hydroquinone. But these, too, are useful only for lightening limited areas where excessive pigment is the result of an abnormal process; they are not useful for lightening *normal* dark skin. Also, the effectiveness of hydroquinone varies from person to person and in different skin areas of the same person. Occasionally, hydroquinone may *increase* pigmentation or cause complete loss of pigment (leukoderma).

After application of hydroquinone, exposure to the sun should be avoided, as sunlight counteracts the action of the drug; that is, it promotes the production of melanin.

BLEPHAROPLASTY (EYELID CORRECTION)

The technique of this PLASTIC SURGERY procedure, which is often performed in conjunction with a FACE-LIFT, is quite simple: it consists of removing an ellipse of skin from the upper eyelid and then a small strip of skin from the lower, with an incision on the outer side coinciding with one of the "crow's feet." Finally, once the surgeon has made sure the corrections on the lids of one eye match those on the other, he finally sutures the incisions with silk and nylon threads.

What is not simple, though, is deciding on the length of the incisions, drawing a steady curve, and measuring the exact amount of skin to be removed: too little would not correct the defect; a few millimeters too much and the eye might look distorted or, worse, not be able to close properly. Also, inside both the upper and the lower lid are three pockets of fatty tissue lying next to one another; any combination of these little lumps can protrude as the result of a weakening of the membrane that contains them, giving the eye a tired, old look, even in young people. In correcting the eyelids, therefore, some of this protruding fat also has to be trimmed. And again, removing the exact amount is of enormous importance, especially from the lateral pocket in the lower lid. An overcorrection would provoke an unattractive depression.

Sometimes cutting excess skin from the upper eyelid is not enough; even before planning a blepharoplasty, a surgeon must decide whether the defect is indeed in the upper lid or rather in a drooping eyebrow. The latter can be elevated by excising a modified ellipse (wider toward the temple) directly above the brow, with the final suture line lying within the brow's upper line. But for eyelids suffering from chronic EDEMA (retention of liquid) there is very little that can be done at all: the puffiness will reappear shortly after the operation.

For these operations, most surgeons prefer local ANAESTHESIA combined with preoperative sedatives. The operation lasts about one and a half hours, and the sutures are usually removed after four or five days; however, if the scars are not completely healed, a special adhesive tape is applied across them for a few additional days.

BODY CYCLES

Any biological event that recurs at a predictable interval—such as the rise and fall of body temperature, the fluctuation of hormone levels, the alternating of sleep and alertness, the monthly MENSTRUATION of women—can be considered a body cycle.

The time it takes to complete a cycle is called the *period* and is often represented by the Greek letter τ. A period may last anywhere from a microsecond (one-millionth of a second) to a year. Brainwaves or ENZYME rhythms, for instance, are calculated in microseconds, while the period of menstruation is about twenty-eight days.

Many of our physiological functions follow a so-called circadian rhythm (from the Latin *circa dies*—around a day), a daily rhythm of activity and rest. However, individuals have somewhat different biological rhythms, as "each person is . . . a unique composite of subtle inherited characteristics, who is moreover shaped by his experience," in the words of Gay Gaer Luce, the author of *Body Time*.

Although scientists still know very little about most of our body cycles, they are beginning to understand the ways the various cycles intermesh, how the human body is transformed hour by hour as its metabolism and vital organs fluctuate rhythmically, and how vulnerable the cycles are to illness, drugs, anxiety, east-west travel, and the environment in general.

Few people have a sense of their own cycles, but many of us know at least something about our daily rhythms—almost everybody can discover, for instance, at which time of day he functions best and when it is best for him to work, rest, eat. The often rigidly regulated time divisions dictated by industrialized societies—with jet travel, night or round-the-clock work—often interfere with the body cycles of many people, who forever find themselves out of tune with their own metabolisms. It is therefore probable that many people would not have to resort to stimulants or tranquilizers, or be the victims of innumerable, inexplicable PSYCHOSOMATIC DISEASES, if they weren't forced to compensate for their internal desynchronization.

BODY ODORS

Individual body odors are mainly caused by the secretion of the apocrine glands—specialized sweat glands found almost entirely in the hairy underarm area—which, unlike the eccrine glands, are activated only by emotional stimulation and emit a complex, organic secretion containing ammonia, PROTEINS, CARBOHYDRATES, lipids and inorganic IRON. The secretion is at first odorless but after about six hours is decomposed by bacteria on the skin to create the characteristic underarm odor.

Mouth odor—halitosis—is usually caused by local decomposition of particles of food, especially fibrous meat caught between teeth and not reached by the TOOTHBRUSH.

In other parts of the body—on the feet, for instance—bacteria break down rubbed-off skin cells in the moist, confined environment of the shoes, producing the equally characteristic foot odor. Another odor is that of vaginal secretions, which readily decompose once they reach the air.

And finally there are odors related to a person's diet, activities, occupations, clothes and personal hygiene, regardless of sex: men and women produce about the same amount of aprocrine secretion and odor.

In general, body odors are little more than a nuisance. However, sometimes they can be symptomatic of more serious problems, for, in many disorders, unusual substances that can generate odors are secreted by the body. Some of these odors can be of help to a physician in formulating a diagnosis. Also, a doctor is immediately alerted when, for instance, a patient is exaggeratedly perfumed or deodorized. For one, the feeling of being "unclean" is not uncommon in certain people whose neurosis is to reject their own bodies (or those of others). Or else the patient may be aware of some unusual odor and try to neutralize it for fear of being embarrassed.

As for halitosis, it may be due to something more serious than poor oral hygiene: it could signal a periodontal disease, caries or gingivitis. More dramatically, odors may help a physician to recognize an emergency, for people in coma and those with severe HYPERTENSION, poisoning, diabetes, and so forth all have distinctive odors.

On the other hand, there is little unpleasant odor from a healthy and hygienic person; in fact, a human body's natural odor, even without the help of deodorizers and perfumes, not only can be pleasant but is part of the body's sexual attraction, not dissimilar in principle from the mating mechanism of most animals.

BOTULISM

Botulism is an acute food poisoning caused by the ingestion of food containing the toxin secreted by a bacterium called *Clostridium botulinum.*

Poisoning by botulism is extremely rare. Although the bacterium is common in the environment, it is usually harmless, because it cannot grow—and therefore cannot produce toxin—in the presence of oxygen. If, however, the bacteria get into an airless container without being destroyed by proper cooking (at least six minutes of boiling) they can multiply and become deadly.

Modern methods of commercial food canning have greatly reduced the threat of botulism in those products. In recent years, most instances of botulism have been found in home canning.

Danger signals: bulged or heaved-up lids; leakage of contents; bubbling or boiling over of contents when the can is opened.

The contents of such cans should never be tasted or thrown away, but rather delivered to the Food and Drug Administration for tests.

BRASSIERES

At the turn of the century, Charles R. Debevoise, a Frenchman, introduced a revolutionary feminine garment which he called a *brassière* —a bust bodice with shoulder straps which freed women from the close-fitting, boned and laced corset of the 1800s.

The term brassiere crossed the Atlantic and is still used in the United States, while in France it was abandoned first for *bandeau* (which, too, is now used by the American bra industry for short-line brassieres) and then for the current term, *soutien-gorge*.

For a few years in the 1920s, brassieres were designed to flatten bosoms, to give them the then fashionable boyish look. But already in 1922 the "uplift" bra had begun to appear, designed to give breasts a more natural—or even fuller than natural—contour.

In the 1930s, the first foam-rubber padded bras were introduced—the famous falsies—which reached their highest success in the 1940s and early 1950s, when most young women wished to resemble Jane Russell, Marilyn Monroe and other full-bosomed movie stars.

The 1950s brought the development of the cup-size structure, the use of nylon, and the contemporary underwire—a curved piece of wire outlining each cup. But it was only in the 1960s that the bra finally became what it should have been all along: a garment designed for the purpose of shaping less-than-perfect breasts so as to make them appear firm, proportionate, and as natural as possible.

Not everybody needs to wear brassieres; women with small, naturally firm breasts are hardly affected by aging, pregnancy, LACTATION, crash DIETS, menstrual disorders, heredity, strenuous EXERCISE, or gravity, which usually cause larger and more fragile breasts to sag and lose their youthful contour. The main reason why most breasts sag is that they don't have major muscles of their own; there is only a thin layer of connective tissue between the mammary glands and the chest muscles over which the glands are "slung." This thin layer tends to overstretch and break down, often with extraordinary rapidity. Except for a lucky few, then, women should wear brassieres most of the time to protect the delicate structure of the breasts from the continuous action of gravity and physical activities. Also, well-fitting brassieres often retard or avoid the formation of STRETCH MARKS.

To find the right size bra, a woman must consider the following basic factors: 1) size of breast; 2) size of cup; 3) position; 4) separation.

Size of breast—Bra sizes come only in even numbers, such as 32, 34, 36. To determine the right size, measure the ribcage under the bust with a tape measure and add 5 inches. For instance, if a woman measures 29 inches underbust, she is size 34 (29 inches plus 5 inches). If she measures 30 inches, the perfect size for her would probably be 35, but since odd sizes are not available (unless the bra is custom-made), she usually fits best into the next size: 36. If a woman measures 33 inches or more, only 3 inches are generally added instead of 5 inches.

Size of cup—Cup sizes range from A to D. (The smallest is AA; the largest, DD.) The right cup can be determined by measuring the chest at the fullest part of the breast. If the measure is the same as the bra size, the cup is an A; with every additional inch the cup size increases. For instance:

$$
\begin{aligned}
\text{Bra size } 34 + 0 &= \text{A} \quad \text{cup} \\
+ 1 &= \text{B} \quad \text{cup} \\
+ 2 &= \text{C} \quad \text{cup} \\
+ 3 &= \text{D} \quad \text{cup} \\
+ 4 &= \text{DD} \ \text{cup}
\end{aligned}
$$

Cups should always be filled out comfortably; if they wrinkle—despite accurate measurements—a woman should choose a *smaller* size, or a different style, or both. If the breast overflows the cup, or if the bra fits only with the hooks in the outside row of eyes, a *larger* size (or a different style, or both) is the best choice. Sometimes, all that is needed is a different fabric.

Position—A well-designed bra should lift a sagging breast to the right position—approximately halfway between the top of the shoulder and the waistline. Shoulder straps help keep the bra in place, but shortening them will not raise the bustline. Too tight straps merely cut into the flesh and cause the bra to raise in the back.

Separation—In choosing a bra style, a woman should be aware not only of the shape of her breasts but also of the distance between them. A woman whose breasts are very close and tend to bunch together in front should always choose an underwire bra, which helps keep the breasts separate. Conversely, breasts with a too pronounced cleavage will look better in a so-called push-up or push-over brassiere, that is, one with a padding in the lower part of the cup only, which will push the breasts up or closer together without actually increasing their size.

Brassieres are available in a variety of styles and fabrics. Bali, one of the most successful bra manufacturers in the United States, is currently producing more than fifty different kinds of bras. The basic types of bra are: 1) soft-cup; 2) stretch; 3) contoured; 4) padded; 5) strapless; 6) underwire.

Soft-cup bras—These bras are unlined and should be worn almost exclusively by women with small, well-shaped breasts that don't need a lift. They are comfortable, light, and slightly accentuate the breasts' shape.

Stretch bras—Also called one-size-fits-all, these are very light, completely elasticized, including the shoulder straps. They are very comfortable, especially for women with sloping shoulders. However, since they take their shape from the breasts, they give minimum support, and unless the breasts are firm, the cups tend to collapse and expand horizontally.

Contoured bras—Contoured bras are lined with a thin layer of polyester, which helps equalize breast size and gives support and shape. It is a good choice for women wearing in-between sizes.

Padded bras—These bras actually add to the dimension of the bust. They are fashioned with an insert of fiberfill throughout the cup, thicker in the center and tapering off at the sides.

Halter bras—These are conventional bras with detachable shoulder straps, which can be either fastened around the neck or crisscrossed on the back, when the style of a particular dress requires naked shoulders.

Strapless bras—This type of bra usually has a lined cup to insure a good bustline definition. How it manages to stay in place without shoulder straps is a mystery to the layman and a source of pride for the manufacturer.

Front-closing bras—These fasten in the front, either with a hook or with a tiny plastic lock. Originally designed only for nursing women, they have become quite popular because of their smooth back, and because they eliminate most of the bending and twisting when putting on a bra.

Underwire bras—Underwire bras were designed to lift, support, and separate full or sagging breasts from beneath the bosom, relieving the tension applied to the shoulder straps. However, early underwires were cylindrical, heavy and generally uncomfortable. In the last eighteen years, the S&S Industries, Inc., America's leading manufacturer of underwires, has developed and patented a flat, thin wire coated in soft plastic, to which in 1969 it added cushioned tips. The new underwire is featherlight and flexible, and it gently hugs the ribcage without the slightest discomfort. Underwire bras gather each breast from the side and center front and contain it within the cup. If the breasts are large, the underwire helps distribute the tissue more evenly and prevents it from accumulating near the underarm or in front. If the breasts are small, the underwire slightly increases their projection, often making padding unnecessary.

Both soft-cup and underwire bras are manufactured in two versions: the *bandeau* (short line) and the *long line*. The latter, which can be mounted on a band a few inches wide or extend to the waistline, is sometimes favored for high-waisted dresses; also, it somewhat slims the midriff while giving support to the bust. However, it should be long enough to avoid bulges at the waistline and should stretch enough to be comfortable when sitting.

In the last ten years, major bra manufacturers such as Bali and Warner have developed bras, called, respectively, Ski-Bali® and Full Comfort®, with extended, partly elasticized top cups which help to cover and keep in place the special SILICONE paddings required by women who have recently undergone MASTECTOMY.

In the early 1970s cups made of preshaped fabric were introduced. Though the techniques are still being improved, the advantages of molded bras are extraordinary; for one, they eliminate seams altogether, making bras look and feel as smooth as natural skin.

The best way of putting on a brassiere is first to slip the straps over the shoulders and grasp both sides of the bra. Next, lean forward, letting the breasts ease into the cups. Then straighten up and, without letting go of the fabric, slide both hands to the back of the bra and hook it, making sure the band is low on the back. The straps should be adjusted, and the nipples should coincide with the center of each cup.

Among the most popular fabrics used for brassieres are:

Cotton—The classic, natural fiber that is absorbent, cool, durable, and unharmed by DETERGENTS. Cotton bras are still the choice for women allergic to certain synthetic materials.

Nylon—A synthetic fiber that is elastic, flexible, practically unshrinkable, easy to wash and to dry. However, it does not absorb perspiration.

Polyester—The generic term for soft, resilient synthetic fibers such as Dacron® and Fortrel® that are cool, nonallergenic and easy to wash.

Rayon—A synthetic fiber often used in blends; absorbent, nonstatic.

Spandex—The generic term for a strong, resilient synthetic fiber that has made possible sheer and very light stretchable fabrics such as Lycra® and Vyrene®. It can be dyed, and recently it has been used in blends with nylon, polyester and other fibers for molded bras.

Tricot—A knitted fabric made of yarns woven in a series of loops, which gives it a certain elasticity without the fabric's actually stretching.

Not all brassiere styles are appropriate for every woman; two women wearing the same size may look and feel better in different styles because their bodies are built differently. Yet, finding one well-fitting bra is not enough: every woman should own several types of bras for different kinds of clothes and different occasions. "Some women become extremely attached to one specific bra," observed Joya Paterson, vice-president of S&S Industries, Inc. "I myself often hang up a dress and its own bra on the same hanger. Besides, breasts change—they swell during MENSTRUATION, for instance. Not to speak of the more permanent changes occurring after a diet or with menopause. It would be like wearing the same makeup all the time, regardless whether it is worn in the brightest sun or in artificial light; by a redhead or by a brunette; with a T shirt or with a sequined evening gown."

BREAST CANCER

Breast lesions include anomalies in development, inflammations connected with pregnancy and lactation, and various types of growths—CYSTS and tumors. The latter can be *benign, premalignant,* or *malignant* (cancerous). Of all breast lesions, breast cancer is not only the most dangerous but also the most common of all kinds of cancer in women.

A typical cancer cell—a result of the presence of defective genes, or of the effects of radiations, certain chemicals, or viruses.

Cancer may occur in almost any tissue or organ of the body, in different forms in different tissues, and often in different forms in the same tissue. The characteristics common to all forms of cancer are their continued growth not under the normal control of the body and their tendency to spread to other tissues and form additional tumors, or metastases. We do not know why the body is not able to control the growth of cancer cells. It is this potentially unlimited growth of cells that serve no useful function in the body that makes cancer so different from other diseases, in which the basic problem is the injury or death of groups of cells.

Cancer cells expand locally by invasion and spread to distant organs along lymphatics, blood vessels or through body cavities, eventually killing host tissues or organs.

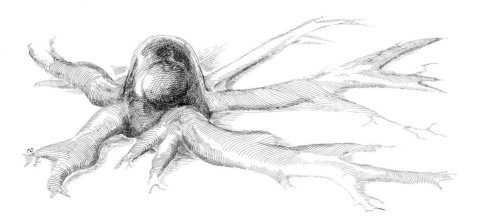

Malignant means that the new growth is made up of cells tending to infiltrate the surrounding tissues and give rise to METASTASES, i.e., the spreading of the disease from one organ to another not directly connected to it. Breast cancer can spread by way of either the bloodstream or the lymphatics, the thin-walled vessels that meander from the breast to the lymph glands (or nodes), most of which are located in the armpit. If the cancer cells get into the blood, they can travel anywhere—to bone, lung, or brain. However, breast cancer in the early stages does not ordinarily reach the bloodstream; spreading through the lymphatics is much more common.

Despite advances in surgery, radiography and chemotherapy (anticancer drugs), there are thousands of new cases of breast cancer every year in the United States, and the mortality rate has remained practically the same for the past thirty years.

Breast cancer usually manifests itself in women over forty, with 75 percent of the cases occurring in women between forty-five and fifty-five. After that age, the incidence increases throughout the lifespan. Besides age, the following factors seem to play a role in the incidence of breast cancer:

Sex—Breast cancer occurs one hundred times as frequently in women as in men.

Fertility—The relative risk of cancer is higher for infertile women.

Age of first pregnancy—Women pregnant after twenty-five have a risk double that of those women first pregnant before twenty.

Nursing—Women who nurse for long terms (thirty-six months) have less risk than those nursing less than three months.

Cysts—Though most cysts are *not* premalignant, some cystic diseases of the breast increase the risk of breast cancer.

Cancer of the ovary, uterus, etc.—Cancers in other organs show a hormonal relationship with breast cancer.

Cancer of the other breast—The risk of developing cancer in the second breast after the first one has been removed is about five times higher than the normal risk of initial breast cancer in the general population.

Sidedness—Breast cancer in women is more likely to develop in the *left* breast. (In men the reverse is true.)

Family history—Women with a mother or sister who has breast cancer have an increased chance of developing it.

Race—Among women in the United States, breast cancer seems to be more frequent in whites. Japan has the lowest incidence of breast cancer in the world, while Denmark has the highest.

Obesity—Obese and stocky women seem to be more prone to breast cancer than slender ones.

Most breast tumors are detected by the patient; only a few are noted by the physician during routine examination, which is often too cursory to detect very small nodules. Yet a woman has better chances for recovery if the breast cancer is detected *before* it becomes palpable. Indeed, this is practically the only thing breast cancer specialists agree on: the earlier a cancer is detected and treated, the greater the chances of survival.

The techniques for early breast cancer detection include MAMMOGRAPHY, THERMOGRAPHY, XEROGRAPHY and a very accurate examination of the breast. None of these techniques is itself conclusive, but their combination can help the physician make an accurate diagnosis or at least alert him to any abnormality.

Basically, a malignant tumor has a hard consistency, an irregular shape, and is generally located in the upper, outer side of the breast, while benign tumors are usually firm but soft, well delineated and mobile. However, the only conclusive proof of malignancy is a BIOPSY, the removal and microscopic examination of a small amount of the affected tissue. If the nodule is malignant, the entire breast and all the tissues that have been directly or indirectly affected by it are usually

This is a thermogram—one of the modern methods of spotting early breast cancer. Thermography is a process that converts the temperature pattern in the breast tissue into a photographic image. Since breast cancer is associated with an elevation of temperature in the skin over the lesion, a thermogram can often record even a small lesion quite accurately. *Courtesy of the American Cancer Society.*

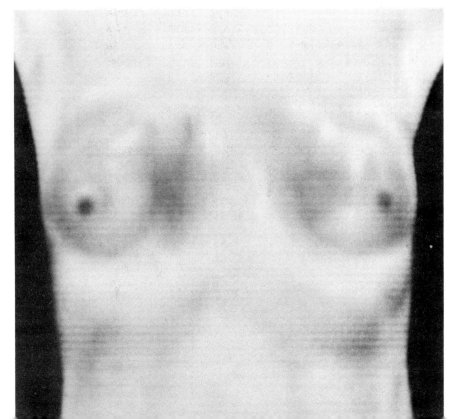

removed on the spot—a delay of even a few weeks could be fatal—with a surgical technique called MASTECTOMY. Postoperative treatment often includes radiation therapy and hormone therapy.

To most women with breast cancer, survival is the most important consideration. But for many people, fear of death or relief at having escaped it is something abstract—certainly not a feeling one can sustain day after day. In fact, some women prefer to gamble on survival rather than lose the breast and live with the mutilation and dysfunctions they associate with mastectomy. Often it is this fear, and not ignorance, that keeps a woman from regular check-ups or, worse, induces her to conceal her disease until it is too late.

In the past, the aesthetic value that the breast has for many women (and men) has hardly been perceived by conscientious cancer surgeons, whose only concern was that of saving the patient's life. Even the idea of explaining the nature of the operation to a bewildered patient and her relatives seemed a waste of time to some surgeons. As for the mechanics of mastectomy, the incisions were usually large and very visible, criss-crossing the chest with little concern for such things as low-cut dresses or bathing suits.

In the last few years, however, cancer specialists have begun to place more emphasis on performing acceptable biopsy and mastectomy incisions, on understanding the advantages and limitations of different procedures, and on selecting the technique offering the best functional *and* cosmetic results for each type and stage of breast cancer. Above all, surgeons have begun to consider, even before performing mastectomy, the possibility of BREAST RECONSTRUCTION after surgery. For a breast cancer specialist this means not only competence in handling the disease but also a respect for every scrap of untainted tissue; it also means, when possible, a discreet *horizontal* incision (rather than the classic *vertical* one) and always a miniaturist's precision with sutures. In a word, deference to beauty, which for the moment only plastic surgeons are being trained to carry into the operating room.

Treatment of breast cancer, many specialists feel, has been developed to the maximum. As of 1974, surgery, radiation, hormones, and chemical drugs have reached their limit of efficiency. The only field open in the cure of breast cancer is immunotheraphy.

Prevention of breast cancer is no longer impossible. Injection of an inactivated breast tumor virus has been shown to completely protect mice against a live virus that produced multiple tumors in mice not protected by this injection. Since a virus has been isolated in the milk of women with breast cancer and in some without cancer, there is a possibility of developing an immunization against breast cancer virus in humans.

BREAST-CANCER SCREENING

In 1974 the National Cancer Institute and the American Cancer Society began conducting a national screening program, free for women thirty-five years of age or older, to detect breast cancer at an early stage.

At various clinics scattered around the country, physicians and specialized technicians give women a physical examination, including MAMMOGRAPHY, THERMOGRAPHY and/or XEROGRAPHY.

Among these centers are:
College of Medicine and Dentistry, Newark, New Jersey
Duke University Medical Center, Durham, North Carolina
Ellis Fischel State Cancer Research Center, Columbia, Missouri
Emory University–Georgia Baptists Hospital, Atlanta, Georgia
Georgetown Institute, Washington, D.C.
Good Samaritan Hospital and Medical Center, Portland, Oregon
Guttman Institute, New York, New York
Iowa Lutheran Hospital, Des Moines
Medical College of Wisconsin, Milwaukee
Mountain States Tumor Institute, Boise, Idaho
Pacific Health Research Institute, Honolulu, Hawaii
Rhode Island Hospital, Providence
St. Joseph's Hospital, Houston, Texas
St. Vincent's Medical Center, Jacksonville, Florida
Temple University–Albert Einstein Medical Center, Philadelphia,
    Pennsylvania
University of Arizona Medical Center, Tucson
University of Kansas Medical Center, Kansas City
University of Louisville School of Medicine, Louisville, Kentucky
University of Oklahoma Health Science Center, Oklahoma City
University of Pittsburgh School of Medicine, Pittsburgh, Pennsylvania
University of Southern California, Los Angeles
Vanderbilt University School of Medicine, Nashville, Tennessee
Virginia Mason Research Center, Seattle, Washington
Wilmington Medical Center, Wilmington, Delaware

BREAST RECONSTRUCTION

BREAST CANCER never results from reduction or augmentation mammaplasty. On the contrary, a woman who has undergone MASTECTOMY because of breast cancer can often benefit from a PLASTIC SURGERY method of breast reconstruction.

Mastectomy is usually performed by a general surgeon whose main goal is, understandably, to remove, as soon as detected, the malignant growth and all tissues that have been affected by it. Until recently, many surgeons would not concern themselves with the psychological trauma that breast mutilation almost always causes in women, especially younger ones, other than reassuring patients that the dangerous growth had been removed in time and urging them to resign themselves to a relatively minor mutilation.

This is not to suggest that all cancer specialists have been insensitive to women's feelings or ignorant of modern procedures in their own profession. Still, until recently, it was indeed difficult for a woman who had undergone mastectomy even to discover that such a thing as breast reconstruction existed. More women will become aware of this procedure in the near future; right now there are hundreds of women who are undergoing or have recently undergone uncensurable but standard mastectomies and who have the right to hope that they may be able to undergo breast reconstruction.

Unfortunately, when a radical mastectomy has left little more than scar tissue surrounded by tight, fragile skin—or worse, when RADIOTHERAPY has burned the tissue irreparably—the only solution a plastic surgeon can offer is a laborious, many-stage procedure of skin grafting, in which skin has to be brought from other parts of the body, thus creating more scars. The results of such an operation are not often proportionate to the time, discomfort and pain involved.

However, in other cases, when the skin has softened and there is enough to work with, the incisions have healed well, and there are no swellings, plastic surgeons can offer a better solution than resignation and padded brassieres: SILICONE prostheses, similar to those used for augmentation mammaplasty.

Among the plastic surgeons whose names in the last several years have become increasingly linked to the treatment of breast problems is Dr. Reuven K. Snyderman of Princeton, New Jersey. The breast-shaped implants Dr. Snyderman and his colleagues use are prolonged, in the upper part, into a flap, which provides a cushioning where the removal of the chest muscle has left a depression almost more objectionable, to some women, than the removal of the breast itself. Improved implants, which will also provide a filling for the armpit defect, are being perfected now.

The method of insertion is similar to that used for enlarging a small breast. One difference is that the surgeon does not try to match the other breast perfectly. Until the skin stretches, the implant has to be very small, lest undue tension of the skin provoke rejection. After about six months, the implant can be changed for a larger one, but if the untainted breast is particularly large and drooping, the surgeon can obtain a really attractive result—and good symmetry—only by reducing this breast rather than attempting to use a larger prosthesis in the other.

The operation lasts less than one hour, and the patient usually may leave the hospital after four or five days. At a later stage, the surgeon can also rebuild the nipple, using tissue from the other breast's nipple or from tissue taken from the outer vaginal area. Yet most patients, Dr. Snyderman noted, seem more concerned with regaining volume rather than with visual symmetry, and even young women rarely come back to have the nipple rebuilt.

Almost unanimously, doctors say that implants never stimulate a recurrence of a malignant tumor. But even if properly and completely removed, certain forms of malignant tumors might appear in the second breast; often it is only a matter of time.

Usually, the most satisfying breast reconstruction of all is that following a subcutaneous mastectomy, because this has left intact the skin and the nipple.

BUBBLE BATH

Bubble baths, which may be in the form of powders, granules, beads, liquids, gels, tablets, capsules, cakes or crystals, are designed to fill the tub with a fragrant foam that will also act as a slight detergent and prevent the forming of a soap ring in the tub.

A good bubble bath is one that, using only a small amount, and without the need of too much water pressure, produces a copious foam that is stable at various temperatures and in the presence of hard and soft water, soap, and dirt.

The major complaint about bubble baths is instability of the foam, mostly because some people use it together with soap, as they think that the bubbles alone won't cleanse.

Some bubble baths contain VITAMINS, chlorophyll, medicinal herb extracts or LANOLIN, but these ingredients really do not seem to add anything of extra benefit to the bath.

The best time for a person to use soap is after the bubble bath—it will then be easier to remove the foam from the tub.

BUNIONS

Bunions are misaligned toe joints which become swollen and tender. The basic cause is weakness of the muscle structure, but heredity and ill-fitting shoes may also contribute to them.

Aside from choosing more comfortable and wider shoes to avoid irritation, and wearing pads to remove pressure from the area, one can do little about bunions.

An enflamed joint of the big toe may also indicate gout, which, of course, calls for entirely different treatment.

CALORIES

Calories are not food but units for measuring energy. One calorie is the amount of energy required to raise the temperature of one kilogram of water (slightly more than one quart) by one degree centigrade—from 14.5° to 15.5°.

To say that a tablespoon of honey, for instance, contains one hundred calories means that the honey, when oxidized in the tissue of the body, will release that amount of energy to be expended in bodily activities.

Various forms of energy are interchangeable: one can measure in calories the energy *spent* in activity and the energy *acquired* with food. Energy expended in most types of activity is proportionate to a person's body weight. In other words, a heavy person burns up *more* calories performing the same type of physical activity than a lighter person.

Calories are all alike, regardless of their source: all foods and all beverages, except water, sugar-free drinks, black coffee and tea, are turned into calories for body use. One pound of body fat has approximately the energy value of 3,500 calories.

The body needs a number of calories each day to maintain its weight. Part of the calories are expended daily just to keep the body's organs functioning—the so-called "minimum calorie need," which is proportionate to the body's size, composition, age. Men generally have a higher minimum calorie need than women, because they are larger and have a greater proportion of muscle tissue and less fat. Women during pregnancy and lactation, as well as adolescents, also have a higher-than-average minimum calorie need.

The additional number of calories spent each day depends on a person's activities and on the length of time spent at them—one hour at a desk obviously consumes fewer calories than one hour playing tennis. The following table shows the number of calories expended in different kinds of activities:

Sedentary activities, such as reading, writing, eating, typing —80 to 100 cal. per hour

Light activities, such as cooking, walking slowly —110 to 160 cal. per hour

Moderate activities, such as gardening, walking moderately fast —170 to 240 cal. per hour

Vigorous activities, such as waxing, walking fast, bowling, golfing —250 to 350 cal. per hour

Strenuous activities, such as swimming, dancing, skiing —350 or more cal. per hour

CARBOHYDRATES

Carbohydrates are a group of organic substances that contain carbon, hydrogen and oxygen. They have retained their old name, when they were thought to be hydrates of carbon.

The best known carbohydrates are *sucrose* (ordinary sugar), *dextrose* (used for foods, drinks, intravenous feeding), *starch* and *cellulose.*

Simple sugars are called *monosaccharides;* chemically more complex ones are called *disaccharides, trisaccharides,* and *polysaccharides.*

Together with PROTEIN and FAT, carbohydrates are an essential element of food, as they furnish energy and heat to the body. Many foods contain all three—protein, fats and carbohydrates—but usually one predominates, which provides a basis for classification. The carbohydrate portion of the diet is taken in the form of starch, such as potatoes, bread, pastry and sugar.

Although protein, fats and carbohydrates all supply energy, each one behaves in a characteristic manner and has its own peculiar function. Carbohydrates are especially useful because they so promptly supply energy for muscular work and exert some control over the metabolism of fat. Thus, impaired consumption of carbohydrates, as in diabetes, disturbs fat metabolism in such a way that toxic by-products—ketones— are found·in large quantities in the liver, which produce ketosis and, if not treated, diabetic coma.

Following digestion, carbohydrate foods are converted into dextrose, the primary sugar that alone can be utilized by the body. Dextrose is then carried to the liver, where, after several complex steps, it is converted into glycogen and stored. Subsequently, as required by the body, glycogen is reconverted into dextrose and returned to the blood stream. This regulation is automatic and adjusted so that the percentage of sugar in the blood—which depends on a delicate balance between dextrose supply from the liver and utilization (combustion) of sugar by the tissues—is essentially constant. In a healthy body, the entire circulation of blood contains only about five grams of sugar, with the lowest level before breakfast and the highest about half an hour after meals, falling back to normal within two hours.

CARCINOGENS

"A carcinogen is a chemical, physical or animate agent which is capable of producing cancer in any organ or tissue of any species following exposure to it in any dose and physiochemical state when given by any route, either once or repeatedly." This is the official definition given by the International Union Against Cancer, a group of cancer specialists.

This means that carcinogens are not ordinary toxins: even for the most powerful toxin there is a safe dose called "no-effect level," meaning that exposure at this level produces no effect because the dose is small enough for the body to isolate or excrete the toxin, or metabolize it into a nontoxic form. But there is no safe dose for a carcinogen. No matter how minute a dose, no matter how rarely administered, it may cause cancer in susceptible people, and its effects are cumulative and irreversible.

Many scientists are convinced that in the case of carcinogens, laboratory animals' reactions are a reliable guide to reactions in humans. However, some disagree, arguing that there is a "no-effect level" of carcinogens. Further, they believe that substances which are carcinogens when *injected* are not necessarily dangerous when *ingested,* or vice versa.

Examples of carcinogens are tobacco; ultraviolet light; chronic irritation, such as that caused by an ill-fitting denture; and, still controversial, DDT.

CAROTENOIDS

Carotenoids are a family of organic chemical compounds which constitute the yellow, orange and red pigments of many flowers, fruits and vegetables.

All carotenoid colors have similar chemical structures, but as their chemistry varies so do their properties. No one knows how many carotenoids there are in nature; some believe that there may be as many as two hundred, of which about ten are considered provitamins—precursors of VITAMINS. In the case of carotenoids, it means that the human body chemically converts some of them into VITAMIN A.

Among the carotenoids known to be provitamins are alpha-, beta-, and gamma-carotene—sometimes spelled carotin—and cryptoxanthin. Of these, beta-carotene provides the greatest amount of vitamin A. Theoretically, one molecule of beta-carotene could yield two molecules of vitamin A, but this efficiency of conversion is not normally achieved by the human body.

Carotene, then, is the pigment that makes carrots carrot-colored; that gives color to tomatoes, sweet potatoes, apricots, peaches, oranges, butter, egg yolk. In certain leafy vegetables, such as spinach, the green chlorophyll masks the yellow of the carotene. A proof of the presence of carotene in the green leaves of plants is seen when the leaves of trees turn yellow in the fall.

Carotene content in foods varies a great deal: some contain ten times more than others. Summer milk, for instance, contains twice as much carotene as winter milk because of the change in the cows' feed from fresh to dry grass.

When large quantities of carotene are present in the blood, a person may show a pigmentation of the skin resembling that of jaundice. This condition is called carotenemia. The discoloration is caused by deposition of carotene in the skin.

In 1963 beta-carotene was synthetized for the first time by the chemists of Hoffmann–La Roche, one of the leading pharmaceutical companies in the United States. After careful studies showed that this substance produced no side effects, Hoffmann–La Roche marketed the synthetic beta-carotene as a nutritional FOOD ADDITIVE and as a safe artificial color for such foods as margarine, cheese and ice cream. In pure form, beta-carotene is deep violet-red and has powerful coloring properties: three grams of the pure crystals are enough to color half a ton of margarine to its well-known yellow shade.

CASTILE SOAP

Castile soap is a fine, hard, neutral soap, usually white but sometimes marbled or green, made of olive oil and sodium hydroxide (soda lye). It is named after the region of Spain where it was originally made.

It also refers to any of various hard soaps made partly from olive oil together with other FATS or oils such as coconut oil.

CELLULITE

Cellulite, the French word for cellulitis, which has an entirely different meaning in English, was first "discovered" in Sweden around the turn of the century and over the years has come to refer, among European women, to a peculiar kind of ugly, bumpy fat located on the abdomen, hips, thighs, arms, knees and ankles. In the early 1970s this mysterious substance—sometimes called *peau d'orange* (orange skin) because of the puckered texture the affected areas acquire when squeezed between thumb and index finger—crossed the Atlantic, and its name has entered the vocabulary of American women. Men, incidentally, don't seem to suffer from cellulite.

One reason for the popularity of the term could be that, from a woman's point of view, it seems slightly less depressing to be the victim of cellulite than to be plain fat or have "riding breeches," the unflattering, homely English expression for those lumps of fat impervious to DIETS, MASSAGE or EXERCISE.

No recognized expert on obesity and dieting, however, will admit that cellulite is anything different from plain fat. When examined under the microscope, they say, the fat cells of cellulite are identical to those of any other human adipose tissue. This may very well be true; on the other hand, it is worth noting that the AMA has simply dismissed cellulite as another continental fad, without investigating it. The fact, for instance, that only women are subject to this kind of puckered and localized fat deposit could have something to do with female hormones. Also, these fat deposits often seem to be unrelated to obesity and to persist even after the rest of the body has slimmed down after a diet. Either fact, from a woman's point of view, should be worth investigating.

The only physicians who do not ignore cellulite are the plastic surgeons. Some even lend it medical status by calling it lipodystrophy, the medical term for any disturbance of fat metabolism. And the "riding breeches" are a trochanteric lipodystrophy, the trochanter being the area of the hips and thighs. Plastic surgeons also offer a solution for it—a surgical solution, of course. With a technique that is relatively simple but that nonetheless amounts to major surgery requiring a high degree of

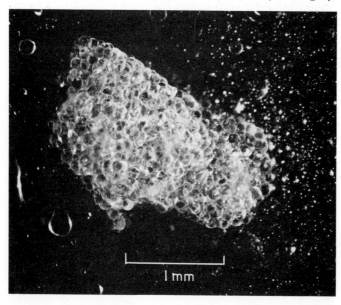

Fragment of adipose tissue surrounded by oil droplets obtained by needle aspiration. *From* Handbook of Physiology. *An illustration of "Metabolism of Human Adipose Tissue in Vitro," by Dr. Jules Hirsch, Waverly Press, 1965.*

1 mm

skill, plastic surgeons all over the world—including the United States—can remove large portions of fat tissue from thighs and abdomen and give them a more graceful contour.

But the real believer in cellulite is a French doctor, Pierre Dukan, who in 1971 wrote a book called *La Cellulite en Question*, published by Editions de la Table Ronde in Paris. Dr. Dukan cannot be reached, and there is no mention in his book of any hospital, clinic, or medical school to which he may be affiliated. Yet his name now has a certain underground status in this country ever since he was extensively quoted in a book called *Cellulite: Those Lumps, Bumps, and Bulges You Couldn't Lose Before*, written by a Mme. Nicole Ronsard, the owner of a beauty salon in New York City.

Under the microscope, Dr. Dukan writes, cellulite indeed looks like any other adipose tissue, except that the cells are "gorged with water and waste material" and stuck to one another by several adherences that make the cellulite look like a sponge. Tendency to cellulite, Dr. Dukan continues, may be hereditary but can appear at any age—suddenly, after an accident or a long illness, or gradually, after years of bad eating and drinking habits, constipation, poor circulation, or taking birth-control pills.

Cellulite can be solid or soft. The former appears to be almost glued to muscles and skin and hurts when massaged. The skin is usually dry, fragile, often wrinkled, with stretch marks and varicose veins, prone to bruises at the slightest blow. However, solid cellulite, according to Dr. Dukan, is easier to treat, because it is usually found in young women in good general health. Soft cellulite is looser and occupies large areas, and while it does not compress veins and nerves like the solid cellulite, it is nevertheless just as deleterious to circulation. It is found in fragile, middle-aged women who abuse diuretics and crash diets, and who suffer from irregular menstruation.

MASSAGE is bad for cellulite, Dr. Dukan believes: it is traumatizing and may worsen bad circulation. Exercise, too, while beneficial for reducing normal fat, does nothing for cellulite. As for SAUNA, it is neither good nor bad. A sound cure for this disturbance consists of a diet rich in protein and low in salt, and of drinking large quantities of purified water. A strictly supervised hormone treatment is also recommended. But it is Dr. Dukan's firm belief that in the near future cellulite will be conquered by ENZYMES, because of their power of inducing chemical reactions in living tissue. Multiple injections of certain enzymes, plus injections of heparin (an anticoagulant drug used in the prevention and treatment of thrombosis and injuries to blood vessels), could break down these fat deposits and transform them into normal fat, which would then melt away with regular diet and exercise.

CERUMEN (EARWAX)

Earwax, a yellow, waxlike substance secreted from the so-called ceruminous glands in the external ear, provides a film along the ear canal to prevent dirt particles, and even insects, from reaching the eardrum. Because earwax is slightly antiseptic, it also helps to protect the external ear from infection.

Normally, the top layer of the earwax dries, flakes off, and is carried to the outer ears by the motion of the jaws while eating and talking. Too much earwax, however, can encourage infection by providing a shelter in which bacteria and fungi can grow. When excessive earwax blocks the ear canal, it causes hearing loss, dizziness, and ringing in the ears.

There are many causes for earwax accumulation, the origins of which are still obscure. It is assumed, for instance, that people secrete more earwax when they feel anxious or fearful, and that when the ceruminous glands are irritated by rubbing the ear with a hard, pointed object, they can release even more wax. Other possible causes are a skin condition known as seborrheic dermatitis, in which excessive amounts of skin particles become mixed with the wax and increase its consistency; or a canal that is too narrow or tortuous.

Sometimes an overenthusiastic use of cotton-tipped applicators results in the deposition of small fibrous strands of the cotton in the canal, where the earwax subsequently becomes enmeshed. After lodging in the ear canal for a while, the wax loses its water content by evaporation and becomes firmer and ultimately quite hard.

Before excessive earwax has completely blocked the canal, the physician can remove it with a curette—a tiny spoon-shaped instrument. When that is not possible, he can remove it with a small jet spray of lukewarm water. If the earwax is dehydrated, it first has to be softened, either with olive oil or other preparations, before being irrigated.

CHEMICAL PEEL

The chemical peel is a procedure (often used as an alternative to DERMABRASION) in which a caustic substance is applied to the face in order to burn the skin's outer layer, the epidermis, and part of the adjoining inner layer, the dermis. The purpose is to eliminate a rough, sun-damaged, large-pored, freckled or blemished skin and restore to it a healthier, younger texture. The removal of a portion of the dermis stimulates the growth of new tissue and helps promote a partial rebuilding of the skin. When it heals, the dermis is slightly thicker, firmer and more resilient, thus plumping up the skin and eradicating fine wrinkles. When the epidermis regrows, it becomes completely and extraordinarily smooth and small-pored.

70

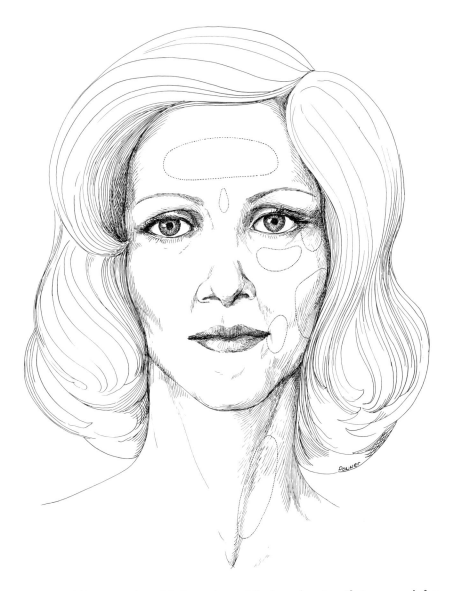

Illustration of the zones of wrinkle formation and the loss of contour that a woman's face undergoes at different ages.

Though such changes are relative to a woman's heredity, complexion, the climate she lives in, and the kind of care she dedicates to her skin, wrinkles and loss of facial contour develop in a rather predictable pattern. In fact, these are frequently used as a criterion for judging a person's age.

Wrinkles (or lines of expression), such as the horizontal lines on the forehead, the vertical frown lines, the lines radiating from the eyelids, or the parenthesis-like lines encompassing the mouth, are generally perpendicular to the long axis of the underlying muscles and are caused by the creasing that accompanies muscular contractions. They are accentuated by smiling, grimacing, squinting, frowning and pursing the lips and become permanent when the aging skin loses elasticity.

Loss of contour (or lines of dependency), such as eye bags, double chin, or drooping jowls, are due to the effect of gravity on loose skin and fatty tissue.

The cross-line pattern of the aging skin is partly due to the intersection of lines of dependency and lines of expression.

CHEMICAL PEEL

Chemical peel has only a limited usefulness in treating the problems of aging tissue, because it tightens loose skin only slightly. But after a FACE-LIFT—which improves the general contour of the face—a chemical peel is ideal to smooth out the fine wrinkles on the upper lip, the forehead, and the eyelids, which are generally unaffected by a face-lift.

As a rule, women with fair skin, fine creases and only slightly sagging skin are ideal candidates for a chemical peel. Those with a more olive complexion may be less satisfied, because the treated areas of the skin could turn a lighter or darker shade than the surrounding skin.

The caustic used for a chemical peel is a solution of phenol (or chloracetic acid), distilled water and a few drops of croton oil and liquid SOAP. The solution is administered with ordinary cotton applicators, with care taken to apply it only to the areas where it is needed, especially around the eyes to prevent it from splashing on the conjunctiva, the delicate membrane that lines the eyelids and covers the eyeball.

Before the treatment, the patient is given a mild sedative to attenuate the solution's burning sensation; this burning rapidly subsides, however, because of the local anaesthetic property of phenol. For several minutes the skin appears white, as if frosted, then turns dark red. Waterproof adhesive tape is applied over the treated area and left in place for approximately forty-eight hours (the longer it remains, the deeper the penetration of the peeler), then carefully removed. An antiseptic powder is dusted on and reapplied several times during the following twenty-four hours, while a thick crust forms. About one week later, the crusts will lift, leaving a pink-colored skin that pales down in about six to twelve weeks. But the maximum benefit of a chemical peel is fully realized only after four to five months, during which time a person should not expose the skin to either direct or indirect sunlight.

The entire face must be treated initially, to avoid contrasting areas, but local touch-ups may be needed later. If unskillfully performed, chemical peel could cause toxic reactions, scars, blotchy discolorations of the skin, or an unattractive ruddiness due to an abnormal enlargement of small blood vessels. But even when the peel is entirely successful, "the skin never looks entirely normal again," as Dr. Bedford Shelmire, Jr., writes in *The Art of Looking Younger*. "The new skin often has a slightly artificial look about it, as though it might be of some synthetic material. This is due to the fact that the regenerated portion of the inner layer consists entirely of scar tissue and therefore lacks the tone and pliability of the original article. It is also much less durable than normal tissue."

However, the overall improvement of the skin after a professionally performed chemical peel is often so astonishing that scores of women (and men) gladly exchange a leathery, splotchy, wrinkled face for one that is ever so slightly artificial.

CHILBLAIN

The blains or sores resulting from exposure to extreme cold often appear first at the big-toe joint and cause inflammation and intense itching. A mild case can be treated with warm bathing of the foot and rubbing with a boric acid or LANOLIN ointment. But severe cases can be serious indeed and should be brought immediately to the attention of a podiatrist.

CHIROPRACTIC

Chiropractic is a system of healing based on the theory that the nervous system controls all other systems and all physiological functions of the human body, and that disease is caused by abnormal functioning of the nervous system—in other words, that interference with the nerve control of these systems impairs their functions and induces disease by rendering the body less resistant to infection or to other exciting causes.

Chiropractic attempts to restore normal functions of the nervous system by manipulation and treatment of the structures of the human body, especially those of the spinal column, and by utilizing physical therapy when necessary. Chiropractors have long claimed extraordinary results—often confirmed by grateful patients' testimonials—with such conditions as HEADACHES, ASTHMA, neuralgia, bursitis, BACKACHE, ARTHRITIS and digestive and circulation disorders. However, people should always first consult a physician to rule out the possibility of a serious underlying disease.

In this country, chiropractors earn their degrees from schools of chiropractic rather than from medical schools. Their training includes four years of instruction in basic anatomy, physiology, biochemistry, microbiology and pathology, and in the interpretation of X-ray films. The New York State Chiropractic Association calls chiropractic "the largest drugless healing profession in America" and points out that although it came into being only in 1895, "the removal of nerve pressure was practiced as a health treatment as far back in history as the time of the early Egyptians, Hindus and Chinese."

The medical profession, however, has dismissed chiropractic as completely unscientific and potentially harmful to health. At best, most physicians feel, chiropractors are sophisticated masseurs who should concern themselves mainly with the problems of POSTURE. For years the American Medical Association has denounced chiropractic as quackery and as a cult, and chiropractors have charged that organized medicine is afraid of competition. The long and bitter debate became particularly intense in the mid-1960s after the passage of the Medicare law, with chiropractors claiming the right to be reimbursed under the program of medical insurance for the elderly and organized medicine opposing such recognition. This debate led to several government studies, which culminated in 1973 in an amendment that included chiropractic in Medicare programs.

As of 1974, the National Institutes of Health are planning a study of the fundamental concepts of chiropractic, under the auspices of the National Institute of Neurological Diseases and Stroke.

CHOLESTEROL

Cholesterol is a fatlike, pearly substance found in all animal FATS and oils; in the bile, the blood, the kidneys, and nerve tissue; and in milk and egg yolk. (Contrary to popular belief, there is *no* cholesterol in chocolate, olive and coconut oils, or nuts.) Cholesterol is an active element in brain metabolism. It is used by the adrenal glands, testicles and ovaries in the production of certain HORMONES. It is absorbed in the intestinal tract from fats in the food, and is manufactured by the liver. When it forms crystals in the gallbladder, cholesterol results in gallstones.

In 1973, the American Medical Association's Council on Food and Nutrition announced that the average level of blood fats—cholesterol, triglycerides and phospholipids—was found to be "undesirably elevated" in most Americans, both men and women. The Council recommended, among other changes in life-style and diet, that the consumption of saturated fats be reduced in favor of polyunsaturated fats, because the latter were found to lower high levels of cholesterol in the blood—hyper-cholesterolemia—thus reducing, in part, the risk of atherosclerosis, the blocking of arteries by fatty deposits in the walls of the arteries, which in turn causes insufficient blood flow to the heart and, ultimately, heart attack or heart failure.

This diet recommendation was in part based on reports that coronary disease is much less common in the poorer nations of the world and had shown a remarkable decrease during the famines that occurred in Europe after World War I and during World War II. Cholesterol, however, is probably only one of the factors contributing to the risk of coronary disease, together with high blood pressure, tobacco smoking, diabetes, tension and sedentary habits.

Indeed, the so-called "cholesterol hypothesis" is being actively investigated, though it remains controversial. In fact, much of the lay public's confusion about cholesterol is owing to the fact that cholesterol has been singled out as the villain by commercial advertisements and news reports. Many people have altered their diets without consulting a doctor, unaware that the relation between cholesterol and heart failure is still, in part, a theory, and that altering drastically the levels of this important, ubiquitous substance in their bodies may be harmful.

So far, investigators have been able to demonstrate only that:
1) the level of cholesterol in the blood is a good indicator of the risk of developing coronary disease;
2) the level of cholesterol can be lowered by switching from saturated to polyunsaturated fats in the diet.

However, there is no proof yet that:
3) cholesterol levels are *directly* related to the development of heart disease;
4) or that a reduction of cholesterol in the diet reduces the subsequent risk of heart disease.

CHROMOSOMES

Chromosomes are several small bodies which are present in the nucleus of a cell. Normally the chromosomes lie extended in the cell's nucleus as thin threads, but when the cell is going to divide, they contract into V-shaped short rods, easily visible under the microscope.

Lying in a certain order along the length of the chromosome are the genes, or hereditary units, which are constant in number in each species. Some chromosomes are associated with the determination of sex. During cell division, each chromosome is split into two identical halves, so that the genetic material can be equally distributed between the newly formed cells.

In the human being there are forty-six chromosomes, or twenty-three pairs, at the time the cell divides. The human sex chromosomes constitute one unequal pair consisting of the X chromosome and the Y chromosome. If the individual is a man, the sex chromosomes consist of one X chromosome and one small Y chromosome (Xy); if it is a woman, they consist of two X chromosomes (XX).

One chromosome in each of the pairs comes from the individual's mother and the other from the father.

CLEANSERS

Cleanser is a generic name for any skin-cleansing agent that acts by loosening particles of dirt, oily skin secretions, dead cells, bacteria, sweat and makeup from the skin's surface. There are five types of skin cleanser: oily or greasy cleansers; COLD CREAMS; SOAPS; DETERGENTS, and rinsable cleansers, or washing creams.

Oils and greases—The oldest forms of cleanser. Oils and greases effectively remove the film of dirt without irritating the skin. However, they are "heavy," tend to mix with the dirt, and are difficult to completely remove from the skin.

75

Cold creams—These are essentially water-containing greases which act much the same as oils and greases.

Regular soaps—Soaps, whether in bar form or in liquid form, have been effective cleansers for ages. The only drawback is that they can cause skin irritation, especially if used too often, left on the skin too long, or rinsed improperly.

Detergents—The word "detergents" refers to hundreds of synthetic substances derived mostly from petroleum. They range from exceptionally mild to irritating for delicate or very dry skin.

Rinsable cleansers—These are similar to soap in that they are creams or lotions containing a soaplike substance. Many women use rinsable cleansers as if they were cold creams and merely *wipe* them off, leaving a film that will mix with new dirt and makeup and eventually cause irritation, dryness and coarseness of the skin, encouraging the formation of blackheads and blemishes. But if removed quickly and rinsed repeatedly, these cleansers are almost as thorough as soaps and are considerably milder.

CO-ENZYMES

Co-enzymes are the nonprotein components of certain ENZYMES, without which metabolic reactions cannot take place. Many VITAMINS, for instance, act like co-enzymes in many biochemical processes.

Co-enzymes have a considerable influence on enzyme activity, which is reduced in case of co-enzyme deficiency. The latter can also lead to reduction in the *efficiency* of the enzyme by reducing the production of apo-enzymes, the portion of an enzyme that requires the presence of a co-enzyme to become a complete enzyme.

COLD CREAM

Cold cream is the prototype of all modern cosmetic creams. Its original formula, slightly less old than the biblical unguents, consisted of a mixture of beeswax, olive oil, water, and rose petals. Its name is probably due to the fact that, when applied to the skin, the evaporating water produced a cool feeling. The wax and oil were meant to cleanse and soften the skin, the rose petals to give the cream a pleasant scent.

Though modern cosmetic creams and lotions no longer resemble the original cold cream, the term "cold cream" is still used for water-containing greasy CLEANSERS. Indeed, its basic formula (wax, oil, water) and purpose (to cleanse and soften the skin) are still the same.

COLLAGEN

Collagen is a gelatinous PROTEIN, the chief constituent of the connective tissue and the organic substances of skin, bones, and cartilage. All tendons, which attach muscle to bone, and ligaments, which attach bone to bone, are primarily collagen.

Since the body tissues are constantly being replaced, there must be something—an ENZYME—that attacks and breaks collagen down, the same enzyme that destroys it in abnormal amounts in certain diseases, such as peridontal diseases, in which bone and supportive tissue around the teeth are lost and the teeth come loose.

Collagen represents 75 percent of the dry weight of the skin. As people grow older, the skin becomes thinner and less resilient, because of structural changes in the collagen: its molecules (which form a rigid, rodlike structure packed together and cross-linked with compounds called aldehydes that prevent them from sliding past one another) become less elastic as the cross-linkages increase in number. Changes in the collagen may account for diseases of the arteries and the thinning of bone structure (osteoporosis)—the problems of old age.

The human digestive system contains an enzyme, called collagenase, which breaks down the COLLAGEN in meat so that it can be digested. Collagen from animal tissue is converted to gelatin after prolonged boiling in water. At ordinary temperature it forms a jelly that becomes liquid when heated and re-solidifies on cooling.

COLOGNE (TOILET WATER)

There is no real difference between cologne and toilet water. The word cologne refers to the German town of Köln (Cologne), where a mixture of citrus oils (lemon, orange, bergamot), lavender, and sometimes rosemary oil used to be manufactured under the name Eau de Cologne. The most famous brands are "4711" and "Jean Marie Farina."

Toilet water was considered a less concentrated form of any type of perfume. The distinction has blurred, so that a weak solution of perfume in alcohol and water may be referred to in the current practice as either cologne or toilet water.

COMMON COLD

Americans apparently suffer between 230 and 500 million colds every year—which, incidentally, induces them to buy at least one billion dollars' worth of over-the-counter cold remedies a year.

"Coughs and sneezes spread diseases," our mothers used to say while teaching us to cover the mouth with a hand. But later we learned that

CHART OF SYMPTOMS
TO HELP PATIENTS TO DISTINGUISH BETWEEN
A COMMON COLD AND "SOMETHING ELSE."

	COMMON COLD	ALLERGIC RHINITIS	SINUSITIS	BRONCHITIS	INFLUENZA	PHARYNGITIS
Duration of illness	At least 5–7 days	Weeks or months	Days; months, if not treated	Variable	About 10 days	Symptoms will clear with or without treatment after about 3 days
Cough	Dry, clear mucus (if any)	None, unless caused by postnasal drip	None	Severe; with purulent sputum	Severe	Cough should be treated for 10 days
Fever	Low-grade (if any)	None	Over 100° F. Variable	Over 100° F. Variable	Over 100° F. Perhaps as high as 104° F.	Over 100° F. Variable
Discharge	Clear, copious nasal mucus	Clear nasal mucus	Thick, yellow nasal discharge	No nasal discharge	Purulent nasal discharge, perhaps sputum	None
Pain	None, except a few aches before or at onset	None	Pain over the involved sinuses	In chest, on coughing or drawing deep breath	Generalized aches	In throat
Sore throat	Should be gone within 3 days	None	None	None	Yes	Red, inflamed
Other			Sore throat may occur as a result of sinus drainage		Diarrhea, vomiting (uncommon)	Headache; abdominal pain; nasal speech; breath odor

From *Patient Care*, September 15, 1974.
Copyright 1974, Miller and Fink Corporation Darien, Connecticut. All Rights Reserved.

those polite gestures were useless, as colds are caused by airborne viruses, called rhinoviruses, which float about in the air.

According to a team of doctors, led by Dr. Jack Gwaltney, at the University of Virginia School of Medicine in Charlottesville, common colds are far more likely to be transmitted by direct skin contact, such as a handshake, or even by touching virus-contaminated surfaces than by a cough or a sneeze. Rhinoviruses, in turn, can be transmitted by the hands to almost anything a person touches. This means that a person can develop a common cold by touching the mucous membranes of his nose or eyes with fingers that have contacted an infected surface. Rhinoviruses survive hours after the drying of the moisture that contains them.

Incidentally, rhinoviruses are not transmitted by kisses, presumably because the viruses would reach the mucosa of the pharynx, while infection will occur *only* when the mucosa of the eyes and the nose is reached.

Another partial misconception is that common colds are caught because of cold weather. True, people catch more colds during the winter than during other seasons, though low temperature and dampness in themselves do not cause the infection. What predisposes people to colds is a depletion of humidity in the environment. Winter air is more than cold—it's *dry*. Cooling air reduces its ability to hold moisture; conversely, by heating cold air, its capacity for humidity is increased. Unfortunately, most home heating systems do not provide enough moisture for the nose, which must warm and humidify the air we breathe before the air enters the lungs. The back of the nose is lined with tiny mobile lashes called cilia, which are covered with a film of mucus. The cilia act as a filter that rids the respiratory tract of dust and other particles that may carry rhinoviruses. Both the humidifying and the filtering action of the nose requires a great deal of moisture to function. The nose structure produces about one liter of moisture a day, but a dry environment uses up most of it, causing the nose passages to become dehydrated and irritated. When the mucus dries on the cilia, it thickens, becoming an excellent culture medium for bacteria.

The basic treatment for the common cold has not changed for years: it still consists of ASPIRIN, fluids, and rest. Decongestants, antihistamines, and cough medicines will help relieve the symptoms. Large doses of VITAMIN C are more effective in lessening the severity and the duration of the common cold if taken as a prophylactic, that is, *before* it starts.

CONDITIONERS

The term conditioner is an extremely general word: it may be applied to almost every hair or nail product on the market—from SHAMPOOS to nail polish—to which one or more ingredients have been added in order to coat the outer surface of either the hair or the nail plate with a protective film.

Among the most effective hair or nail conditioners are those containing PROTEIN, usually a kind called collagen protein.

The use of hair conditioners results in each individual hair being coated with a film of protein, which, incidentally, increases the thickness of each hair, giving the impression that there is more hair than there actually is. This protein film also serves to protect hair from the damage it may suffer as a consequence of HAIR WAVING or COLORING.

Under the microscope, the outer layer of the hair shaft, the CUTICLE, looks as if it is covered with tiny fish scales fitting one on top of the other. The free ends of these hard, shiny scales point upward toward the direction of hair growth and contain SEBUM, which gives hair its luster. The chemicals in hair preparations can roughen, loosen or destroy the cuticle scales, exposing the middle layer, the cortex. The ideal conditioner would be one that could replace the natural proteins washed out or chemically removed from the cortex, but, for the moment, conditioners can hardly affect the cortex.

The inner layer, the medulla, is the least accessible to conditioning treatments. Even with conditioning products based on CHOLESTEROL and LANOLIN, which most closely duplicate the action of natural sebum, it is difficult to establish the degree of absorption of these compounds.

Nail conditioners are usually painted on the bare nail. As with hair conditioners, such preparations serve to fill in the tiny imperfections in the nail plate, though they do not influence the growth pattern or the character of the nail itself. Nail polish may be applied over these conditioners.

CONGENERS

Congeners are chemicals responsible for differences in flavor, aroma, and color among alcoholic beverages. Some are distilled out of the fermenting mash along with the alcohol; others are added to the brew by the charred oak of the barrels, which also extract some of the natural congeners. Still others are deliberately added by the manufacturers, as in liqueurs.

Bourbon, rye, rum and brandy contain the most congeners, while vodka has one of the lowest contents of all.

Scientific researchers investigating the role of congeners in hangovers recently discovered that the higher the content of congeners in a liquor, the more severe the potential hangover. Thus, the popular belief that vodka won't cause hangovers may well be scientifically true.

CONTACT LENSES

Contact lenses are thin, light lenses made of acrylic plastic, designed to fit over the cornea for the correction of vision defects as a substitute for prescription glasses. They are about 9 mm in diameter, slightly smaller than the average cornea (12 mm), and they float on a thin film of tears. Since they move with the eyes, contact lenses allow a greater field of vision than glasses and do not cause distortions, as the eye is always looking through the center of the lens.

Contact lenses correct a wide range of visual defects and provide excellent visual sharpness for people with NEARSIGHTEDNESS. This sharpness is often superior to that achieved with eyeglasses, because glasses are thick at the edge and thin in the center, making things look smaller and distorting light passing through the centers. To get a clear picture of what is around him, a person with glasses must constantly turn his head. Contact lenses have none of these drawbacks. Moreover, contact lenses are often better than glasses for astigmatism, a condition that results from irregularities in the curve of the cornea. Some light rays passing through the irregular portions of eyeglasses are bent slightly out of focus, so that parts of the image become fuzzy and distorted. The layer of tears that contact lenses hold against the cornea fills in the irregularities, correcting the astigmatism. Contact lenses are useful, too, after cataract surgery when they can take the place of the removed crystalline lens of the eye.

Not everyone can adapt to contact lenses, and most people need time before they can overcome their initial discomfort. Also, conditions such as HAY FEVER that cause excessive eye-watering make regular contact lenses unwearable, though some people may be able to switch to SOFT CONTACT LENSES. And some diseases that affect the cornea or cause chronic inflammation of the eyelids or the conjunctiva—the membrane lining the inner surface of the eyelids—may preclude the wearing of contact lenses altogether. But under normal conditions, once a person has adjusted to contact lenses, he may never want to go back to eyeglasses.

Contact lenses are manufactured in different colors, which may enhance or even change the eyes' natural color. They are stored in an antiseptic solution and should be handled with clean, dry hands, free from soap or cream residues. Women are advised to wear the lenses *before* applying makeup: they will not only see better what they are doing but also avoid coating the lenses with traces of COSMETICS.

Prescriptions for contact lenses should be revised as often as those for glasses, and the lenses should be professionally cleaned and polished at least once a year.

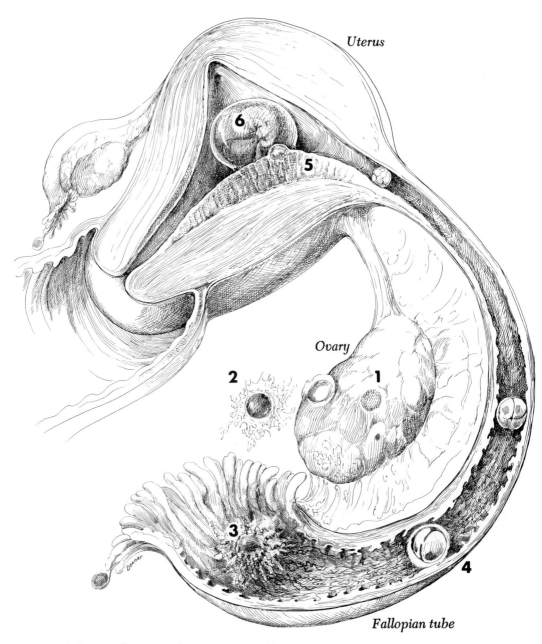

Uterus

Ovary

Fallopian tube

A drawing illustrating the various steps of human conception.

1) The egg cell develops in the ovary.
2) The mature egg is released from the ovary during ovulation and passes along the Fallopian tube.
3) The egg is met by several spermatozoa, which have been swimming toward it from the uterus, and is entered by one.
4) The fertilized egg continues to advance toward the uterus.
5) The egg implants in the uterus lining, the endometrium.
6) The egg begins to develop into an embryo inside the uterus.

CONTRACEPTION

At present, no contraceptive method is perfect for everybody. Until the promised once-a-month shot of PROSTAGLANDINS, the extraordinary new hormonelike drug, becomes available, a woman can only try the method that is best for her, that gives her the highest level of protection and that least interferes with her health and sexual pleasure. This involves thinking realistically about her feelings toward sex and the conditions under which she makes love (with whom, how often, etc.).

Techniques of birth control currently available have proven satisfactory for a majority of women. However, in certain cases contraceptives seem to fail. Lack of information is almost never the main reason, psychiatrists observe. Certain women, for instance, feel that the use of contraceptives is a sign of promiscuity and are affronted when a gynecologist suggests them. Some find it repulsive to fit their own diaphragm; others misuse the contraceptive or "forget" to use them, as a means of self-punishment or in order to punish or gain control over a sexual partner. Still others are not emotionally prepared to face any form of responsibility.

There are four categories of contraceptive methods: *nonfunctional, chancy, functional,* and *permanent.*

Among the better-known nonfunctional contraceptives are:

Douches—To douche right after intercourse with any ingredient, from the mythic Coca-Cola to the most powerful spermicides, cannot prevent pregnancy, because long before a woman can reach the bathroom thousands of spermatozoa have reached the uterus—unreachable by any douche.

Feminine hygiene sprays—Many products are sold as aids to "feminine hygiene." In some cases, advertisements hint at "birth control power." Needless to say, they do *not* prevent pregnancy.

The following contraceptive methods can be considered chancy:

Vaginal foam, cream, or jelly—These products try to prevent the semen from reaching the uterus, but they do not always succeed. They are sold with a special applicator that measures the right amount, and they should be applied no more than a half hour before intercourse. If a woman makes love again later, she needs another dose.

Vaginal foaming tablets—These are easy to use but not always effective. The tablets should be moistened (they work only when moist) and immediately inserted deep into the vagina at least five minutes before intercourse, so they have time to dissolve. The foam thus produced covers the neck of the uterus just as vaginal foam does. A tablet loses its effectiveness one hour after insertion.

Vaginal suppositories—These are small, cone-shaped, waxy materials containing a spermicide. A suppository should be inserted ten

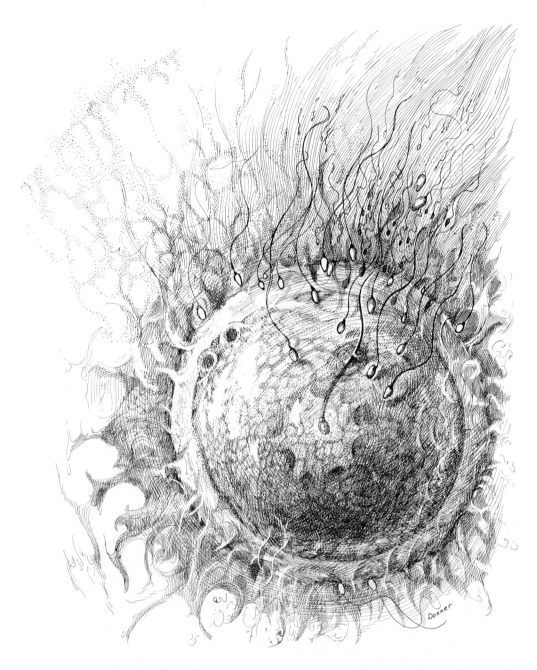

A many-times-enlarged mature ovum is seen surrounded by an envelope of follicle cells called the *corona radiata*. During maturation, the innermost cells secrete a gelatinous substance that coats the ovum with a protective film.

After the ovum leaves the ovary, the *corona radiata* becomes detached, and this allows the sperm to come close to the ovum. Only one in a million spermatozoa—presumably the strongest and fastest—can penetrate and fertilize the ovum, though several bore through the gelatinous envelope.

How the ovum turns away all spermatozoa but one is still a mystery; one theory is that the first spermatozoon to come in contact with the ovum provokes a reaction in the cell membrane which causes the other spermatozoa to be rejected.

minutes before intercourse so it can melt at body temperature. It, too, loses effectiveness after one hour and has not proven reliable enough to be recommended widely.

Coitus interruptus (withdrawal)—This refers to intercourse voluntarily interrupted by the male partner in order to prevent his semen from reaching the uterus. Withdrawal often fails because of carelessness or poor control, or because some sperm is released *before* the man's climax.

Rhythm method—The rhythm method is based on the fact that there are only certain days in every month when intercourse can result in pregnancy: the day before and the day just after ovulation, when the EGG CELL is released from the ovary. Theoretically, by avoiding making love during the "unsafe" time, a woman can prevent pregnancy. But, for the present, it is next to impossible to tell exactly when is the unsafe time. Even with the supervision of a gynecologist, daily measuring of temperature (body temperature drops at the time of ovulation and abruptly rises twenty-four hours later) and a month-by-month record of menstrual periods, it is difficult to predict ovulation. Furthermore, sperm can survive two days, which means that the egg cell can be fertilized about forty-eight hours *after* ovulation—to say nothing about what happens to the spontaneity of a

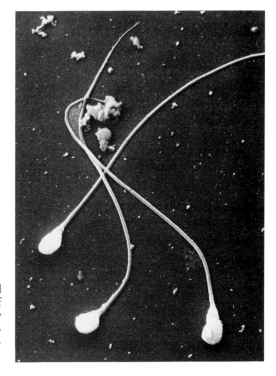

An electron micrograph (original magnification: 7,000 times) of three human spermatozoa taken by Dr. David M. Phillips of the Population Council, Rockefeller University, New York City.

relationship when it is subjected to this kind of calculation. However, the rhythm method is being restudied. A group of women participating in one such study was trained to detect patterns of cervical secretions as a method of distinguishing fertile from infertile days. During *fertile* days, the secretion is clear and slippery; during *infertile* days, it is dry and flaky.

Breast feeding—A new baby gives its mother some natural protection against becoming pregnant, but apparently for much less time than the traditionally "safe" six weeks after delivery (or ABORTION).

Condoms—The condom, or prophylactic, is a nonprescription, disposable device used by the male. Traditionally made of a thin sheet of latex, it is now made of lamb gut. It is meant to fit over the penis in order to hold the semen and keep the sperm from entering the birth canal. The condom can be used only on the erect penis, and it should be put on before intercourse, since, as already mentioned, some sperm is released long before climax. Enough space should be left at the tip to make room for the semen when it is released. It must be removed before the penis relaxes, for it could easily slip off and spill the semen into the vagina. The chances of a condom's breaking are minimal (in the United States they are periodically checked by the FDA for quality), but stretching may weaken them. The condom has been—and still is—ridiculed as old-fashioned and even sordid. As for physicians, many wish that condoms were more popular, because they provide an excellent protection against venereal diseases. However, unless it is used in conjunction with vaginal foam or jelly, the condom is considered a chancy method of contraception.

For a description of functional contraceptives see CONTRACEPTIVE PILL; DIAPHRAGM; INJECTABLE CONTRACEPTIVE; INTRAUTERINE DEVICE; PROSTAGLANDINS.

For a description of permanent contraceptives, see TUBAL LIGATION; VASECTOMY.

CONTRACEPTIVE PILL

The contraceptive pill, often called simply The Pill, is one of the most extraordinary, most talked-about medications of the last fifty years. As of 1973, The Pill is used by more than eight million American women, and for the time being it is the most effective of all means of female contraception, short of sterilization, of course.

Although The Pill is available under numerous brand names, most oral contraceptives contain two female sex hormones, estrogen and progestin (the synthetic progesterone), designed to prevent pregnancy essentially by suppressing ovulation, i.e., interfering with the interaction of the pituitary gland with the ovaries and probably causing other changes in the uterus lining.

The most common types of The Pill are: 1) the "combination" pill, in which the hormones estrogen and progestin are combined in one pill that is taken for about twenty days a month, with one week off; 2) the "sequential" pill, in which a pure estrogen pill is taken for fourteen or fifteen days and an estrogen/progestin pill for the remaining five or six days of the cycle.

With the "combination" or the "sequential," a woman may forget to take one tablet, in which case she should take one as soon as she remembers. If she misses as many as three, she should stop taking them, use other contraceptives, and start afresh the following cycle.

"Combination" pills such as Ovulen® may contain equal parts of estrogen and progestin. Enovid-E ®, on the other hand, is an "estrogen-dominant" pill, while Demulen® is a "progestin-dominant." A gynecologist may prescribe one or the other of these various types of "combination" pills, depending on a woman's tolerance of *synthetic* hormones or on her deficiency of either of the *natural* hormones. While most women do well on most of the products available, some may complain, for instance, that an "estrogen-dominant" pill makes them gain weight, feel nauseous, swell their ankles, give them HEADACHES, make contact lenses suddenly feel uncomfortable. "Progesterone-dominant" pills may cause increase of appetite, predisposition to moniliasis (vaginal infection), FATIGUE, ACNE or hair thinning.

For young women who are taking the pill for the first time, there is a relatively new, low-dose "sequential" marketed by Parke-Davis with the name of Loestrin 1.5/30 ® (the figures indicate that the pills contain 1.5 mg of progestin and 30 mg of estrogen).

A gynecologist may forbid altogether the use of The Pill to a woman who has or has had a thromboembolism (blood clot). Too, women who suffer from kidney disease, mental depression, ASTHMA, HYPERTENSION, diabetes or epilepsy may have their conditions worsened by The Pill.

At the beginning of 1973, a new type of pill, sometimes referred to as the Mini-Pill, was made available in this country under two brand names: Micronor®, made by Ortho Pharmaceutical Corporation, and Nor-Q.D.® made by Syntex. The Mini-Pill contains a small amount of only one synthetic hormone, progestin, and is taken every day of the year without interruption. Apparently, Micronor® is a little less effective than either the "combination" or the "sequential." In practice, this means that the risk of pregnancy is increased if a woman forgets to take this kind of pill every single day. Also, Micronor® may produce an irregular, unpredictable bleeding pattern. However, Micronor® is often the choice of women with an excessive production of natural estrogen. But the most important quality of the Mini-Pill is that, unlike the "combination" and the "sequential," it does not disorganize ovulation; it only acts on the lining of the uterus, making it unsuitable for implantation of the fertilized egg. The Mini-Pill, then, is the first step toward the contraceptive of the future. Researchers in the field of reproductive science expect that the next great advance in fertility control will be aimed at the last phase of the menstrual cycle; in other words, instead of the interference with ovulation which currently occurs with The Pill (which still produces a number of side effects, especially when taken for a long time), contraception will be obtained by preventing either the egg's early development or the implantation of the egg cell in the uterus.

In the fall of 1973, the FDA approved the use of yet another oral contraceptive called diethylstilbestrol, better known as DES, or morning-after pill.

DES is a synthetic estrogen which acts on the lining of the uterus and apparently alters the speed with which the egg cell moves in the genital tract. It has been proven reasonably effective when administered within twenty-four to seventy-two hours after intercourse in the dose of 25 mg, twice a day for five days. However, DES is not 100 percent effective, especially if taken *after* seventy-two hours. More important, if a woman is *already* pregnant, DES may be dangerous to the fetus.

Incidentally, for some years DES has been one of the most controversial growth stimulants for cattle. In 1972, the FDA finally banned its use as an animal-feed additive to prevent it from entering the human food chain, because experiments showed that this hormone promoted cancer in five species of animals. Cattlemen protested violently, for DES increased the cattle's weight so significantly that, for one, it saved the cattlemen millions of dollars' worth of feed.

Naturally, there are many and complex differences between animal and human cancers; however, the consensus of the medical community as of 1974 is that DES should be reserved for emergency situations—rape, incest, and for those cases in which a physician feels that a patient's physical or mental well-being may be endangered by pregnancy. In the opinion of certain gynecologists, DES's major value is psychological; it makes a woman feel that *something* is being done to help her, rather than leaving her to worry for weeks until a regular pregnancy test can be made.

COSMETIC ALLERGY

ALLERGY to cosmetics may affect various organs of the body, but the most common forms are allergic conditions of the skin, hair and nails.

COSMETICS, at present, are quite safe; all the major lines now exclude those substances that are likely to cause trouble, though the word "hypoallergenic" that is added to the labels of many cosmetics is no extra guarantee and might be banned soon. Of course, there are still many people who cannot use one or more specific items in a line of makeup. The problem is usually caused by ingredients such as PERFUMES or preservatives. But no one particular brand is better for the skin than another.

Eye makeup and eye shadows may cause dermatitis on the skin around the eye, irritation of the eyelids or of the conunctiva, the lining of the eye and the lids.

Face powders seldom cause reactions, because orris root—a common allergen—is not used as an ingredient in the United States.

Lipstick, probably the most used of all cosmetics, may produce an allergic reaction. Often, the ingredient to which people are sensitive is the dye in the so-called indelible lipsticks.

Hair dyes, bleaches, SPRAYS, STRAIGHTENERS and WAVERS are the major hair cosmetics which could cause allergic reactions. There are various kinds of hair dyes, and the dyes more likely to produce a reaction are also the ones that produce the best colors: the oxidation dyes. A federal law requires that a patch test be done before each application of oxidation-type hair dyes, but in practice this is done only at the time of the first application, if ever. Most people, customers and hairdressers alike, find it a time-consuming, overly cautious procedure—until one becomes sensitized, that is.

Other types of dyes, such as hair rinses and progressive dyes, very seldom cause allergy.

Bleaches, when properly applied, rarely affect the scalp or the adjacent skin, but if carelessly used they may cause irritation and even hives.

The same is true for straighteners and wavers: they may cause dermatitis (which heals rapidly) only if improperly used.

Perfumes, too, may sometimes provoke allergic reactions. The most common type of reaction is called Berlocque dermatitis: a dark streak running down from where the perfume was applied. Something similar happens with those perfumes that contain a sunlight sensitizing ingredient.

Nail polish often causes dermatitis, but usually on the skin near the eyes or the nose—where a woman with freshly polished nails may touch herself—rather than on the fingers. On the other hand, base coats usually affect the nail bed itself. In the most severe cases, the nail may hurt and even become loose. ARTIFICIAL NAILS, too, can sometimes cause allergic inflammation of the nail bed.

ANTIPERSPIRANTS may cause allergic reactions almost as often as hair dyes. The main skin irritation occurs because the antiperspirant seals in bacteria in the tiny cuts that happen while shaving the underarm.

SOAPS containing deodorants can cause reaction to sunlight—the so-called photodermatitis, which is similar to allergic contact DERMATITIS, exept that, in addition to the chemical, radiant energy is needed for the formation of the photocontact allergen.

In general, a cosmetic that is responsible for an allergic reaction is easier to identify than other allergens; or, at least, it is often easier to avoid, by simply switching to a similar product of another brand.

COSMETICS

Cosmetics, in the words of the Food and Drug Administration, are "articles intended to be rubbed, poured, sprinkled, or sprayed on . . . or otherwise applied to the human body . . . for cleansing, beautifying, promoting attractiveness, or altering the appearance."

This is true enough, but the FDA's definition does not mention the fascination involved in the ritual of "making up." Regardless of the end result—for often the awareness of one own's physical imperfections may be imaginary, or, worse, the application of cosmetics may emphasize real imperfections—cosmetics are so much a part of human beings' perception of themselves that they never were or will be a fad, or even a luxury. Cosmetics, in a sense, are a necessity; especially now, when the line of demarcation between makeup and curative measure is beginning to blend, and sophisticated customers are learning, for instance, that skin care and adornment are two sides of the same issue. Also, many realize that several expensive cosmetics are either made of very inexpensive raw materials or could be substituted for by "kitchen" ingredients with the same results. But then, expensive, exotic skin oils smell better than plain olive oil, and the container of an expensive lipstick is more elegant than a cheap one, even if the quality of the lipstick is probably the same.

Emphasis on a particular kind of cosmetic may shift because of trend-setting of fashion magazines, which in turn may reflect the personal innovations of famous actresses, models, or socially prominent women. In general, though, this is something that concerns only the cosmetic industry. In other words, in one season manufacturers may record a drop in lipstick sales and, simultaneously, an increase in the sale of eye shadows and rouge, which means that for a while pale lips, rosy cheeks and dramatically shadowed eyes are in vogue. Next, maybe, "earth colors" or a pearly complexion with vivid lips may be preferred. Essentially, however, cosmetics change very little, and nothing really new is expected to come along "to take the female by storm," in the words of a cosmetic market expert.

For those women who use and love cosmetics but are uncertain, for instance, of which combination of shades and textures are best for them, or are unaware of such things as the tone of their complexion or the importance of different kinds of light, basic guidelines for the proper use of cosmetics are always useful and often welcome. Fashion magazines can and do publish lists of suggestions—"if you are a brunette with green eyes . . ."—over and over without fear of becoming repetitious.

But truly sophisticated women know that there are no rigid rules for applying makeup, as there aren't in any form of art—of which makeup is a form, however modest and ephemeral. For these women, cosmetics can indeed create a delightful and ever-changing illusion of beauty, not too different from the promises of advertisements. They know how to distinguish between "sheen" and greasiness; how to put on a veil of face powder rather than look as if they had fallen into a talcum jar.

It would be nice if aesthetics were the only problem with cosmetics. Unfortunately, this is not so. Because of their vast use, and because they are made of a variety of chemical ingredients, cosmetics present many of the problems typical of drugs and FOOD ADDITIVES. For years, however, cosmetics and SOAP were exempt from nearly all regulation applied to drugs and food, and only in 1968 did the National Commission on Product Safety estimate that annually thousands of persons suffered adverse, sometimes serious, reactions to cosmetics. Eventually, the FDA

1) A model giving the last touch to her coloring-pencil-only makeup.

2) The finished work.

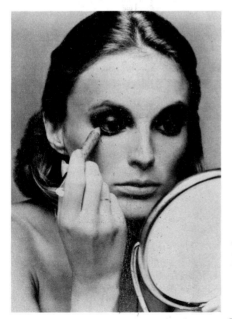 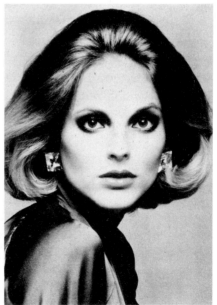

Courtesy of Elizabeth Arden, New York City.

91

ordered cosmetic manufacturers to list ingredients on all labels. This allows consumers with known ALLERGIES to avoid products that could cause hypersensitive reactions. The regulation, effective as of March 31, 1975, requires that a label list the cosmetic's ingredients—except FRAGRANCES and flavors—in decreasing order of prevalence. (Previously, manufacturers could voluntarily register cosmetic formulas with the FDA and request the agency to observe the confidentiality of trade secrets.)

Still controversial is the use of the terms "hypoallergenic" or "dermatologically tested," which manufacturers have been using on certain cosmetics for many years. The terms have meant different things to different people—consumers as well as manufacturers. Some consumers, for instance, have understood the term to mean nonallergenic, when actually it only means that the product is less likely to cause adverse reactions. There is no known way yet to produce a cosmetic which will not adversely affect someone somewhere. The cosmetic industry itself has proceeded with its own varied criteria for what should be considered hypoallergenic. Some manufacturers simply omit from their products

Pablo Manzoni, the creative director of Elizabeth Arden, making up a model with coloring pencils. Except for mascara and foundation, a woman's entire makeup kit could be in that handful of multicolored pencils.

Creamy, manageable, encased in soft wood, able to be sharpened with almost any type of pencil sharpener, coloring pencils are probably one of the most charming cosmetic-industry gimmicks—one that was adopted so quickly by so many manufacturers that the original "inventor" must have given up the impulse of patenting his idea the minute he first doodled a coloring pencil in his mind.

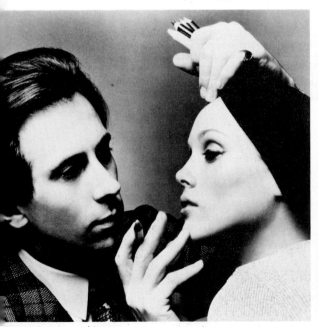
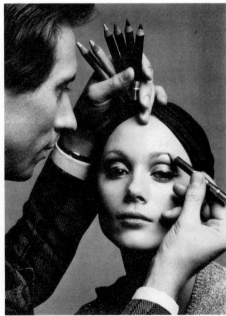

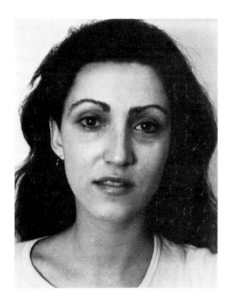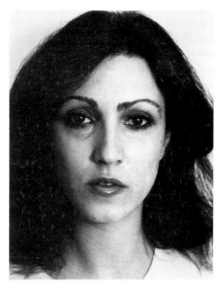

Left: A young woman in front of her mirror, with an expression of slight disappointment that even the most beautiful women feel when confronting their own clean faces in the raw morning light.

Right: The same woman after making herself up—seven minutes in all—with mascara, two eye shadows, two tones of blusher, lip gloss, and a touch of cover stick.

Applied with a light hand and carefully blended, the cosmetics do not impose their own texture; they merely bring into focus her lovely, fine features.

perfumes or other ingredients they believe may cause problems. Others perform PATCH TESTING with the finished products; still others use the term hypoallergenic on the basis of a low rate of allergic reactions. Those who do carry out clinical testing differ greatly in the number and type of people they use for tests—tests on *normal* people do not prove the safety of cosmetics for *allergic* people—and probably no manufacturer tests its products in comparison with products that do not make such claims. And finally, the term hypoallergenic may well be misleading and its use soon forbidden altogether, since most manufacturers have already removed common irritants and allergy-causing ingredients from *all* their products.

To make things even more complicated, some adverse reactions to cosmetics may have nothing to do with allergy. A mascara, for instance, that is perfectly safe when first opened could, if not kept clean or if misused, grow harmful bacteria and cause an eye infection.

Cosmetic ingredients, some of which are industrial secrets, can be divided into the following categories:

Acids and alkalis—The most commonly used acid in cosmetics is citric acid; the most common alkali, ammonium carbonate. Too much or too little of either ingredient may irritate the skin.

Buffers—Buffers are chemicals added to a cosmetic formula in order to control its pH, i.e., the degree of its acidity or alkalinity. They are used as an alternative to adding acids or alkalies to the formula.

Color additives—The most important ingredients of cosmetics, and the most likely to cause allergic reactions. The colors have to be certified as harmless and suitable for use, but only recently has it become possible for the FDA to chemically analyze the types and quantities of color additives used in cosmetics.

Flavor additives—The same additives are often used for both food and drugs. They are derived from a variety of spices and essential oils and are used mainly for lipsticks, dentifrices and mouthwashes.

Fragrances—Often a complex formula, as a single scent may contain dozens of fragrances. Fragrances are an important ingredient of cosmetics, as a pleasant smell is often the only reason why a person chooses a particular cosmetic.

Moisture regulators—Chemicals such as glycerin, which keep the cosmetic from drying out; or chemicals such as calcium silicate, which prevent cosmetics from absorbing moisture from the air.

Preservatives—Substances such as certain alcohols and essential oils used to protect cosmetics from decomposition due to the multiplication of bacteria and fungi. They have to be colorless, odorless, nontoxic, nonirritant, stable, and easy to mix with the other ingredients of the compound.

Surface-active agents—Also called surfactant, that is, products that make it easier to effect contact between the skin surface and a cream or lotion. They may help mix water and oil, or keep a mixture smooth and uniform, and so forth.

CRAB LICE (CRABS)

Crab lice, better known as "crabs," are a species of parasitic insect infesting the human body mainly in the pubic hair, though they can be found on eyebrows, eyelashes and underarm hair. The insects, and especially their eggs, cling to the pubic hair with clawed legs, causing a wild itching and occasionally skin eruptions. They presumably can be picked up from public seats and toilets, but more frequently by sexual contact with a person who is infested. Crabs can be cured by shaving the pubic area and applying an insecticide ointment.

CURETTAGE

Curettage refers to the scraping of a body cavity by means of a curette—a slender spoon-shaped knife—to clean its surface, to obtain material for BIOPSIES, or to remove a lesion, a growth or a foreign body.

CURLING IRON

A curling iron is a rod-shaped metallic instrument that, when heated, is used to curl or wave hair. The old-fashioned curling iron required heating by direct flame; the modern version is heated by an electric current. With either device, the hair is curled by the heat given off by the metal.

Most electric curling irons generate dry heat; a few are equipped with a manually controlled shot of mist. The best ones have cool tips, so that they can be placed on a dressing table while heating.

If the heat is too low, the hair will not be curled properly; if the heat is too great, the hair may be damaged, become fragile and dry. Generally, if the curling iron is hot enough to burn one's fingers, it will burn hair, too. However, the heat generated by most electric curling irons is low enough to be relatively safe. On the other hand, the results are not so satisfactory or long-lasting as some advertisements claim: it takes a while to learn how long to hold the iron on the hair and how much hair to wind at a time. The best use for a curling iron is for quick touch-ups between regular hair settings or for correcting a few unwanted natural curls.

CUTICLE REMOVER

Cuticle remover is a liquid, cream or gel that softens nail cuticles faster but not better than soaking them in warm, soapy water.

As in the case of cuticle creams and oils (designed to keep cuticles soft), which could be replaced by any good MOISTURIZER, cuticle removers are not particularly useful. In fact, excessive use may cause irritation.

CYSTITIS

Cystitis is an inflammation of the urinary bladder, the organ in which urine is stored until evacuated. Cystitis is caused by bacteria or irritants and is more common in women than in men, because, for one thing, the woman's bladder is adjacent to the vagina, which makes it vulnerable to internal trauma. For instance, during intercourse, a vigorously thrusting penis may exert pressure through the vaginal wall and against the bladder.

More important, the woman's urethra—the passage that conducts urine out of the bladder—follows a straight course only $1\frac{1}{2}$ inches long (in the man, the urethra runs a long, curved course 8 or 9 inches long), which provides an easy access to bacteria and vaginal secretions.

With cystitis, the inflamed bladder swells and stretches as if it were filled with urine. This leads the nerves of the bladder muscle to signal this expansion to the brain as a continuous urge to urinate, though the bladder may be empty. The pressure exerted during futile and frequent attempts to urinate only increases the inflammation and the discomfort.

Mild cases of cystitis require only a medication containing an antiseptic and some ingredients soothing to the bladder. More serious cases are treated with sulfonamides (sulfa drugs) or ANTIBIOTICS. Since relief usually comes after one or two days, many women tend to stop treatment before they have used up the entire prescription. This is a mistake, since the bacteria, at that point, have merely decreased in number; and if the medication is discontinued, the remaining bacteria will multiply after a few weeks and often develop immunity against that particular dose, or even type, of drug.

Cystitis may be recurrent, but if treated at the very first sign of bladder irritation it may not require a doctor's attention. A woman can cure herself by drinking abundantly and urinating frequently, never allowing the bladder to become too full, and by scrupulously and frequently washing, rinsing and drying the vaginal area, especially before intercourse.

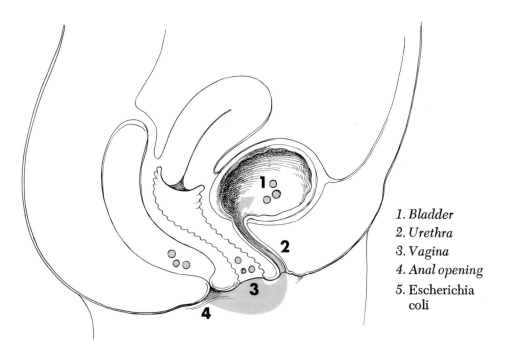

1. Bladder
2. Urethra
3. Vagina
4. Anal opening
5. Escherichia coli

Above: Cross-section of the female pelvis. The female urethra is only one and one-half inches long, and its opening is in front of that of the vagina. This provides the most frequent route of bacteria to the bladder, resulting in cystitis—an inflammation of the bladder walls.

Right: A microscopic view of the bacteria *Escherichia coli,* the organism chiefly responsible for cystitis.

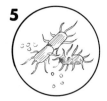

CYSTS

Any closed capsule with a characteristic membrane containing a liquid or semiliquid substance that develops abnormally in the human body—often in the skin or mucous membrane—is called a cyst.

Cysts often appear in the ovaries and in the sebaceous glands, as in severe cases of ACNE. Cysts are the most common lesions of the female breast. They may appear when, for instance, the milk ducts become dilated.

Sometimes cysts disappear spontaneously, but often they have to be excised or burned off (cauterized). Doctors often can tell whether a lump in the breast is a cyst or BREAST CANCER just by touching it, but in general only an accurate BIOPSY by a pathologist can tell for sure.

If a cyst is well defined, globular, mobile and larger than $1\frac{1}{2}$ cm in diameter—macrocyst—it is best treated by inserting a hypodermic needle in it and aspirating all the fluid it contains. This technique is relatively painless, requires no hospital stay and, most important of all, leaves no scars. A Pap stain test (which is similar in technique to the PAP SMEAR TEST used for cervical cancer detection) will then establish whether the fluid contains abnormal cells. And after a few days, MAMMOGRAPHY of the breast should be performed for additional screening for cancer.

If the cyst is very small—microcyst—too small to be steadied for the aspiration technique, it is best treated with conventional cauterization.

In the past, physicians were reluctant to aspirate cysts because of the fear of needling what might be a malignant tumor. However, with the increasing experience in evaluating breast lesions, doctors have learned to recognize gross, simple cysts of the breast.

D

DANDER

Dander refers to minute scales from hair, feathers or skin that may act as allergens.

DANDRUFF

Dandruff is the most common of scalp diseases characterized by excessive scaling of the scalp. The flakes are either oily and yellow or dry and grayish white and appear in patches. A person may have noticeable dandruff on one side of the head and much less on another part. The temples and the crown of the skull are common locations for dandruff.

Dandruff diminishes in the summer and increases in the winter, but in general it is a steady process characteristic of an individual, much as is hair growth.

A minimal scaling of dandruff can usually be controlled by washing at proper intervals or by using an antidandruff preparation. But occasionally the symptoms become quite severe, and there may be redness and inflammation together with itching and flaking of the scalp. Dandruff does not affect hair roots, but since it itches, scratching may damage the hair near the scalp and cut the scalp, which in turn may cause a bacterial infection that may accelerate hair loss, though there is no evidence that dandruff can cause baldness.

These symptoms may also appear in other areas: the sides of the nose, around the ears, or on the chest. Dermatologists refer to this condition as seborrheic dermatitis and, in general, do not clearly differentiate between dandruff and seborrheic dermatitis in the belief that dandruff is merely a low-grade version of the latter. But some distinguished dermatologists, such as Dr. Albert M. Kligman of the University of Pennsylvania School of Medicine in Philadelphia, believe that there is *no* relation between the two conditions. People can suffer from seborrheic dermatitis *without* having dandruff.

One of the major functions of the outer layer of human skin is to provide a tough, resilient barrier to protect the tissues beneath it. The outermost barrier is called stratum corneum, a layer of hardened, dead cells about twenty to forty cells thick, which are constantly being worn, scraped, or rubbed off. New cells, manufactured at the base of the epidermis, gradually move to the surface and replace the lost ones. Along the way they slowly harden and die. This normal process of skin-flaking has led many people to consider that dandruff is more a normal condition than a pathological one. However, it has been discovered that the processes in the normal scalp are orderly and complete, and the flakes peel away only a few layers thick, while in the scalp with dandruff the scaling is in much disorder, the life cycle of the cell is not always completed before it leaves the scalp, and the flakes may be twenty to fifty cell layers thick. Underneath the incipient flakes, the stratum corneum is thinner than normal.

This phenomenon could be explained by assuming that the process of cell birth and migration is being greatly accelerated in the case of dandruff. However, this has not been proven; in fact, the causes of dandruff are still unknown, though many theories have been proposed—everything from hormonal imbalance to poor hygiene, tension, ALLERGY, disturbance of the sebaceous glands, and deficiencies in the diet. The most popular theory is that the bacteria and fungi that live on the scalp cause it. Again, there is no evidence; nevertheless, some manufacturers have tried to develop treatments based on the hypothesis that dandruff is infectious in nature.

Any good SHAMPOO can provide some control over dandruff, because, as it is used fairly often, it cleans the scalp and rids it of itching and flaking. But often these symptoms return in just a few days, and unless the hair is washed every two or three days (it takes from one to three days for the scalp to generate a new supply of dandruff) conventional shampoos are usually not the answer. Incidentally, too frequent shampooing sometimes has a drying effect, which may also cause flaking. Some medicated products—containing such ingredients as sulfur, tar, salicylic acid, selenium sulfide or zinc pyrithione—seem to be more effective, repressing the return of noticeable dandruff symptoms for five to seven days.

DENTAL FLOSS

Dental floss is a flat waxed thread used to clean between the teeth and under the gum margins where a TOOTHBRUSH cannot reach. This helps to prevent the accumulation and growth of microorganisms which can form a substance called PLAQUE, the chief cause of gum bleeding and infection (pyorrhea).

Though most people find their own way of using dental floss, the easiest way seems to be the one illustrated in oral hygiene pamphlets. Break off a length of about 18 inches. Wind one end two or three times around one of the middle fingers; wind the other end around the other middle finger. This leaves a length of about 3 inches between the two hands. Holding the floss taut, use the thumbs and the forefingers to guide it gently between the teeth and slide it just beneath the gum margins. With an up-and-down motion scrape it on the side of each tooth.

In using dental floss one should not try to force it or snap it between the teeth—the gums are sensitive and can be easily slashed.

Dental floss should be used at least once a day, preferably before brushing. Unwaxed floss is sometimes recommended because it presumably doesn't slide off the teeth, thus facilitating the scraping of plaque from the tooth surface.

DENTAL IMPLANTS

Dental implants are the modern solution for people who have struggled with full or partial dentures for years, or for those whose teeth are beginning to loosen because of decay, infection, or loss of bone support.

A denture can be unsightly and uncomfortable. After a while it inevitably becomes "too big" for the jaws, because jawbones subjected to a denture's stress and constant friction literally melt away in time. Also, pain becomes unbearable when a reduced jawbone exposes the nerve canal.

Dental implants are a relatively new discipline, and oral implantology is not yet recognized as a specialty, though as of 1975 it is taught in more than forty dental schools in the United States alone.

There are three basic types of implants: *subperiosteal, intramucosal,* and *endosteal.* With the exception of the subperiosteal, most implants are made of titanium, a very light metal that not only is inert, i.e., does not provoke chemical reactions, but is also resilient and elastic so that it can be shaped without breaking.

Each type of implant is based on a totally different concept of design and function. The choice of the right type for a specific dental problem is perhaps the most difficult step in an implant. For a skillful implantologist, the techniques themselves are relatively simple: they are usually performed in the office, under local anaesthesia, and the pain is minimal, as nerve endings are seldom involved. However, a successful and lasting implant depends almost entirely on the proper diagnosis.

Subperiosteal implant—The most common indication for this procedure

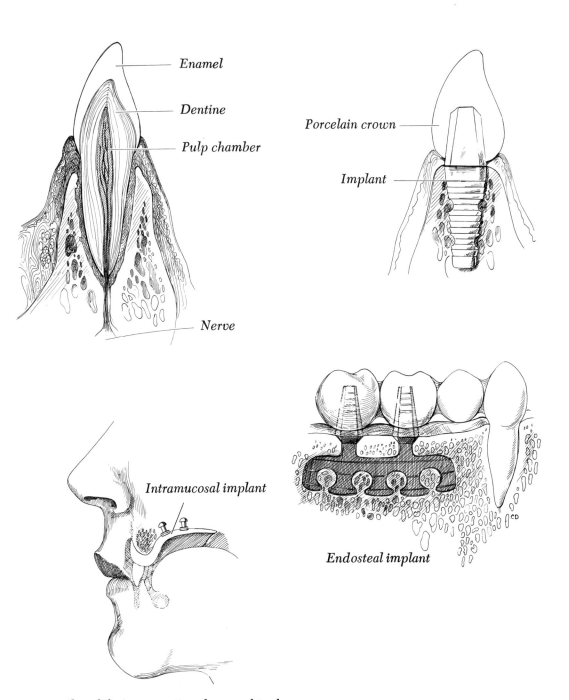

Enamel

Dentine

Pulp chamber

Nerve

Porcelain crown

Implant

Intramucosal implant

Endosteal implant

Above left: A cross-section of a normal tooth.

Above right: A vitreous-carbon implant, used for the replacement of single teeth or for securing a loose full denture.

Below left: An intramucosal implant, used to improve an unstable, loose upper denture.

Below right: An endosteal blade implant, used for patients who are missing several or all of their posterior teeth on one or both sides.

is a severely atrophied, edentulous (toothless) mandible, which occurs in people who have worn lower dentures for many years and have difficulty speaking or chewing. The subperiosteal implant, consisting of a vitallium (a chrome-cobalt alloy) lattice, is placed underneath the gum on the cortical bone (the denser stratum of the jawbone), since the softer alveolar bone, which normally supports the roots of the teeth, has disappeared.

Four posts, connected to the underlying framework, protrude through the gum, which quickly heals around them. Later, a bridge is made to fit over the four posts. The frame inside firmly supports the posts, which in turn keep the bridge in place. The new teeth are kept 1 mm from the gum so as not to cause pressure on the soft tissue.

Intramucosal implant—This is the best procedure for the maxilla. An implantologist can improve an unstable, loose upper denture by fastening on its base a series of small titanium snaps. The denture is then pressed briefly against the gum, on which the snaps leave their marks. Quickly, the implantologist stains the marks with surgical ink and then prepares in the gum little holes the size of the snaps. The same day, the denture is snapped in place, the snaps fitting snugly in the matching holes. Within two weeks, healing is completed. The denture is secure and can still be removed for cleaning.

Endosteal blade implant—This implant serves the same function as the subperiosteal, yet it is used in completely different circumstances. It is most useful for a patient who, for instance, is missing all of the posterior teeth on one or both sides, or where there are wide spaces between remaining natural teeth. A dentist might put in a partial denture, but there is no place in the back of the mouth on which to hook it, and soon it pulls loose the front teeth to which it is fastened.

Unlike the subperiosteal, which rests *on* the bone, the blade implant is anchored *into* the bone, with the entire blade-shaped portion buried below the surface of the jawbone, except for a thin post protruding through the gum, which functions as an artificial tooth on which the doctor can later construct a fixed bridge.

Another type of endosteal implant is the vitreous-carbon implant, made of a plasticlike material cured at extremely high temperature. A grooved vitreous-carbon plug is tapped into a hole drilled into the jawbone. A stainless steel post is then fitted into the plug and covered with a temporary plastic crown until the tissue heals and the bone grows solidly into the grooves of the implant. Later, a permanent crown is placed on the steel post. When enough healthy bone is present, this technique can be used for the replacement of single teeth, eliminating the need for a bridge.

DENTAL SEALANT

In modern dentistry, the term sealant is used to describe an adhesive liquid resin brushed over the chewing surfaces of posterior teeth to keep decay-causing bacteria and food particles out of vulnerable pits and grooves.

The sealant, which was first introduced in the 1960s by Michael Buonocore, a Rochester, New York, physician, is usually made of some industrial adhesive, such as polyurethanes, and can be applied quickly, safely, and without anaesthesia. The tooth enamel is first cleaned of debris with a polishing brush and pumice. Each tooth is then air-dried, isolated with cotton rolls, and conditioned with a solution of phosphoric acid and zinc oxide, and the sealant is painted on each tooth surface with a fine camel's hair brush. Finally, the sealed teeth are exposed for a few seconds to ultraviolet light, which will polymerize—harden—the sealant, thanks to an ultraviolet-light-sensitive catalyst dissolved into the adhesive just before use.

The sealant is transparent, and the underlying enamel can be easily checked by the dentist. It usually remains intact after a single application, though sometimes it wears off and has to be reapplied after a few months. Some investigators, however, feel that even if the sealant is not permanent, it reduces the incidence of caries, especially in children. Others disagree; still others feel that the sealant, if applied on all decay-free pits and grooves and reapplied at every annual checkup, will prevent caries altogether.

Recently, the sealant has been mixed with a fluoride additive, with the purpose of providing tooth enamel with a long-term application of fluoride, the chemical compound whose microscopic presence in the drinking water has been found to increase resistance of teeth to decay. So far, despite communal water fluoridation or the use of dietary supplements of fluoride (a compound of fluorine), the pits and grooves of posterior teeth have remained as susceptible to caries as they have always been, and researchers are now investigating whether people might benefit more from fluoridated teeth than from fluoridated water.

DENTIFRICE (TOOTHPASTE)

Dentifrice is a preparation used to clean and polish the surface of teeth. It is composed of an inorganic, mild abrasive, a detergent, a flavoring substance, a sweetener, a humectant, a binder, and a preservative.

A dentifrice can be manufactured in paste, powder, liquid, or tablet form. Combined with the mechanical action of a TOOTHBRUSH, it contributes to the elimination of PLAQUE and reduces tooth and gum decay and mouth odor.

DERMABRASION

Since the 1950s, extensive research has been conducted for a therapeutic toothpaste. Substances such as chlorophyll, the green coloring matter of plants, and more recently urea and fluorine have been added for the purpose of neutralizing the bacteria responsible for dental caries, but as of 1974 nothing significant has yet been developed.

Among the most unsuccessful attempts at therapeutic toothpaste was one containing penicillin, which failed because of ANTIBIOTICS' capacity of producing resistant strains of bacteria in the organism. Also, the suppression of certain bacteria may be followed by overgrowth of other microorganisms, including fungi.

For the moment, then, taste is perhaps the most important factor in the selection of a toothpaste. As for the manufacturer, to develop an acceptable flavor for a toothpaste is a task as delicate as that of a perfumer striving to create a new fragrance. A good toothpaste has to have a well-rounded, smooth flavor with an initial impact and a lasting, pleasant aftertaste. More important, each ingredient must be compatible with the others and remain essentially unchanged during the toothpaste's so-called shelf life.

DERMABRASION

Dermabrasion is a cosmetic surgery technique which consists of sanding the skin—usually of the face—with a rotating wire brush or a steel bur. Dermabrasion is used to smooth scars, reduce surface irregularities, and even out ridges and other aftereffects of ACNE or chickenpox. It is also helpful in removing so-called *traumatic* tattoos—foreign material that sometimes is driven into the skin during an accident. (*Aesthetic* tattoos are more difficult to eradicate with this technique, because the pigment is located much deeper within the skin.)

Irregular scars often can be improved by dermabrasion, which equalizes the margins and eliminates elevations. Fine wrinkles, such as the "pruning" that appears around the mouth with aging, can also be improved, even if only temporarily.

Dermabrasion is carried out with a motor-driven instrument, the dermabrader, which revolves at a high speed and is controlled by varying the pressure on a foot pedal. Attached to the dermabrader is a tiny cylinder of sandpaper or wire brush. The cylinders of sandpaper are available in several sizes: the larger ones are used for sanding broad flat surfaces, while the smaller ones help in planing narrower surfaces, such as around the nose. The wire brush is needed for *deep* planing; for more *superficial* sanding, a smooth cylinder, called diamond fraise, is used.

Local ANAESTHESIA is achieved by freezing the skin with ethyl chloride. This method temporarily hardens the skin and yet preserves its usual surface contour. The effect of ethyl chloride, however, is so short that abrasion can be performed only a few square centimeters at the time. Other local anaesthetics have the disadvantage of altering the skin configuration, and when used, the doctor marks the ridges and depressions with surgical ink so that they can be identified.

Bandages are applied and the patient can go home, if not out in the world. After a few days a crusty surface develops, which is then smeared with some mineral oil or COLD CREAM to help remove the crust and lubricate the surface beneath, which tends to be dry. The crust will shed in about one week, leaving a pink surface—the new layer of epidermis that has formed over the raw dermal surface—which soon fades, depending on the patient's type of skin. Powder and makeup can be applied after the abraded surface has healed, but it is important to wash the area well each day and to lubricate it. Direct or indirect sunlight should be avoided for several months after abrasion because it may produce discolorations and dark, uneven spots.

The face and scalp respond better to dermabrasion than any other area of the body. The back of the hands do moderately well, while the chest and upper and lower arms do poorly, as do legs and feet. People with dark skin do not profit much from dermabrasion, as the treated areas often become darker than the normal adjacent skin.

Still, dermabrasion is a sound and often extremely successful procedure. Improvement is achieved because once the dermis—the inner layer of the skin—has been thinned by this technique, it never regains its original thickness. And the new layer of epidermis which grows over it is considerably smoother and more even-colored than the old one.

DERMATITIS

Any skin inflammation or eruption, typically marked by reddening, swelling, oozing, crusting, or scaling, is called dermatitis.

However, dermatitis is a generic term; there are many types. The most common are:

Allergic contact dermatitis—This is caused by contact with a sensitizing substance, allergen, to which a person has become allergic, such as POISON IVY, RAGWEED, COSMETICS, or nickel in earrings. It tends to spread upon brief exposure to a very small amount of the allergen. PATCH TESTING is for the moment the only reliable method for diagnosing allergic contact dermatitis. Incidentally, it is important that the proper solution be used for the patch test to avoid a *false-positive* or a *false-negative* response in the patient, which could mislead the physician in his diagnosis.

DERMOGRAPHISM (SKIN WRITING)

Atopic dermatitis—Also called eczema, this condition usually develops in children with a family history of ALLERGY, but it can also appear in adults. Eczema tends to localize in the neck, wrists, and sometimes on the face. It results from the skin's coming in repeated contact with chemicals, natural or synthetic.

Contact dermatitis—This is a reaction produced by contact with generally irritating or toxic substances. It is an extremely common condition, especially among workers in industry who handle acids, solvents, and rubber, and among housewives whose hands are constantly in contact with soap, detergents, bleaches, oven cleaners, floor polishes, and excessive moisture. Ironically, overtreatment of contact dermatitis is even more common and often more severe than the dermatitis itself. Some patients try self-medication, for instance, using wrong medications such as mercurial compounds, tars, or some of the many "caine" medications—benzocain, for example—or switching rapidly from one drug to another when the first one doesn't seem to work.

Seborrheic dermatitis—Commonly called DANDRUFF, this condition is related to the body's oil glands and their secretions.

Avoidance of irritants or allergens is, as usual, the best cure for all forms of dermatitis (except dandruff). Treatment starts with plain water compresses followed by application of calamine liniment (for contact dermatitis). For more severe cases of eczema or poison ivy dermatitis, the dermatologist may prescribe corticosteroids, ANTIBIOTICS, antihistamines and sedatives.

DERMOGRAPHISM (SKIN WRITING)

Dermographism refers to a condition in which certain areas of the skin react exaggeratedly to scratching, stroking, and the smallest pressure from clothes—such as belts, brassiere straps, girdle seams or hooks—by developing red, itchy welts and streaks that resemble the writing pattern.

The cause of dermographism is unclear, though it could be a symptom of some ALLERGY, as it often occurs in connection with other allergic reactions. On the other hand, it may suddenly occur for no apparent reason and become chronic or persist for a while.

Dermographism is unpleasant but harmless; it cannot be cured, but dermatologists can prescribe medications for the welts and itching.

DETERGENTS

Unlike SOAP, which is a single chemical entity yielded from animal and vegetable fats, detergents vary greatly in chemical composition, as they are synthetized from hundreds of different substances derived mostly from petroleum.

The major advantage of synthetic detergents is that they do not combine, as soaps do, with the minerals (chiefly calcium and magnesium salts) found in hard water to form an unattractive and insoluble curd on skin, bathtubs or fabrics.

While some dermatologists feel that a white, unscented soap such as Ivory® is the best choice for cleansing delicate and not-so-young skin, detergents are considered excellent for young people's oily skin and are often the base of medicated cleansers used in the treatment of ACNE. Also, detergents have almost entirely replaced pure soap in household cleansers and in most SHAMPOOS. Here, too, they avoid the dull film of insoluble calcium and magnesium salts that soaps tend to deposit on hair shafts.

Often, detergents and soaps are difficult to distinguish—they both can be manufactured in cakes, and both foam. Also, some products are combinations of soap *and* detergent. However, words such as "soapless" or "nonalkaline" are often included in the labels of synthetic detergents.

Recently, a major cosmetic manufacturer has claimed that a new synthetic cleanser, based on so-called amphoterics—substances that have the capacity of reacting chemically both as an *acid* and as a *base*—are just as effective as, and milder than, the purest soap.

DIAPHRAGM

The diaphragm is a small, lightweight dome of soft rubber used by women to prevent conception. The rubber is stretched over a flexible ring, which allows the diaphragm to be compressed when it is inserted deep into the vagina and then released to seal the cervix.

The diaphragm must fit exactly, and different women need different sizes. Only a physician should prescribe the exact size of diaphragm needed by a woman. Size may change after childbirth, weight change, or a pelvic operation, and the diaphragm should be checked by a doctor any time a woman gains or loses more than ten pounds.

Diaphragms must always be used with a spermicidal jelly applied on the inside of the dome and around the rim. It can be inserted as early as two hours before intercourse and must be left in place for at least six hours afterward. The diaphragm does not interfere with a man's or a woman's sexual pleasure, though some men insist that they can always feel when a diaphragm is in place.

The idea of a mechanical device used by women as a physical barrier to sperm is as old as the most ancient of cultures. It was a moistened sponge or lint soaked in honey in Egypt; disks of oiled bamboo tissue in the brothels of China; half a squeezed lemon in eighteenth-century Italy. The modern form began to emerge in Holland at the end of the nineteenth century. It was made of vulcanized rubber and was called pessarium. But only in 1932, when the first spermicidal jelly was approved by the medical profession, did the diaphragm become the safe, effective, widely used CONTRACEPTIVE it is today. The modern diaphragm was the first contraceptive device to transfer to women the initiative of preventing conception. It meant that it was now acceptable to "premeditate" sex, rather than wait to be reluctantly swept off their feet by seduction, as respectable Victorian women were expected to do.

As the diaphragm's popularity has declined somewhat, both the pejorative and the favorable connotations of the diaphragm have been transferred to oral contraceptives.

DIETS

The science of nutrition, which is barely sixty years old and still has a long way to go, has been accompanied by a series of "miracle" diets that usually promise quick and painless weight reduction. Most of these diets state or suggest that calories don't count, "as long as the calories consumed are, so to speak, the promoter's pet calories," as Dr. Jean Mayer, professor of nutrition at Harvard University, recently observed.

One of the first diets to be widely publicized was the eighteen-day Hollywood diet of the 1920s, which was based on a heavy consumption of citrus fruits, an average intake of six hundred calories a day, and a promise of five pounds a week loss. Next came an era in which diets concentrated on just a few foods.

Literally every few months we witness the revival of one or another mutually contradicting diets—high protein, high fat, high carbohydrate, mashed potato, grape, champagne, lollipop, whipped cream, six glasses of water a day, the "Air Force diet," the "Boston Police diet," the "No-Willpower diet," the "Pray-Your-Weight-Away diet," the "Drinking Man's diet," the Stillman diet, the Mayo (no relation to the Mayo Clinic) diet, the no-diet diet, and so on.

Diets, then, whether *perpendicular* (depending on one ingredient) or *horizontal* (allowing the dieter to eat all normal food but strictly limiting quantities), come and go, and eventually come back, sometimes under a different name. They all are successful for a while, but none of them works for long. This is just as well: they won't have the time to become harmful as, for instance, crash diets. Anything from the all-the-coffee-and-cigarettes-one-can-stand diet to total fasting can cause serious complications besides being psychologically destructive, as most crash dieters rapidly gain their weight back.

A *real* diet is well balanced and varied. It restricts the intake of calories while supplying considerable proteins, moderate carbohydrates, and little fat. A reducing diet should simply be a temporarily restricted version of proper eating habits, accompanied by daily exercise.

Real diets, of course, are not miraculous but rather boring and difficult to respect. A seemingly endless sequence of three-ounce hamburgers, miserly portions of fresh vegetables, butter-free baked potatoes, half glasses of wine, artificially sweetened coffee, and transparent slices of toasted bread, with lots of celery (at 7 calories per stalk), is not an inviting proposition.

The truth is that *all* foods contribute calories, and there will be no loss of excessive fatty tissue unless the body expends more energy than it consumes. A pound of fat is the equivalent in energy of 3,500 calories; each time a person eats 3,500 calories more than he expends, he *gains* one pound. Conversely, by eating, let's say, 1000 calories a day and expending 1,500, a person will *lose* one pound in a week. Anyone who is overweight—true obesity requires professional help—and is determined to go on a diet by himself should first count *all* calories (including those of snacks, drinks, and "nonfattening" foods); measure portions; reduce salt and cut down drastically on sugar; and chew slowly, with long pauses between mouthfuls.

For those who find it difficult to stick to a self-imposed diet but, again, are not obese, the modern solution is a supervised reducing program based on behavior modification, i.e., the unlearning and relearning of eating habits. Essentially, such programs include a well-balanced diet, exercise, and a training of "thin behavior" based on two standard concepts of the so-called behaviorist school of psychology: 1) all behavior, including harmful behavior, is learned; 2) behavior can be changed. Thus, a skillful nutritionist, without necessarily analyzing in depth the psychological background that may cause a fat person to take in large quantities of calories regardless of his nutritional needs, is often able to pinpoint that person's own pattern and rituals of compulsive eating and reeducate him.

Some programs, such as the Center for Psychological Services in Miami, use the so-called aversion therapy, which consists of punishing a patient for indulging in unhealthy habits—in this case, overeating—though it can be used also for heavy smoking, alcoholism and drug addiction. For instance, a patient may be served in the office a large portion of his favorite food—chocolate ice cream, let's say—and asked to eat it while electrodes are attached to the hand that holds the spoon. Each time the patient takes a mouthful of ice cream, he receives a shock intense enough to be painful. Or else he is urged to eat ice cream made repugnant by the addition of salt or quinine.

109

FOODS	Food energy cal	Protein gm	Fat gm	Saturated (total) gm	Oleic gm	Linoleic gm	Carbohydrate gm	Calcium mg	Iron mg	Vitamin A value I.U.	Thiamin mg	Riboflavin mg	Niacin mg	Ascorbic acid mg
Almonds, Shelled—1 cup	850	26	77	6	52	15	28	332	6.7	0	0.34	1.31	5.0	tr
Apple Juice—1 cup	120	tr	tr				30	15	1.5		0.02	0.05	0.2	2
Apples, Raw—1 apple	70	tr	tr				18	8	0.4	50	0.04	0.02	0.1	3
Apricots, Dried—1 cup	390	8	1				100	100	8.2	16,350	0.02	0.23	4.9	19
Apricots, Raw—3 apricots	55	1	tr				14	18	0.5	2,890	0.03	0.04	0.7	10
Asparagus—4 spears	10	1	tr				2	13	0.4	540	0.10	0.11	0.8	16
Avocados—1 avocado	370	5	37	7	17	5	13	22	1.3	630	0.24	0.43	3.5	30
Bacon, Broiled—2 slices	90	5	8	3	4	1	1	2	0.5	0	0.08	0.05	0.8	
Bagels—1 bagel	165	6	2				28	9	1.2	30	0.14	0.10	1.2	0
Bananas—1 banana	100	1	tr				26	10	0.8	230	0.06	0.07	0.8	12
Barbecue Sauce—1 cup	230	4	17	2	5	9	20	53	2.0	900	0.03	0.03	0.8	13
Beans, Dry—1 cup	210	14	1				38	90	4.9	0	0.25	0.13	1.3	0
Beer—12 fl oz	150	1	0				14	18	tr		0.01	0.11	2.2	
Bluefish, Baked—3 oz	135	22	4				0	25	0.6	40	0.09	0.08	1.6	
Bouillon Cubes—1 cube	5	1	tr				tr							
Broccoli, Cooked—1 stalk	45	6	1				8	150	1.4	4,500	0.16	0.36	1.4	162
Butter—1 stick	810	1	92	51	30	3	1	23	0.0	3,750				0
Buttermilk—1 cup	90	9	tr				12	296	0.1	10	0.10	0.44	0.2	2
Cabbage, Raw—1 cup	15	1	tr				4	34	0.3	90	0.04	0.04	0.2	33
Cake, 2-Layer—1 portion	200	2	7	2	3	1	32	39	0.2	80	0.01	0.04	0.1	tr
Cake, With Icing—1 portion	275	3	10	3	4	1	45	51	0.5	120	0.02	0.06	0.2	tr
Candy (Caramels)—1 oz	115	1	3	2	1	tr	22	42	0.4	tr	0.01	0.05	0.1	tr
Cantaloupe—½ melon	60	1	tr				14	27	0.8	6,540	0.08	0.06	1.2	63
Carbonated Water—12 oz	115	0	0				29			0	0.00	0.00	0.0	0
Carrots, Raw—1 carrot	20	1	tr				5	18	0.4	5,500	0.03	0.03	0.3	4
Catsup—1 cup	290	6	1				69	60	2.2	3,820	0.25	0.19	4.4	41
Cauliflower, Cooked—1 cup	25	3	tr				5	25	0.8	70	0.11	0.10	0.7	66
Celery, Raw—1 stalk	5	tr	tr				2	16	0.1	100	0.01	0.01	0.1	4
Cheddar Cheese—1 oz	115	7	9	5	3	tr	1	213	0.3	370	0.01	0.13	tr	0
Chicken, Cooked—3 oz	115	20	3	1	1	1	0	8	1.4	80	0.05	0.16	7.4	
Chocolate, Semisweet—1 cup	860	7	61	34	22	1	97	51	4.4	30	0.02	0.14	0.9	0
Clam Chowder—1 cup	210	9	12				16	240	1.0	250	0.07	0.29	0.5	tr
Clams, Raw—3 oz	65	11	1				2	59	5.2	90	0.08	0.15	1.1	8
Coconut, Fresh—1 (2x2x½") piece	155	2	16	14	1	tr	4	6	0.8	0	0.02	0.01	0.2	1
Cola Drinks—12 oz	145	0	0				37			0	0.00	0.00	0.0	0
Cookies—1 brownie	95	1	6	1	3	1	10	8	0.4	40	0.04	0.02	0.1	tr
Corn, Cooked—1 ear	70	3	1				16	2	0.5	310	0.09	0.08	1.0	7
Corn Flakes—1 cup	100	2	tr				21	4	0.4	0	0.11	0.02	0.5	0
Corn Meal—1 cup	435	11	5	1	2	2	90	24	2.9	620	0.46	0.13	2.4	0
Corned Beef—3 oz	185	22	10	5	4	tr	0	17	3.7	20	0.01	0.20	2.9	

FOODS	Food energy cal	Pro-tein gm	Fat gm	Satu-rated (total) gm	Oleic gm	Lin-oleic gm	Carbo-hydrate gm	Cal-cium mg	Iron mg	Vita-min A value I.U.	Thia-min mg	Ribo-flavin mg	Nia-cin mg	Ascor-bic acid mg
Cottage Cheese—1 cup	260	33	10	6	3	tr	7	230	0.7	420	0.07	0.61	0.2	0
Crabmeat, Canned—3 oz	85	15	2				1	38	0.7		0.07	0.07	1.6	
Cranberry Sauce—1 cup	405	tr	1				104	17	0.6	60	0.03	0.03	0.1	6
Cream, Heavy—1 cup	840	5	90	50	30	3	7	179	0.1	3,670	0.05	0.26	0.1	2
Cream, Light—1 cup	505	7	49	27	16	1	10	245	0.1	2,020	0.07	0.36	0.1	2
Cream, Sour—1 cup	485	7	47	26	16	1	10	235	0.1	1,930	0.07	0.35	0.1	2
Cucumbers, Raw—1 cucumber	30	1	tr				7	35	0.6	tr	0.07	0.09	0.4	23
Danish Pastry—1 portion	275	5	15	5	7	3	30	33	0.6	200	0.05	0.10	0.5	tr
Dates, Pitted—1 cup	490	4	1				130	105	5.3	90	0.16	0.17	3.9	0
Doughnuts—1 doughnut	125	1	6	1	4	tr	16	13	0.4	30	0.05	0.05	0.4	tr
Eggs, Raw—1 egg	80	6	6	2	3	tr	tr	27	1.1	590	0.05	0.15	tr	0
Eggs, Scrambled—1 egg with milk & fat	110	7	8	3	3	tr	1	51	1.1	690	0.05	0.18	tr	0
Figs, Dried—1 fig	60	1	tr				15	26	0.6	20	0.02	0.02	0.1	0
Flour, All-Purpose—1 cup	420	12	1				88	18	3.3	0	0.51	0.30	4.0	0
Frankfurters—1 frank	170	7	15				1	3	0.8		0.08	0.11	1.4	
Gelatin, Dessert Powder—1 pkg	315	8	0				75							
Gin, 100-Proof—1 jigger	125						tr							
Ginger Ale—12 oz	115	0	0				29			0	0.00	0.00	0.0	0
Grapefruit, Medium—½ portion	45	1	tr				12	19	0.5	10	0.05	0.02	0.2	44
Grapefruit Juice, Canned—1 cup	100	1	tr				24	20	1.0	20	0.07	0.04	4.0	84
Grapes, American—1 cup	65	1	1				15	15	0.4	100	0.05	0.03	0.2	3
Green Beans, Cooked—1 cup	30	2	tr				7	63	0.8	680	0.09	0.11	0.6	15
Ham—3 oz	245	18	19	7	8	2	0	8	2.2	0	0.40	0.16	3.1	
Hamburgers—3 oz	245	21	17	8	8	tr	0	9	2.7	30	0.07	0.18	4.6	
Honey—1 tbsp	55	tr	tr				14	4	0.2	tr	tr	0.01	tr	tr
Ice Cream—½ gallon	2,055	48	113	62	37	3	221	1,553	0.5	4,680	0.43	2.23	1.1	11
Jam—1 tbsp	55	tr	tr				13	4	0.3	tr	tr	0.01	tr	tr
Lamb, Cooked—1 chop	400	25	33	18	12	1	0	10	1.5	tr	0.14	0.25	5.6	
Lard—1 cup	1,853	0	205	78	94	20	0	0	0.0	0	0.00	0.00	0.0	0
Lemonade Concentrate—1 can	430	tr	tr				112	9	0.4	40	0.04	0.07	0.7	66
Lemons—1 lemon	20	1	tr				6	19	0.4	10	0.03	0.01	0.1	39
Lettuce, Raw—1 head	30	3	tr				6	77	4.4	2,130	0.14	0.13	0.6	18
Liver, Beef, Fried—2 oz	130	15	6				3	6	5.0	30,280	0.15	2.37	9.4	15
Malted Milk—1 cup	245	11	10				28	317	0.7	590	0.14	0.49	0.2	2
Margarine—1 stick	815	1	92	17	46	25	1	23	0.0	3,750				0
Mayonnaise—1 tbsp	100	tr	11	2	2	6	tr	3	0.1	40	tr	0.01	tr	
Milk—1 cup	160	9	9	5	3	tr	12	288	0.1	350	0.07	0.41	0.2	2
Milk, Dry—1 cup	245	24	tr				35	879	0.4	20	0.24	1.21	0.6	5
Muffins—1 muffin	120	3	4	1	2	1	17	42	0.6	40	0.07	0.09	0.6	tr
Mushrooms, Canned—1 cup	40	5	tr				6	15	0.12	tr	0.04	0.60	48.0	4

FOODS	Food energy cal	Pro-tein gm	Fat gm	Satu-rated (total) gm	Oleic gm	Lin-oleic gm	Carbo-hydrate gm	Cal-cium mg	Iron mg	Vita-min A value I.U.	Thia-min mg	Ribo-flavin mg	Nia-cin mg	Ascor-bic acid mg
Noodles—1 cup	200	7	2	1	1	tr	37	16	1.4	110	0.22	0.13	1.9	0
Oatmeal—1 cup	130	5	2			1	21	22	1.4	0	0.19	0.05	0.2	0
Olive Oil—1 cup	1,945	0	220	24	167	15	0	0	0.0		0.00	0.00	0.0	0
Olives, Green—4 medium	15	tr	2	tr	2	tr	tr	8	0.2	40				
Onions, Raw—1 onion	40	2	tr				10	30	0.6	40	0.04	0.04	0.2	11
Orange Juice, Concentrated—1 can	360	5	tr				87	75	0.9	1,620	0.68	0.11	2.8	360
Oranges—1 orange	65	1	tr				16	54	0.5	260	0.13	0.05	0.5	66
Oysters, Raw—1 cup	160	20	4				8	226	13.2	740	0.33	0.43	60.0	
Pancakes—1 cake	60	2	2	tr	1	tr	9	27	0.4	30	0.05	0.06	0.4	tr
Parmesan Cheese—1 oz	130	12	9	5	3	tr	1	383	0.1	360	0.01	0.25	0.1	0
Peaches, Canned—1 cup	200	1	tr				20	10	0.7	1,100	0.02	0.06	1.0	7
Peaches, Raw—1 peach	35	1	tr				10	9	0.5	1,320	0.02	0.05	1.0	7
Peanut Butter—1 tbsp	95	4	8	2	4	2	3	9	0.3		0.02	0.02	2.4	0
Peanuts, Roasted—1 cup	840	37	72	16	31	21	27	107	3.0		0.46	0.19	24.7	0
Pears, Raw—1 pear	100	1	1				25	13	0.5	30	0.04	0.07	0.2	7
Peas, Cooked—1 cup	115	9	1				19	37	2.9	860	0.44	0.17	3.7	33
Pecans—1 cup	740	10	77	5	48	15	16	79	2.6	140	0.93	0.14	1.0	2
Peppers, Hot—1 tbsp	50	2	2				8	40	2.3	9,750	0.03	0.17	1.3	2
Peppers, Sweet—1 tbsp	15	1	tr				4	7	0.5	310	0.06	0.06	0.4	94
Pies (Approx.)—1 sector	350	3	15	4	7	3	51	11	0.4	40	0.03	0.03	0.5	1
Pineapples, Canned—1 cup	195	1	tr				50	29	0.8	120	0.20	0.06	0.5	17
Pineapples, Raw—1 cup	75	1	tr				19	24	0.7	100	0.12	0.04	0.3	24
Pizza—1 wedge	185	7	6	2	3	tr	27	107	0.7	290	0.04	0.12	0.7	4
Popcorn, with Oils & Salt—1 cup	40	1	2	1	tr	tr	5	1	0.2			0.01	0.1	0
Popsicles—1 popsicle	70	0	0	0	0	0	18	0	tr	0	0.00	0.00	0.0	0
Pork, Fresh, Cooked—1 chop	260	16	21	8	9	2	0	8	2.2	0	0.63	0.18	3.8	
Potato Chips—10 chips	115	1	8	2	2	4	10	8	0.4	tr	0.04	0.01	1.0	3
Potatoes, Boiled—1 potato	105	3	tr				23	10	0.8	tr	0.13	0.05	2.0	22
Potatoes, Fried—10 pieces	155	2	7	2	2	4	20	9	0.7	tr	0.07	0.04	1.8	12
Prunes, Cooked—1 cup	295	2	1				78	60	4.5	1,860	0.08	0.18	1.7	2
Prunes, Dried—4 prunes	70	1	tr				18	14	1.1	440	0.02	0.04	0.4	1
Pudding Mix—1 pkg	410	3	2	1	1	tr	103	23	1.8	tr	0.02	0.08	0.5	0
Raisins—1 pkg	40	tr	tr				11	9	0.5	tr	0.02	0.01	0.1	tr
Rice, Cooked—1 cup	225	4	tr				50	21	1.8	0	0.23	0.02	2.1	0
Roast Beef, Lean & Fat—3 oz	375	17	34	16	15	1	0	8	2.2	70	0.05	0.13	3.1	
Roquefort Cheese—1 oz	105	6	9	5	3	tr	1	89	0.1	350	0.01	0.17	0.3	0
Rye Bread—1 slice	60	2	tr				13	19	0.4	0	0.05	0.02	0.4	0
Safflower Oil—1 cup	1,945	0	220	33	44	114	0	0	0.0		0.00	0.00	0.0	0
Salad Dressing, French—1 tbsp	65	tr	6	1	1	3	3	2	0.1					
Salami—1 oz	130	7	11				tr	4	1.0		0.10	0.07	1.5	

FOODS	Food energy cal	Protein gm	Fat gm	Saturated (total) gm	Unsaturated Oleic gm	Unsaturated Linoleic gm	Carbohydrate gm	Calcium mg	Iron mg	Vitamin A value I.U.	Thiamin mg	Riboflavin mg	Niacin mg	Ascorbic acid mg
Salmon, Canned—3 oz	120	17	5	1	1	tr	0	167	0.7	60	0.03	0.16	6.8	
Sardines, Canned—3 oz	175	20	9				0	372	2.5	190	0.02	0.17	4.6	
Sauerkraut, Canned—1 cup	45	2	tr				9	85	1.2	120	0.07	0.09	0.4	33
Sausages—2 slices	80	3	7				tr	2	0.5		0.04	0.06	0.7	
Sherbet—1 cup	260	2	2				59	31	tr	120	0.02	0.06	tr	4
Shrimp, Canned—3 oz	100	21	1				1	98	2.6	50	0.01	0.03	1.5	
Soup, Canned—1 cup	180	7	10	3	3	3	15	172	0.5	610	0.05	0.27	0.7	2
Soybean Oil—1 cup	1,945	0	220	33	44	114	0	0	0.0		0.00	0.00	0.0	0
Spaghetti—1 cup	155	5	1				32	11	1.3	0	0.20	0.11	1.5	0
Spaghetti with Meat Sauce—1 cup	330	19	12	4	6	1	39	124	3.7	1,590	0.25	0.30	4.0	22
Spinach, Cooked—1 cup	40	5	1				6	167	4.0	14,580	0.13	0.25	1.0	50
Steak, Lean & Fat—3 oz	330	20	27	13	12	1	0	9	2.5	50	0.05	0.16	4.0	
Strawberries, Raw—1 cup	55	1	1				13	31	1.5	90	0.04	0.10	1.0	88
Sugar, Brown—1 cup	820	0	0				212	187	7.5	0	0.02	0.07	0.4	0
Sugar, White—1 cup	770	0	0				199	0	0.2	0	0.00	0.00	0.0	0
Sweet Potatoes, Cooked—1 cup	155	2	1				36	44	1.0	8,910	0.10	0.07	0.7	24
Swiss Cheese—1 oz	105	8	8	4	3	tr	1	262	0.3	320	tr	0.11	tr	0
Swordfish, Broiled—3 oz	150	24	5				0	23	1.1	1,750	0.03	0.04	9.3	
Syrup—1 tbsp	55						14	35	2.6			0.02	tr	
Tangerines, Raw—1 tangerine	40	1	tr				10	34	0.3	360	0.05	0.02	0.1	27
Tartar Sauce—1 tbsp	75	tr	8	1	1	4	1	3	0.1					
Tomato Juice, Canned—1 cup	45	2	tr				10	17	2.2	1,940	0.12	0.07	1.9	39
Tomatoes, Raw—1 tomato	90	2	tr				9	24	0.9	1,640	0.11	0.07	1.3	42
Tuna Fish, Canned—3 oz	170	24	7	2	1	1	0	7	1.6	70	0.04	0.10	10.1	
Veal, Cooked—3 oz	185	29	9	5	4	tr		9	2.7		0.06	0.21	4.6	
Vinegar—1 tbsp	tr	tr	0				1	1	1.0					
Vodka, 100-Proof—1 jigger	125						tr							
Waffles—1 waffle	210	7	7	2	4	1	28	85	1.3	250	0.13	0.19	1.0	tr
Walnuts, Chopped—1 cup	790	26	75	4	26	36	19	tr	7.6	380	0.28	0.14	0.9	tr
Watermelon—1 wedge	115	2	1				27	30	2.1	2,510	0.13	0.13	0.7	30
Whiskey, 100-Proof—1 jigger	125						tr							
White Bread—1 slice	70	2	1				13	21	0.6	tr	0.06	0.05	0.6	tr
Whole Wheat Bread—1 slice	65	3	1				14	24	0.8	tr	0.09	0.03	0.8	tr
Wines, Dessert—3½ fl oz	140	tr	0				4	9	0.4		tr	0.01	0.1	
Wines, Table—3½ fl oz	85	tr	0				4	9	0.4		tr	0.01	0.1	
Yeast, Dry—1 pkg	20	3	tr				3	3	1.1	tr	0.16	0.38	2.6	tr
Yogurt—1 cup	150	7	8	5	3	tr	12	27	2.1	340	0.07	0.39	0.2	2

Adapted from Home and Garden Bulletin No. 72,
United States Department of Agriculture, Washington, D.C.
Prepared by Consumer and Food Economics Institute, Agricultural Research Service

Less ambitious behavior-modification programs concentrate mainly on reinforcing proper eating routines. Patients are asked, for instance, to keep a diary of every bit of food they consume. Then they are taught to eat always sitting down, preferably in the same place—at a table—rather than in front of television, in bed, or while walking. They are encouraged to use small dishes, to practice eating slowly and putting down knife and fork between bites, and to leave the preparation of food to others.

An unorthodox "diet" which doctors do not recommend but which is becoming popular was first tried successfully in 1973 by an English housewife, Mrs. Shirley Turner, who convinced her dentist to put locked braces on her teeth, the kind designed for fractured jaws. A liquid, vitamin-supplemented diet helped her lose one hundred pounds in six months. Since then, a Michigan oral surgeon, Dr. Gilbert Klieff, reported that he has reluctantly put locked braces on about one hundred patients who had read about Mrs. Turner in the papers. Only about 10 percent of Dr. Klieff's patients asked to have the braces removed before they reached their goal. The rest, apparently with only minimal physiological problems, such as a temporary inflammation of the gums, have lost as many as one hundred pounds and are ecstatic.

DIMETHYL SULFOXIDE (DMSO)

DMSO, a strange chemical first discovered in 1866 and practically forgotten until the early 1960s, is now considered one of the most extraordinary and versatile drugs of this century.

In 1962, Dr. Stanley W. Jacob, a professor of surgery at the University of Oregon, almost by accident rediscovered DMSO and quickly realized its enormous and multiform potentials. He demonstrated that DMSO not only is safe but can control pain; relieve inflammation, infections, and burns; kill bacteria, viruses and fungi; reduce muscle spasms, ARTHRITIS, breast cysts; and, when used together with an ANALGESIC, even produce local ANAESTHESIA, as it also functions as a carrier, that is, helps carry other drugs through the tissues.

Dr. Jacob discovered that DMSO has the ability to go right through the skin; the only tissues it cannot penetrate are tooth enamel and nails. It can reach all tissues and organs shortly after being painted or sprayed on the skin, leaving a person with a faint taste of garlic in his mouth.

Having realized DMSO's large margin of safety and its ability to fight both pain *and* inflammation and to relieve muscle spasms, researchers began to use the drug successfully for the treatments of certain chronic HEADACHES, such as the dreadful tic douloureux and the tension headache. DMSO is simply painted on (or injected into) the area where the headache occurs, though the drug spreads through the tissues so rapidly that it could be painted on any part of the body and obtain the same result. Even for those headaches that don't respond directly to DMSO, this can be used as a carrier for other drugs.

DMSO is already a prescription drug in Denmark, Germany, Sweden and Russia. In the United States, however, it is still under investigation at the National Academy of Sciences. Still, Dr. Jacob and other researchers are convinced that DMSO will eventually become an over-the-counter drug—the ASPIRIN of the twenty-first century.

DISCLOSING SOLUTION

A disclosing solution is a purple tablet or a red, fast-dissolving wafer that is chewed and swished around the mouth for sixty seconds before brushing one's teeth, and then spit out or swallowed. They are all safe; one of them, Red-Cote® brand, even has a raspberry taste.

The result is pink gums and teeth, with markedly darker hues and spots, usually along the gums and on the surfaces between the teeth. During the sixty seconds, the disclosing solution has dyed the otherwise invisible film of dental plaque, the microbial mass that is developed constantly in the mouth and adheres tenaciously to the teeth, eventually mineralizing to become hard, razor-sharp deposits of tartar.

With the help of a mouth mirror, a good light, DENTAL FLOSS, and a flexible but sturdy toothbrush, the PLAQUE, which usually escapes a perfunctory toothbrushing, can be removed.

Since the dye is water-soluble, it will disappear in about half an hour. Disclosing tablets should be used every day until one's toothbrushing technique has improved; afterward it can be used occasionally as a spot-check.

DOUCHES

To douche means to wash out the vagina, usually with a stream of lukewarm water or a cleansing solution, such as diluted vinegar.

Although some women regard douching as a routine form of cleanliness, these are seldom necessary for women with *normal* vaginal secretions. Many gynecologists, in fact, feel that douches should not be used at all—especially during pregnancy—except as an addition to medication for vaginal infections or irritations.

When douching is prescribed by a physician, a douche bag is preferable to a syringe, in order to get a steady and slow flow of the solution rather than a sudden spurt. The douche bag is connected to a long rubber tube, which is usually equipped with a flow-regulating clasp and a hard-rubber, perforated nozzle.

DRUG INTERACTIONS

While reclining along the slanting side of the bathtub, with the knees slightly raised and spread apart, a woman should introduce the nozzle gently into the vagina as far as it will go. In order to cleanse all the vagina's folds and creases, she should fill it completely with the solution and hold the solution inside for a while by pressing the lips of the VULVA together around the nozzle with thumb and forefinger, after snapping the clasp shut. Finally she can let the solution gush out and repeat the procedure a few times, until all of the douche solution has been used. The entire area should then be dried thoroughly and the vaginal medication applied according to the doctor's instructions.

DRUG INTERACTIONS

In an era of complex and powerful prescription drugs, physicians are beginning to be more and more concerned with the countless possibilities of drug interactions, that is, the various mechanisms by which different drugs taken simultaneously may neutralize one another's efficacy; combine to produce insoluble substances; or alter one another's absorption, distribution, or excretion from the body. One drug may cause an exaggerated or toxic reaction to another or interfere with normal ENZYME activity in the body.

The possibilities of dangerous reactions are multiplied when interaction occurs between prescription drugs and the so-called over-the-counter (OTC) drugs. There are more than one-hundred thousand different OTC drugs on the market, and many patients as well as physicians consider such products as ANTACIDS, ANALGESICS, sedatives, stimulants, LAXATIVES and antihistamines insignificant when compared with prescription drugs. People are often unaware that many OTC drugs merely contain *smaller* quantities of certain perscription drugs and that the same powerful ingredient may be contained in several different products.

Examples of drug interaction:
1) A prescription drug that is a weak acid would be easily absorbed in the acidic environment of the stomach; but if the patient also takes an antacid, the latter can prevent the prescription drug from being properly absorbed.
2) When ANTIBIOTICS, such as penicillin and tetracycline, are used together, their individual effect is frequently diminished.
3) A prescription drug transferred from its original container into another that once contained a different drug may mix with traces of the latter.
4) ASPIRIN increases the "blood-thinning" effect of an ANTICOAGULANT. For this reason, a patient with heart disease who has been taking an anticoagulant under his doctor's supervision may risk hemorrhage if he uses aspirin for a simple HEADACHE.

116

5) A mixture of a BARBITURATE or tranquilizer and ALCOHOL may not simply add their effects but multiply each other and produce dizziness, blurred vision, and intoxication.

Many potentially dangerous drug interactions are already recognized and understood and can be avoided or minimized by a physician's intelligent adjustment of *dosage* and *frequency*, and by a strict review of a patient's self-medicating habits.

Dr. Gerald J. Aitken, a New Jersey internist, has gone one step further. He has designed a printed form, which folds to pocket size, on which a patient's birth date, ALLERGIES, diet restrictions, previous drug reactions, and all medicines he is currently taking are recorded. This "medicine profile" should be shown to every doctor—"one specialist may have no idea what drugs another specialist has prescribed," Dr. Aitken observed. And every pharmacist who fills a prescription for that patient should enter on the form the name and the dosage of each new medication.

E

EARLOBE PIERCING

The piercing of earlobes for jewelry, though often done informally in the back of a jewelry store, is considered by many as a minor medical procedure, to be performed in a doctor's office, following a number of safety measures that are presumably ignored by a jeweler.

The most important precaution, doctors say, is to have the piercing done with a stainless steel needle. The temporary earring, too, should be stainless steel, because nickel—an element found in most metal alloys, including those of gold and silver—is one of the five most common causes of allergic contact DERMATITIS. Even pure gold earrings are not quite safe following ear piercing, though ALLERGY to gold is much rarer than allergy to nickel.

Moreover, women seem to be much more susceptible to nickel than are men; besides, there is apparently an even higher incidence of the sensitivity in women who wear nickel-containing earrings immediately after their ears have been pierced. A five-cent coin is usually used for nickel patch tests.

Another concern that women should have when considering whether to have their ears pierced is the aesthetic effect: the little hole in each lobe should be not only symmetric with that in the other ear but also perfectly centered.

Some doctors patiently take measurements and mark with surgical ink the place to be pierced. Recently, however, Dr. Raymond L. Garcia, a dermatologist at Lackland Air Force Base in Texas, has devised a quick and infallible new system for piercing ears that involves using a surgical clamp—a sort of tweezers with flat, round base plates, approximately the size of an earlobe—modified by a one-eighth-inch hole drilled through the center of each base plate. The doctor sterilizes and anaesthetizes the earlobe; delicately clamps the earlobe; passes a stainless steel needle through the two holes and the lobe, without having to measure, since the

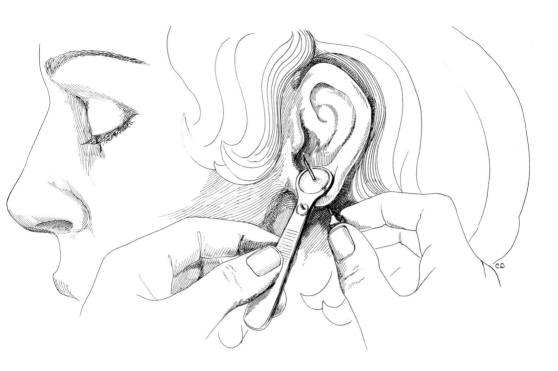

A safe and quick method of earlobe piercing devised by Dr. Raymond L. Garcia, a dermatologist from Texas: a tweezerlike surgical clamp with a tiny hole in the center of each jaw, which is pressed around the earlobe. Without having to measure—since the holes are in dead center—a stainless steel needle is then passed through the holes and the earlobe.

holes are in dead center; inserts a fourteen-karat gold earring in the needle opening; and finally withdraws the needle, leaving the earring post in the correct position.

EARTH SHOES

Earth Shoes are fan-toed shoes, boots or sandals with heels about ½ inch lower than the ball of the foot, thus supposedly promoting a healthier, more comfortable posture than that provided by normal shoes.

The originals were invented in 1957 by Anne Kalsø, a Danish costume designer and yoga expert. She had noticed that footprints on beaches showed the heel sinking deeper than the toes. Later she designed Earth Shoes to promote a straighter spine and improve breathing and circulation.

Despite Earth Shoes' popularity, only a few podiatrists recommend these shoes, and they even warn that Earth Shoes can be harmful to people with flat feet or other foot problems. Others point out that footprints people leave when walking barefoot on a soft surface such as sand are deeper at the heel only initially: once the weight of the body is transferred from the heel to the toes, just before lifting the other foot in preparation for the following step, the toes sink into the sand just as deeply as the heel. More important, when used on hard pavements such as asphalt, it is doubtful whether Earth Shoes indeed can simulate the "earthy" surface on which feet were originally made to walk.

EDEMA (SWELLING)

Edema refers to an abnormal accumulation of fluid in the intercellular tissue spaces of the body, causing puffy swelling, or distention and compression of organs, usually associated with defective circulation.

ELECTRIC CURLERS

Mechanically, electric curlers work like ordinary rollers—circular or round objects used to hold the hair in the curled position until hair, previously softened by water, dries and hardens again in the shape of the rollers. The only difference is that electric curlers are heated before being used and are fastened in place with special hairpinlike holders. Also, in order to make them easier to roll, the curlers are equipped with tiny protuberances.

The curlers are heated within their own unit. When they are ready for use they are no longer connected to the source of electricity, so that they neither are too hot to handle nor present the hazard of electric shock. Some of the latest models are equipped for both dry and moist heat. A CONDITIONER can be added when the mist is turned on.

Electric curlers are safe, but they should be used only occasionally, as they may cause the hair to become excessively dry and brittle. Also, repeated use brings up the hair's natural oil, making it dirty quickly.

Most types of electric curler units need no more than ten minutes to heat; the curlers should be wound in the hair for about five minutes, after which they cool off. The curlers should always be removed slowly, gently, and straight down to prevent the hair from being caught in the curler's "bumps" and breaking. One solution, apparently popular with New York fashion models, is to file off the bumps a little.

Electric curlers are used differently for different kinds of hair. To add body to *fine and straight hair*, small curlers are used in small sections of hair that has been dampened slightly. The curlers are left in until completely cold.

For *naturally wavy hair*, large curlers should be used and removed quickly.

For *tinted hair*, the conditioner should always be used, and the curlers should be removed before they are completely cold.

ELECTRIC HAIR-STYLERS

Electric hair-styler is a generic term for a variety of hair-grooming aids: 1) hand-held hot-air blower; 2) bonnet-type dryer; 3) styling dryer. Numbers one and three are similar in that they have heating coils and blowers. The only difference is that number three has a provision for mounting a comb or brush within the hot airstream, so that the hair can be simultaneously dried and shaped.

Externally, most styling dryers are molded in the shape of a short club that, with its bristled attachments, looks like a giant electric toothbrush. Air is sucked in through the handle end and is heated as it makes its way toward the so-called "business" end, to be blown away through the hair-styling attachment.

Another popular style is flat or slablike on its business end, with a relatively large air-intake grille on one side.

Electric stylers work on the principle that hair tends to hold the shape it's in as it dries. Straight hair may be wrapped around rollers to form curls; conversely, wavy hair may be brushed out under tension and simultaneously dried to straighten it. Whatever the style of the dryer, there are no prompt results unless the hair is drying as it is being shaped. It is a matter of time, but all dryers put out enough heat to shape hair. How long it takes to reach the point at which hair is dry enough (slightly damp) to be shaped depends on the length of the hair and the power of the dryer.

None of the available dryers yet conveys the perfect drying combination of air flow and air temperature (200° F. to 220° F.), which incidentally has a bad effect on ears, scalp, and neck unless the dryer is moved about briskly. The other solution—more air at a lower temperature (150° F. to 180° F.)—has a drawback, too: the vigorous air flow blows the hair around and undoes the set. Some dryers are equipped with a switch. When the hair is wet and heavy, it can stand hot and breezy air; and when it starts to dry, the air flow and temperature can be reduced.

Most women use electric hair-stylers in the bathroom, which can be dangerous because of the high humidity. Fortunately, dryers usually don't leak electricity. Still, it is best not to wet the attached comb or brush.

Electric hair-stylers are generally equipped with a thermostat which acts when the internal temperature becomes excessive. The grille should be kept free from lint or hair: internal temperature may rise if the air flow is partially blocked.

Dryers should never be set down when still running: the vibration may cause it to creep over an edge and fall. Before using a dryer, a woman should apply MOISTURIZER to the face and throat, and direct the hot blasts only to the hair.

ELECTRIC SHAVERS

Many women find a safety razor more than adequate for shaving their legs and underarms, but some, finding it difficult to shave around the shinbone and disliking to dabble with lather, prefer electric shavers.

Again, many find men's electric shavers perfectly acceptable, though there should be such a thing as an ideal electric shaver for women: light, quiet, simple to operate and to clean, equipped with an on/off switch, and nonirritating to the skin, especially under the arms.

However, the ideal electric shaver for women is still to be designed, and the ones available now are basically similar to those designed for men by the same brand; the only difference is that they are fancier-looking and sometimes more expensive.

Some of the better brands, such as Lady Norelco®, have adapters for power outlet sockets in foreign countries (120 volts in the United States; 220 volts abroad).

All electric shavers work best when clean; most are supplied with a brush.

ELECTROENCEPHALOGRAPH (EEG)

The electroencephalograph—EEG for short—is a complex electronic device used in sleep research laboratories to measure, by recording electric currents developed in the brain, what happens in a person's body when he sleeps.

A number of tiny electrodes are taped to a sleeper's head and body; each transmits a specific message—variations in blood pressure, pulse, respiration, body temperature, eye movement and muscle tone—along multicolored electric cables to a control room. There the messages are fed to a giant amplifier—the EEG polygraph—that drives a row of inked pens, beneath which moves a strip of graph paper. Each pen, driven by a signal from a section of the brain, swings upward when the electric charge is *negative* and downward when it is *positive*. The up-and-down movements are traced on the paper as waves—the visible signs of the brain's electric activity. Each wave shows a change of voltage in the sleeper's brain: the *height* of a wave indicates how high the voltage is, the *number* of waves shows how rapidly the voltage is changing.

Each stage of NORMAL SLEEP shows its characteristic brain waves: small and narrow for Stage I; growing rapidly larger for Stage II; higher and slower for Stage III, very large and slow for Stage IV; irregular and small during REM sleep, the stage during which people dream.

After a night spent in a sleep laboratory, a volunteer sleeper leaves behind about half a mile of records, which researchers can interpret to determine, for example, whether the sleeper is depressed, anxious, or an alcoholic, has vivid dreams or nightmares, or has taken sleeping pills or an unsuitable dosage of a prescription drug.

Once researchers had established, through the EEG records, the consistency and the rhythmic sequence of sleep stages, they were also able to find out whether *all* sleep stages are necessary for a healthy, sound sleep. They discovered that when they awakened volunteer sleepers for several nights in a row as soon as the EEG machine signaled the beginning of a REM sleep period, the sleepers became irascible and anxious and invariably lapsed into REM sleep almost the moment they closed their eyes. Also, they continued to spend longer periods in the REM stage, until they seemed to have compensated for their "dream deprivation."

The same thing happened when the volunteer sleepers were deprived of Stage IV (Delta sleep), though their reaction during the day was one of depression and lethargy and complaints of an undefinable malaise.

By the early 1970s, sleep researchers had defined eight major sleep disorders that can be detected on EEG records:
1) Protracted time needed to fall asleep.
2) Too long or too short Stage IV sleep.
3) Too long or too short REM sleep.
4) Abnormal sequence of sleep stages, such as skipping of stages or unpredictable progress.
5) Unusually long or short periods spent at any stage of sleep.
6) Early awakenings.
7) Multiple awakenings during the night.
8) Awakenings in the middle of nightmares.

Any illness, physical or mental, is reflected in some alteration of sleep patterns. Depression, for instance, can affect sleep stages in many different ways, the most common being reduction of Stage IV, early awakenings, and shifts from one level of sleep to another with abnormal rapidity. Indeed, EEG records of a severely depressed person can be so disorganized that researchers may find it difficult to interpret them.

EEG machines and sleep laboratories are already quite advanced, although they are still used essentially for research only. In the near future, however, sleep analysis might become part of a patient's check-up and might presumably become a routine method for diagnosis of INSOMNIA, for which the proper treatment could then be formulated without relying solely on potentially dangerous hypnotic drugs.

ELECTROLYSIS
When the passage of an electric current through a substance is accompanied by chemical changes that are independent of the heating

effects of the current, the process is known as electrolysis, and the substance is called electrolyte.

But electrolysis more commonly refers to a technique for the permanent removal of superfluous hair, which consists of inserting a fine electric needle into the hair FOLLICLE until it reaches and destroys the papilla, the source of nourishment of the hair. Only the destruction of the papilla ensures the permanent removal of a particular hair.

The electricity originally used for electrolysis was galvanic current, a reduced form of direct current, i.e., one flowing evenly and continuously in one direction throughout the entire circuit and producing a chemical action. The needle absorbs hydrogen from the cells of the papilla, thus disintegrating it and preventing it from reproducing again.

In the last several years, the galvanic method has been virtually replaced by the short-wave process (electrocoagulation), for which a modified high-frequency electric current is used. The basic procedure and the end result are essentially the same as electrolysis; however, the advantage of the short-wave process is that it coagulates the papilla in one-fifth of a second, rather than disintegrating it at the considerably slower rate of fifty seconds to three minutes for each papilla. This means that more hair can be removed in one session with less irritation to the tissue. Also, since short-wave equipment is provided with electronic timers that shut off the current automatically after a few seconds, the danger of scars because of excessive electricity is completely eliminated.

The electrologist holds the needle lightly between the thumb and the index finger of one hand; with the other he gently stretches the skin around the hair to be removed so as to facilitate the insertion of the needle. He slides the needle gently into the follicle at the same angle the hair grows out of the skin. He then presses a foot pedal to send the current through the needle.

If the hair to be removed is thick, the electrologist may have to insert the needle twice. The hair is then gently drawn out of the skin with tweezers. In order not to irritate the skin, since electrolysis is not altogether painless, an expert electrologist will not remove in the same session hairs that grow too close together. Finally a soothing lotion is applied to the skin, as well as an antiseptic powder or antibiotic cream, with instructions to the patient not to rub or use regular makeup on the area for at least twenty-four hours.

Sometimes, if the follicle is somewhat twisted either because of very curly hair or because the hair has been repeatedly depilated, or if the electrologist has been excessively cautious and has failed to destroy the papilla, the hair may regrow after electrolysis, and the treatment has to be repeated.

Various types of home electrolysis devices are advertised for permanent removal of hair by self-treatment. These devices usually consist of a tube, which is used as a handle, and contain batteries to provide the electric source. A needle extends from the tube (or from a cord) and transmits the current. However, dermatologists usually discourage people from trying these devices. For one thing, inexperienced users find it difficult to determine the direction of the hair follicle, the location of the papilla, and the amount of current needed to eliminate the hair without producing scars.

The most common areas in which superfluous hair is found are the upper lip, the chin, the eyebrows, the lower abdomen and the upper thighs. The breasts and the underarms are more sensitive and may develop a rash for a few days after electrolysis. When the superfluous hair grows through a mole, a dermatologist should first examine the mole for possible malignancy. If the mole is benign and the patient wishes to have it removed for aesthetic reasons, dermatologists usually do so *after* a reputable electrologist has removed the hair. If the mole were removed *before*, it would be difficult, if not impossible, for the electrologist to locate the papilla (which is usually deeper than the mole itself) because of the scar tissue.

Among the best schools in the world for electrologists is the Kree Institute of Electrolysis, Inc., in New York City, named after Paul M. Kree, a brilliant technician and inventor who in 1916 perfected the first safe electric needle for electrolysis. The institute is at present headed by Garo Artinian, who succeeded Mr. Kree and under whose direction the technique of electrolysis has been further developed.

ELECTROSURGERY

Electrosurgery is an electronic cutting technique which is being used more and more—among other specialties—in dentistry and oral surgery for the purpose of correcting speech problems and removing diseased or excessive tissue for better fitting dentures.

Instead of the usual steel scalpel or instruments, a fine wire needle or loop called an electrode utilizes the power from the high frequencies of sound waves (like those used in AM or FM radios) to "cut" through the tissue. The cutting is accomplished by a concentration of electronic energy from the active electrode, rather than by the pressure of the instrument against the tissue.

Many surgical procedures can be done more quickly and efficiently with electrosurgery because the high-frequency current can pass through the living tissue without causing shock or excessive heat (as does, for instance, electrocautery). Also, it minimizes bleeding and scarring and is self-sterilizing. "With this instrument, one can remove a fraction of a millimeter of tissue at a time, and have exact control of depth, contour, and shape," said Dr. Daniel Strong, a New York dentist. He was one of the first practitioners in this country to use electrosurgery in dentistry.

Among the procedures for which electrosurgery is used are gingivectomy and frenectomy.

Gingivectomy—An operation that trims the gingiva (gums). Many unattractive smiles are due to front teeth embedded in fleshy gums. They are normal size and perfectly healthy, requiring nothing but to be cleared of the gum overgrowth and recontoured.

Frenectomy—An operation that cuts the frenum, the small vertical membrane under the tongue connecting it to the floor of the mouth. When the frenum is too short, a person may become "tongue-tied" and be unable to bring the tongue past the edge of the lower teeth, a condition which usually results in a speech defect.

Electrosurgery is also used to remove diseased gum tissue and scar tissue caused by ill-fitting dentures, without leaving new scars. Healing is rapid and the discomfort is minimal.

EMOLLIENTS (VANISHING CREAMS)

Emollient creams are essentially variations of the basic COLD CREAM formula—a mixture of oil and WATER—modified to help the skin feel softer and smoother rather than to cleanse it.

Any of a large variety of oils can be used, as practically all oils serve the same purpose: to coat the skin's roughened, scaly surface with a smooth film that flattens the dry flakes, and to retard the evaporation of water. However, the most aesthetically convenient are oils with a high melting point, because they feel less greasy and when rubbed on the skin seem to vanish—which is preferable when used underneath makeup during the day.

At the moment, the most common name for emollients is MOISTURIZERS.

ENZYMES

Enzymes—once called ferments—are soluble, organic protein compounds produced by a living organism. They act as catalysts, that is, they are capable of accelerating or producing biochemical changes (digestion, for example) in specific substances called substrates without themselves being changed.

Enzymes are extremely elaborate compounds; biochemists still disagree on their definition and exact functions. Hundreds have been identified, and more are being discovered all the time.

Enzymes are named after their respective substrates, to which the ending *-ase* is added. For example, *lipase* (lipos = fat + -ase) is a fat-splitting enzyme occurring in the liver, stomach, etc. And *protease* is an enzyme that digests proteins.

Certain enzymes, such as those active in digestion, are called *extracellular* enzymes because they are released from the cells that produce them; but most are found *within* the cells, where they are involved in processes by which tissue is built up or broken down.

EPILATING WAX

Epilating wax is one of the methods of temporary removal of superfluous hair from the upper lip, the chin, the legs and the arms.

A wax composition is applied in molten state and allowed to solidify, causing the hair to become enmeshed in a plastic mass. Once it has solidified, the waxy film is stripped away and each hair is uprooted with it, with only an occasional follicle destroyed by repeated treatments.

Removal should be performed in the direction of the hair growth and should be firm and swift, in order to minimize discomfort. Indeed, waxing may be painful and cause some skin irritation, especially if the wax is too hot.

Waxing is the only technique of temporary depilation that is not usually done at home: the very caution a woman would instinctively apply in stripping away the adhesive wax film by herself would render waxing ineffectual. Another drawback is that, since waxing is most effective when the hair is relatively long, women often become impatient and shave the hair between waxing treatments.

On the other hand, when performed by a skillful operator in a beauty salon, waxing can be an excellent depilatory technique removing hair from below the skin surface and therefore ensuring a smooth, hair-free skin for several weeks.

EPISIOTOMY

Episiotomy is an operation in which an obstetrician makes a small incision at the time of delivery to enlarge the opening of the vagina when it is too small to allow the baby to emerge. Tissue in the birth canal may be torn during the process of birth itself, so it is preferable that the incision be neat, straight and fast-healing instead of a ragged tear.

Episiotomy is performed by cutting part of the perineal tissue (the area between the anus and the external genitals) either straight back or diagonally on one side. Successive episiotomies can be made in slightly different locations.

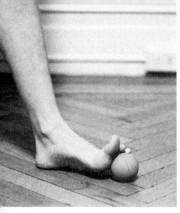 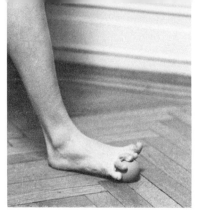

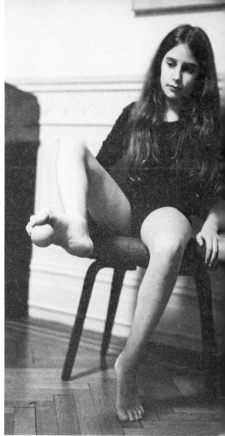

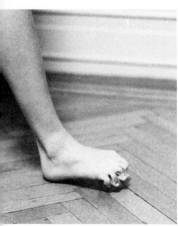 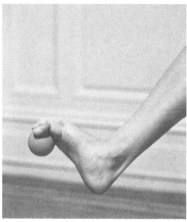

Top left and center: One of Carola Trier's youngest and most serious pupils, Anne, 12 years old, is shown here in the first position of foot exercise. The leg is straight, and a rubber ball is placed under her lifted toes.

Bottom left: Anne is instructed to widen her toes and wrap them around the ball.

Bottom center: After several tries, Anne is able to lift her leg and hold the rubber ball with her toes for a few seconds.

Right: Anne finally has mastered the exercise and nonchalantly poses with her toes securely wrapped around the ball.

What young monkeys do instinctively becomes here an excellent exercise for all humans, as well as part of a ballerina's basic training: she needs strong and prehensile feet for her future toe-dancing.

EXERCISE

It is impossible for the human organism to maintain normal functions without sufficient physical activity. Properly planned and regulated exercise helps the body to develop and maintain a good level of health and physical fitness. In particular, proper exercise can:

1) control weight, as a complement for DIETS;

2) control muscular and mental FATIGUE resulting from the stress of activities and responsibilities;

3) prevent a number of illnesses, such as disease of the heart and the circulatory system, and build resistance to both physiological and PSYCHOSOMATIC DISEASES;

128

4) be of significant importance during convalescence and for rehabilitation (*passive* exercise—which requires the supervision and help of an instructor—is used to regain muscle tone, to relax, and to provide neuromuscular reeducation. *Active* exercise, involving the use of the body's musculature against some force—such as gravity—is designed to strengthen muscles, improve endurance in weakened muscles, restore or maintain joint motion, and teach movement patterns that will reestablish control lost through injury.);

5) be of aid to pregnant women for an easier childbirth;

6) improve POSTURE, which in turn helps to develop body coordination, balance and flexibility; prevent double chin, protruding abdomen, sagging shoulders, etc.;

7) help internal organs to function more efficiently by improving circulation;

8) release nervous tension;

9) retard aging, as sedentary people tend to deteriorate physically much earlier than active people.

There are various types of exercise, and each achieves one or more results:

1) Running and jumping, as well as throwing or kicking a ball, are forms of exercise in which the body achieves *muscular power*, resulting from the combination of strength and speed of movement.

2) Isometric exercises, in which the body is held in a static position during muscular contractions, and isotonic exercises, in which the body is lifted or propelled in some direction, achieve *muscular strength*.

3) Successive movements such as handstands, pushups or walking, performed over a period of time, improve *endurance*.

4) Successive movements of the same type, at a fast rate, such as running or skating, improve *speed* and *breath coordination*.

5) Tennis, soccer, and dancing develop *agility* and *coordination*.

6) Bending, twisting, flexion and extension movements are designed for *flexibility*.

In choosing an exercise program, a person should first decide what his goals are—improvement of physical fitness, maintenance of general health, or appearance—and determine the extent of his physical capacities as limited by age, weight, and body type. The time of day for exercise should be chosen according to one's inclinations and timetable. Exercise can be performed anytime, except shortly after eating (up to one hour). Once a certain time is chosen, it is easier, psychologically speaking, to keep up with the program if the schedule is respected.

Each exercise session should begin with a period of warmup—stretching and flexing the extremities to relax the muscles, and breathing deeply

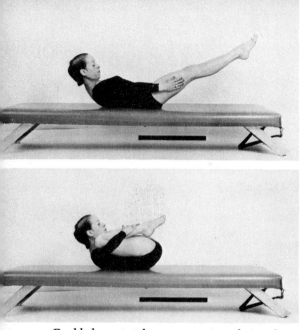

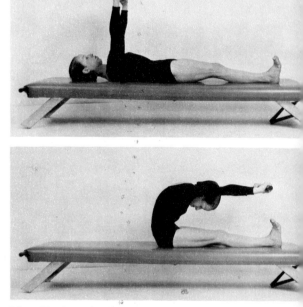

Double-leg stretch, an exercise designed to strengthen the lower back and the abdominal muscles and to relieve tension in the lower back. The double-leg stretch should always be done slowly, at the beginning of a session, and should be repeated 5 to 6 times.

Mrs. Trier performing the *roll-up*, an exercise involving the abdominal muscles, the tendons in the back of the knees, the spine, and the entire musculature of the back, from head to toe. The roll-up should be repeated 3 to 5 times.

This is the *jack-knife*. Once the legs are kicked straight up in a "jack-knife" fashion, this exercise promotes the articulation of the vertebrae by pressing them one by one against the surface of the mat, while lowering the back. The jack-knife also promotes muscle flexibility in the back and releases tension throughout the entire back musculature. It should be done slowly, 3 to 5 times.

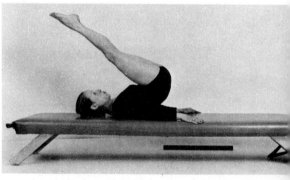

Carola Trier, photographed while performing some of the classic exercises of contrology, the physical-culture system developed by the late Joseph H. Pilates, the famous gymnast. The purpose of contrology is to employ every muscle and tendon in the body, not by strenuous athletics, but by stretching, tensing, flexing, and bending the body, as well as breathing properly throughout the exercises. Its goal is to develop a high level of strength and beauty under control of the mind.

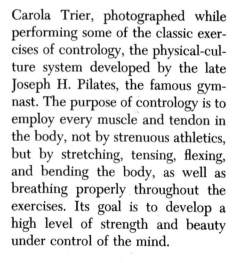

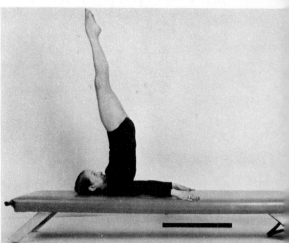

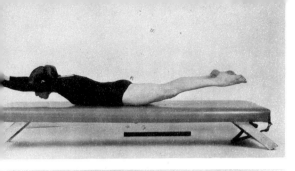

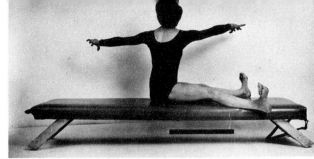

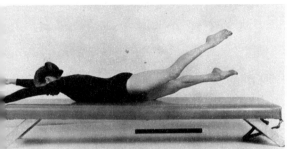

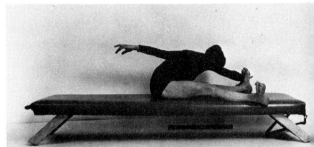

Dry swimming, an exercise that promotes coordination of muscles and movements from fingertips to toes. It also enhances the spine's flexibility and the tensile strength of the back muscles. A dry-swimming session includes 10 movements, alternating arms and legs. It should always be performed at a moderate rhythm.

The diagonal motions of the *saw* are useful in reducing the waistline and lengthening the torso, while at the same time stretching the entire back. It should be done slowly, 5 times each session.

The *rolling-back* exercise promotes the flexibility and articulation of the back. Once mastered it is the equivalent of a relaxing massage. It should be repeated about 5 times.

Control stretch represents the culmination of mental and physical control and coordination. As performed by Mrs. Trier, it is as beautiful and seemingly effortless as a ballet figure.

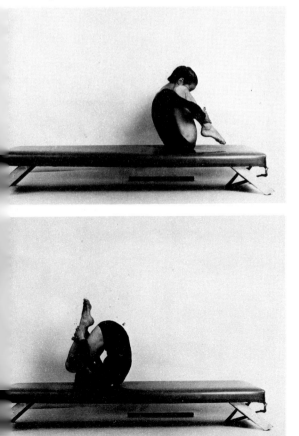

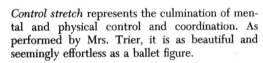

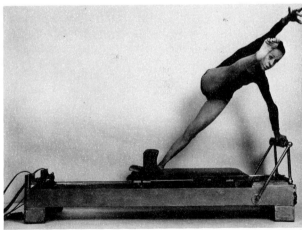

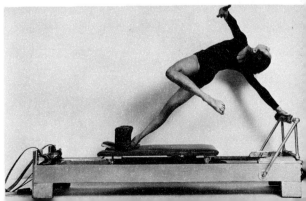

and rhythmically to increase the circulation and supply the blood with fresh oxygen. The exercise itself should always be performed in a progressive fashion: from simple to more complex. Only after successfully and painlessly accomplishing the simple exercises can one progress to the more difficult ones. Exercise programs should be determined by a trained instructor who can evaluate individual needs and rhythms.

Exercise should be performed at regular intervals—at least three or four times a week. Sporadic and too energetic exercises are more detrimental than no exercise at all. Also, it is best to exercise often and lightly—better four times a week for half an hour than once a week for two hours consecutively. Sometimes exercises are more efficient and more pleasant if performed to music, either as a background or as a rhythm.

When first exercising without instruction, most people are rather unfamiliar with their own bodies, and their attempts to breathe correctly and to consciously direct unfamiliar movements of their muscles may be awkward. However, a skillful instructor can in a short time lead an individual to gain awareness of his body and, eventually, total mental control over it.

"The basis for proper exercise," Carola Trier, a well-known New York instructor, never tires of explaining to her pupils, "is to educate the body to return to instinctual movements of balance and harmony, such as we see in babies and animals. Many of us have forgotten these movements through social misconceptions of posture, plain bad habits, 'comfortable' ways of doing things, and avoidance of daily movements that are no longer necessary in an industrial society."

EXFOLIATION

Exfoliation refers to an extremely mild form of skin peeling, more like a deep cleaning than an actual chemical peel.

Exfoliation products can be lotions, gels or creams, which are applied to the skin, allowed to dry, and then massaged off. Their action plus the friction of the massage removes a superficial layer of dead cells, giving the skin a clean, shiny, more transparent look.

Exfoliation should be followed by moisturizing. It can be safely done at home *only* with a product that has the mildest kind of peeling effect. Any deep peeling should be done by a dermatologist or a cosmetic surgeon.

F

FACE MASQUES (FACIALS)

Face masque or facial refers to a popular beauty treatment in which a variety of preparations, generally containing water, alcohol, aromatics, a CLEANSER and a base (which determines the type of masque), can be applied to the face and neck and shortly after washed or peeled off for the purpose of cleaning, soothing and refreshing the skin.

Because of the alcohol, and because of the water's rapid evaporation, most face masques have an instant cooling effect followed by a sensation of warmth and of tightening of the skin. And when the masque is removed, the skin not only is clean and refreshed but has a rosy and almost transparent tone.

There are four basic kinds of masques:

Clay masque—The base is mineral clay; it hardens on the skin and has the ability to absorb oil and dirt. Recommended for oily skin.

Moisturizing masque—The base may be some jellylike moisturizer sometimes mixed with protein; besides a cleansing, it adds moisture. Recommended for very dry, slightly dry, and normal skin.

Peel-off masque—The base is either a rubber, or wax. It is applied as a lotion or a cream, and when dry it is peeled off in one sheet. Recommended for slightly oily and normal skins.

Massaging masque—The base is some kind of plastic applied as a lotion or cream; when it has dried it is removed in small pieces by rubbing. It is excellent for removing dirt and a superficial stratum of dead cells. Recommended for oily and normal skins.

Masques, however, are neither a *true* skin treatment nor necessary for routine skin care—in fact, some facials are less effective in removing dirt and dead cells from the skin's surface than regular cleansers and THINNERS. Also, some may irritate very delicate skin if done more than once a week. And incidentally, a white of egg applied to the face at home with a pastry brush, allowed to dry and then washed off with lukewarm

133

water, is probably just as effective and soothing as most fancy preparations offered at beauty salons.

The only tangible advantage of a facial is that it makes pores look smaller and erases—albeit temporarily—some of the wrinkles and fine lines from a mature face. This is a result of the slightly irritating action of the aromatic ingredients and the tightening effect caused by the hardening of the base while the water evaporates. When the masque is washed or peeled off, the tiny blood vessels in the skin's inner layer swell a little and leak some fluid into the surrounding tissue, making the skin look plump and rosy for a few hours.

What makes facials popular, then, with both women and men is not the assurance of some permanent improvement of their skin but the pleasant, relaxed, pampering atmosphere of a beauty salon which a facial epitomizes.

FALLOPIAN TUBES

The Fallopian tubes, also called oviducts, are the two long, slender passages extending from the upper lateral angles of the uterus to the region of the ovaries on each side, through which the ova pass from the ovaries to the uterus upon their maturation.

FALSE EYELASHES

Until artifice becomes more acceptable, false eyelashes will never be really popular, cosmetic industry experts feel, and may disappear altogether—except from the stage, where they are needed to correct in part the flattening effect stage lights have on the actors' features.

Yet false eyelashes—both strip lashes and their more recent version, individual lashes—are still manufactured and sold, though at least one reasonably priced brand of disposable lashes-by-the-yard has been discontinued.

Of all makeup techniques, the application of false eyelashes is probably the most difficult to learn. Periodically, fashion magazines publish instructions on how to apply lashes properly. One of the clearest sets of instructions is the following, which appeared in the *Vogue Beauty & Health Guide*, 1973–74.

How to Wear Strip Lashes:
Flex the lashes around a finger so that they will follow the curve of the eye when applied. Look down into the mirror without closing eyes, but open the mouth a little so that the face muscles are pulled down. To look natural, lashes should start one-quarter

of an inch from the inside corner of the eye, since lashes don't normally grow in that corner.

The Lash-by-Lash Routine:
Individual lashes are attached not to the skin but to your own lashes. The effect is to double the thickness of natural lashes, not their number. Apply them when you have at least a half hour to spare. The adhesive must dry completely before makeup is added. First select the lashes you will use—short ones for the inside of the eye, toward the nose; long ones for the center; medium at outer edge. Make sure your own lashes are completely clean and dry, otherwise the adhesive will not take hold. (A plastic glue is difficult to remove and can damage real lashes; a nonplastic product, such as surgical adhesive, will not last so long but can be removed without harm.) With chin up, stand looking down your nose into the mirror so that the eyes are open but the lids lowered. Starting from the inside of the eye, pick up each lash with tweezers, dip base in adhesive, and, using the base as a brush, stroke adhesive all the way down your own lash. Then press the false lash base to the natural lash base. Use non-oily eye makeup and non-oily makeup remover. Your new lashes will last about a week; however, if you want to remove them before then, a pad soaked in oily makeup remover and stroked down the lashes will usually do the trick. Do not use individual lashes on lower lids—the natural lashes there are too fragile. Substitute strip lashes cut into small pieces. Mascara is not necessary or advisable —it can't be cleaned off without the lashes coming off too.

FATIGUE
The temporary drain of energy caused by too much work, not enough sleep, skipped meals, jet lag, or simply the cyclic decline of HORMONE levels in the body at certain times of day is *normal* fatigue. It will disappear after a few hours of relaxation or sleep. However, when the exhaustion persists or occurs after a small expenditure of energy, for instance, or at a time when a person should feel rested, fatigue may be either *organic* or *psychological.*

Organic fatigue can result from infections, malignancies, and vascular, metabolic, or endocrine diseases. Also, it may be caused by the combined action of such drugs as amphetamines, tranquilizers or sleeping pills with ALCOHOL. Amphetamines alone can actually cause fatigue: when the stimulant's quick pick-up wears off, it may leave in its wake an even deeper tiredness.

Psychological fatigue is more complex and elusive, because it often arises out of conflicts and frustrations people are not always aware of. Also, the distinction between normal, organic, and psychological fatigue is blurred. Consider, for instance, the tiredness that accompanies the nervousness and emotional instability of MENOPAUSE; or the tenseness, anxiety and emotional instability of a person suffering from hypoglycemia, the abnormal decrease of sugar in the blood; or the additional energy required to adapt to different time zones, customs, languages, lodgings.

"It is difficult to see how such different things as cold, heat, drugs, hormones, sorrow and joy could provoke an identical biochemical reaction in the body," recently wrote Dr. Hans Selye, director of the Institute of Experimental Medicine and Surgery at the University of Montreal. "Stressful boredom" is often the only cause of chronic fatigue. "Just as our muscles become flabby and degenerate if not used," Dr. Selye continued, "our brain slips into chaos, unless we constantly use it for some work that seems worthwhile to us."

Usually, internists or general practitioners are the first ones to be consulted by people suffering from chronic fatigue. The doctor will begin by giving the patient a check-up that includes urinalysis, a blood count, an X-ray of the chest, and a record of eating habits, sleep patterns, alcoholic intake and previous illnesses and surgery. Should organic causes of fatigue be ruled out, the doctor can be sure that the patient is suffering from a fatigue closely associated with depression. If this is the case, the choice of cure will depend in part on the physician's temperament and his scientific bent. He may recommend psychotherapy or PSYCHOACTIVE DRUGS. Sometimes, as Rosemary Blackmon, a *Vogue* magazine editor, once wrote, "a single question from a doctor you know—it may be as simple as, 'Are you having any *fun?*'—may bring you around. First of all, you're *not* having any fun—that may come as a surprise when you're made to think about it. Secondly, you don't know why."

Indeed, there is no place for fatigue when duty is pleasure, and when work—any work—coincides with play.

FATS

Fat is the generic name for certain animal and vegetable products that are solid at room temperature. It also refers to adipose tissue, which forms soft pads between various organs of the human body, serves to smooth and round out the body's contours, and furnishes a reserve supply of energy.

Fat molecules consist of a tryglyceride, which consists of a triple molecule of glycerol (an organic alcohol) linked to three molecules of various fatty acids (organic compounds of carbon, hydrogen and oxygen).

There are two kinds of fat: *saturated* and *unsaturated*. Saturated fats are those whose fatty acid molecules—stearic acid, for instance—contain the maximum possible number of hydrogen atoms. A fat is unsaturated when the atoms of carbon in the fatty acid molecule—such as the oleic or the linoleic acid—are linked by a chemical *double bond*, which, if broken, would allow the uptake of additional hydrogen atoms.

Unsaturated fats are *mono-unsaturated* when there is only one double bond, *poly-unsaturated* when there are several double bonds. Saturated fats, such as meat and dairy fats, tend to be solid at room temperature; unsaturated fats, most of which are vegetable fats, tend to be liquid. Incidentally, fats are chemically similar to oils, from which they are distinguished roughly by their consistency at room temperature.

Fats in the diet serve as vehicles for the intake of fat-soluble VITAMINS (A, D, E and K). They are broken down in the small intestine with the help of ENZYMES, and their components—fatty acids and glycerol—are transferred through the intestinal walls into the lymph and the bloodstream, which carry them to storage areas such as the liver, to be used as a source of energy for the body's complex functions.

Fat production in the body itself is called fat synthesis. Activated by an enzyme called glycerokinase, the stored glycerol turns into a compound called glycerophosphate, which reacts with the fatty acids in the adipose tissue to form new fat molecules.

FOLLICLES

Follicles are of various kinds. Among the most important are:
1) small cavities found on the skin or within the body, such as hair follicles;
2) small, round, hollow structures within the ovaries, also called Graafian follicles, each of which contains an unripe OVUM, or EGG CELL. Once a month, at the onset of MENSTRUATION, one follicle in either the left or the right ovary (alternating each month) ruptures and its egg cell is released into the uterus.

FOOD ADDITIVES

Food additives are substances, or a mixture of substances, other than basic foodstuff which are present in food as a result of any of the various stages of its production, processing, storage or packaging. Additives may be nutritious or nonnutritious, physiologically active or inert. They may be present in the food *intentionally*—to achieve some modification in the food—or *incidentally*, such as residues of pesticides or of chemicals used to treat animal diseases; or packaging material that "migrates" into the food.

Some additives are used to improve the nutritional value of certain foods; others are used to make the food tastier, to make it look more appetizing, to prevent spoilage, etc.

As of 1974, the food industry in the United States manufactures at least thirty-two thousand different kinds of food items and about three thousand different additives. Following are some of the most common types of food additives.

Acidulants—These are fruit acids added to give a tart taste to soft drinks and jams, and to improve the texture and tartness of processed cheese.

Anticaking agents—Keep table salt and powdered sugar free-flowing.

Antimyotics—Prevent spoilage action of such microorganisms as MOLD, bacteria and yeast in bread, cheese and citrus fruits.

Antioxidants—Prevent rancidity in vegetable oils and FATS, potato chips, candies. Also prevent change in color or flavor caused by oxygen in the air. Apricots, bananas, and pears darken when exposed to the air after being cut or bruised. Two of these antioxidants—butylated hydroxytoluene (BHT) and butylated hydroxyanisole (BHA)—have become controversial since large quantities of them were found to produce changes in the brain chemistry of pregnant mice and abnormal behavior in their offspring.

Bleaching agents—Speed natural bleaching and "maturing" of flour in order to prepare it more quickly for baking. Also used to bleach cheeses such as gorgonzola and blue cheese. Although bleached flour does not have the nutrients of whole grains, so far no harmful effects caused by bleaching agents have been confirmed.

Buffers—Neutralize some natural acids, as in canned tomato soup.

Coloring Agents—A few coloring agents are natural, such as carotene, which is found in carrots and is a source of VITAMIN A. But most are synthetic and are sometimes called coal-tar dyes. They are used in soft drinks, candy, frozen desserts, oranges, pumpernickel bread. There are hundreds of synthetic colors, many of which are controversial. One is Red No. 2, used extensively in soft drinks and gelatins, and to give maraschino cherries their traditional bright red color. In 1972 the use of Red No. 2 was curtailed 50 percent by the FDA, but the decision was reversed in 1974, when the dye was declared completely safe.

Curing agents—Originally used to preserve meats and prevent BOTULISM. Salt and saltpeter (potassium nitrate) were the traditional curing agents, and salt is still used to cure ham and bacon. But for the last fifty years, sodium nitrate has been considered more effective than saltpeter. Modern curing agents are also meant to modify flavor and stabilize or add color. However, sodium nitrates and nitrites, which give the pink color to frankfurters, bologna, corned beef, and smoked salmon, are now controversial because they are considered indirectly carcinogenic.

Defoaming agents—Prevent foaming during processing of such products as bottled orange juice.

Emulsifiers—Prevent separation of oil from vinegar in salad dressings. Also preserve the homogeneity of chocolate candies, as cocoa butter and chocolate tend to separate when exposed to temperature changes.

Firming agents—Prevent canned fruits and vegetables from becoming soft.

Flavor enhancers—These may be spices and natural oils such as ginger, cloves and citrus oils; aromatic chemicals that give ready-to-eat foods the flavor of, for example, cherries or grapes; or chemicals such as monosodium glutamate which enhance the natural flavor of food. Some of these flavoring agents are controversial.

Foaming agents—Used in pressure-packed whipped cream, for example, to preserve its whipped look.

Growth stimulants—These include ANTIBIOTICS, HORMONES and other medications used in cattle and poultry feed to stimulate growth and prevent disease. One of the most controversial is a female hormone called diethylstilbestrol (DES); it has been shown to induce cancer in laboratory animals, and recently large residues of it have been found in meats, milk and eggs.

Humectants—Keep moisture in such items as marshmallows or shredded coconut.

Leavening agents—Make food such as cakes, waffles and muffins light in texture by releasing carbon dioxide through fermentation. Yeast, which used to be the only product available, is still a favorite leavening agent.

Nutrients—Improve the nutritional quality of certain foods: VITAMIN C added to fruit drinks; VITAMIN D to milk; VITAMIN A to margarine; and potassium iodide to salt to supply iodine.

Preservatives—See *Antioxidants* and *Curing agents.*

Sequestrants—Remove particles of substances such as minerals by combining with them and setting them aside, so as to keep color and clarity in water, mayonnaise, canned beans, salad dressing, etc.

Stabilizers—Help keep flavor and a smooth texture in instant chocolate milk, for instance, or in commercial ice cream, to increase viscosity and prevent the water in the product from freezing into crystals.

139

Thickeners—Used to increase the consistency of jams and jellies, and also to compensate for the low-quality ingredients and the inadequate production methods that are sometimes used in the manufacture of ice cream, yogurt and certain cheeses.

Sweeteners—These are synthetic, nonnutritive agents such as saccharine and cyclamates, commonly used in soft drinks. Cyclamates were banned in 1969 as carcinogenic; however, as of 1974 they are being rehabilitated and may soon be back in low-calorie drinks. Saccharine, which has been used for eighty years without evidence of harm to humans, has recently been demoted from the FDA's Generally Recognized As Safe (GRAS) list because of the reported finding of bladder tumors in rats that were fed large quantities of saccharine. This sweetener is undergoing further scientific review but in the meantime is being allowed to remain on the market.

Food additives are indeed a controversial matter. Critics believe, for example, that nitrite is the most toxic chemical in the nation's food supply. They point out that, under certain conditions, nitrate can be converted to nitrite in the stomach; this nitrite can react with some amines (found in beer, processed meat, and drugs such as antihistamines) to form nitrosamines, which in turn may be carcinogenic. The FDA counters by pointing out that without nitrites we would have botulism, a deadly food poisoning.

Monosodium glutamate, a common food additive, has for years been almost universally considered harmless, if not actually beneficial. Yet some people have odd reactions when they eat it—the so-called Chinese restaurant syndrome (CRS), which consists of a burning sensation in the neck and forearms, chest tightness, and headache, all of which subside in about two hours.

Food colorings—of which four million pounds a year are produced—are probably the most superfluous of all additives. And, incidentally, the label "certified color" does not mean that the dye has been tested for safety, but merely that the FDA has checked each batch for impurities. A classic example of the uselessness of color additives is a 1972 experiment in which a supermarket put on its shelves maraschino cherries that had not been dyed with the famous Red No. 2, but were their natural golden yellow color. Customers seemed to have no qualms at all about buying the cherries.

The reason why food additives are so controversial is that their possible toxic and carcinogenic effects are not clear-cut: toxicology and cancer research are still uncertain sciences. There is the possibility of the additives' cumulative effect being stored unchanged in the organism, as well as the possibility of chemical interaction, i.e., the additive may be harmless in itself but may become poisonous if ingested simultaneously with another additive in another food. However, *poison* is a relative term—an overdose of vitamin A may be fatal, while acetic acid, a potent toxin in high concentration, is nothing but vinegar when diluted to a 5 percent acidity! CARCINOGENS, on the other hand, follow a different set of rules: no matter how minute the dose or how rarely eaten, most experts feel, carcinogens may cause cancer in susceptible people. Some researchers, however, disagree; they feel that there *is* such a thing as a safe dose of a carcinogen.

With so many questions unsettled and so much scientific confusion, there really is not much that people can do for the moment, except become critical readers of labels and learn to evaulate the incomplete information they offer, and keep asking for more informative labeling.

FOOD ALLERGY

Many people who suffer from all sorts of chronic and seemingly PSYCHOSOMATIC disturbances are in reality allergic to certain foods.

While allergists are on reasonably safe scientific ground with such allergies as ASTHMA, HAY FEVER and certain drug allergies, they have much less understanding of the mechanisms of food hypersensitivity. One of the main reasons is that the symptoms of bronchial asthma, for instance, are predictable and clearly distinguishable from those of any other respiratory disease. Also, the antigens responsible for asthma—DANDER, dust, pollen—can usually be identified in skin tests. But with food allergies, symptoms and skin tests both are often ambiguous, if not misleading. For one, some potentially allergenic substances may be lost during the preparation of food extract used for skin tests, so that some patients may have definite allergic reactions to certain foods and yet show a *negative* reaction in a skin test. Conversely, some people show a *positive* skin test with foods to which they have no hypersensitivity.

One of the major problems in correlating allergy symptoms with the foods that cause them is the time interval between the ingestion of the food and the appearance of the allergic reaction. Symptoms of food sensitivity—rashes, wheezing, diarrhea, nausea—may appear within minutes, hours, or even days after exposure to the foods in question. With few exceptions, people do not keep a record of *what* and *when* they ate that would allow them to trace the source of a presumably food-related allergic reaction. Some doctors even believe that, in some instances, symptoms of food allergy may not appear until a person has temporarily stopped eating a particular food.

Another problem in determining the cause of a food allergy is the fact that the actual chemical substance responsible for the allergic reaction may be, not the food itself, but a substance that is produced when

ENZYMES break down food during digestion. Also, since most foods are themselves complex chemical compounds, some people may react to only one component, while others may be sensitive to different components of the same food. And finally, there are people who are sensitive to FOOD ADDITIVES or to the insecticides with which fruits and vegetables are often sprayed.

"Faced with such dilemmas," recently wrote Dr. Heinz J. Wittig, professor of allergy and clinical immunology at the University of Florida College of Medicine, "many allergists have shied away from giving much credence to reports . . . of numerous patients' suffering from food hypersensitivities. Instead they tend to adhere to the few unequivocal cases where the causality is obvious (e.g., the appearance of . . . urticaria, within minutes after certain foods are ingested)." Meanwhile, however, Dr. Wittig noted, patients continue to suffer from "more subtle" types of allergy.

The most reliable method of diagnosing food hypersensitivity is still the so-called *elimination diet,* in which all suspected foods are eliminated from the patient's diet for at least one week, and then, one by one, reintroduced in large quantities. Once certain foods have been identified as being responsible for the same symptoms on at least two separate occasions, a permanent diet excluding those foods can be formulated.

Dr. Theron G. Randolph, a food allergy specialist at the Lutheran General Hospital in Park Ridge, Illinois, who belongs to a group of physicians calling themselves clinical ecologists, has developed his own elimination diet. As a clinical ecologist, Dr. Randolph is concerned primarily with today's environment—an elusive jungle of fumes, smells, and manmade chemicals which we breathe, touch, dress in, sleep on, wash and deodorize with *as well as eat and drink.* The relationship between man and his environment—including his diet—is what he calls human ecology. We constantly adapt to the environment, Dr. Randolph observes. Most people adapt well, but some, and apparently their number is growing, either cannot adapt or, having adapted to a point, suddenly break down. In the case of maladaptation to food, the human body becomes "addicted" to the very foods it is allergic to. At first a person is just fond of these foods; later he feels a need for them and experiences a boost each time he eats them; finally he suffers "withdrawal" symptoms when he cannot have them.

Dr. Randolph conducts his tests in a special unit at the Henrotin Hospital in Chicago. The patient is isolated for about two weeks in an environment as controlled as possible, with no gas burners, synthetic materials, disinfectants, cosmetics, perfumes, drugs, or flowers, and with air filters and chlorine-free water in each room. During this time the patient fasts, swallowing nothing but spring water for four or five days, the time needed for all foods to be eliminated from his body. Withdrawal symptoms usually set in after about twenty-four hours: the patient feels depressed, his sense of smell becomes enormously acute, he suffers from INSOMNIA, excessive PERSPIRATION, abnormal pulse. By the third day the symptoms are usually gone, and the patient feels well and often is not even hungry. After five days he is presented with large portions of one food per meal, and his reactions to each type of food are observed. If he encounters a food to which he is allergic, he immediately feels violently sick, for the symptoms are heightened by the body's sudden reexposure to large doses of allergens, which act almost like "overdoses" for the "addict" whose adaptation process had been interrupted by the fasting.

Simple food allergies don't respond to desensitization—the technique used successfully for inhalant allergy—which consists of injections of small quantities of the allergens. However, for many patients who suffer multiple allergies (including food allergy), desensitization, in the words of Dr. Wittig, "will, by decreasing the total allergic load, enhance the benefits to be gained from dietary elimination."

Another experimental technique, called the *provocative-neutralizing method,* whose validity is presently being investigated, has been used for many years, mostly by ENT specialists, to deal with cases of multiple food allergies. The method consists of inducing allergic symptoms by giving a patient an intracutaneous injection of a so-called *provoking* dose of the food extract that has proven to be allergenic and then relieving the symptoms by successive injections of the same food extract, variously diluted, until the proper *neutralizing* dose is found. Once the specific neutralizing dose of each allergenic food for that particular patient is established, all neutralizing doses are mixed together into a single solution and injected twice a week, so that (it is claimed) the patient can eat most or all of the foods he is allergic to, apparently without any allergic symptoms.

Mild allergic reactions to various foods can be treated with *antihistamines, sedatives* or *corticosteroids,* depending on the patient's condition. Severe food allergy symptoms (which, as previously mentioned, could reach the proportions of ANAPHYLAXIS, involving the skin, the respiratory tract, the cardiovascular system, or several systems at once) require immediate injections of epinephrine combined with antihistamines and corticosteroids, again depending on the severity of the reaction.

Since food allergies are often subject to change with time, patients should be examined every year in order to determine whether they are still sensitive to certain foods. Incidentally, frequent and excessive intake of previously innocuous foods may provoke new food sensitivity. Therefore, diets should always be moderate and varied, with a regular, but not too frequent, rotation of food.

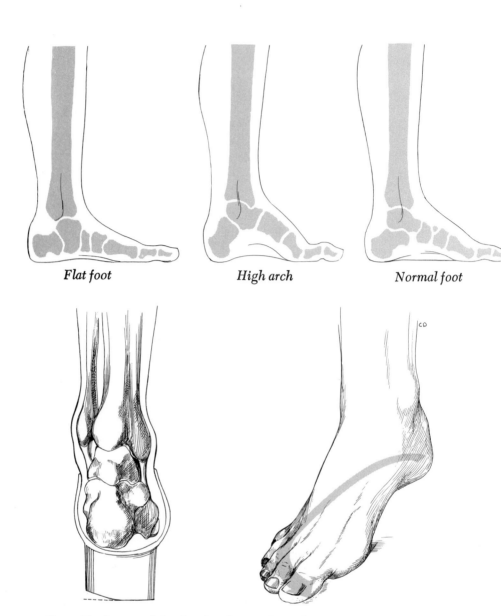

Flat foot　　　*High arch*　　　*Normal foot*

Above: The bottom of the foot has three arches, whose curvature varies considerably from person to person. Two of these arches, called longitudinal, run along the foot; one on the inner side, one on the outer side. The third arch, called transversal, runs across the ball of the foot.

The arches provide the foot, respectively, with the flexibility needed for walking and a proper balance of the body weight.

If the longitudinal arches are lower than normal, the foot is flat. If these have an exaggerated curvature, the condition is called clawfoot.

Below left: A normal foot wears only the outer edge of the shoe heel because of the way the body weight is distributed while walking.

Below right: The heel, which is the first part of the foot to touch the ground, transmits the body weight from the legs to the ground and provides a lever for the calf muscles to act on the foot. As the heel leaves the ground, the weight is shifted forward along the outer side of the foot to the small toes and finally to the big toe, which presses down and pushes the foot off the ground in preparation for the following step.

FOOT COMFORT

No part of the human body seems to work so hard and to be so neglected as the foot. Although feet are in almost constant use, many people tend to take them for granted and pay them little attention until they become a source of discomfort.

The human foot functions essentially in two ways: as a *pedestal* (to stand on) and as a *lever* (to propel the body forward). It is composed of many bones with movable joints between them, which give it the suppleness necessary to act as an efficient pedestal.

In order to act as a lever without collapsing, a structure composed of so many separate segments as the foot has to be shaped as an arch. Indeed, the bones in the foot are placed so that they catch and bear the entire weight of the body on two arches for each foot: one *along* the foot, called the long arch, and one *across* the foot, between the ball and the toes. When it is being used as a lever to propel the body forward, the long arch becomes accentuated, and the foot is held rigidly in this position by the action of the muscles so that it cannot collapse under the body's weight.

These two functions demand somewhat opposite requirements: the first, a flat and supple foot; the second, a rigid, arched one. In order that the same foot may carry out both functions adequately, it must be supple and well controlled by good muscles; its exact shape is of secondary importance.

The toes contribute to both functions of the foot by taking their share of the body's weight and, when only one foot is on the ground during each pace in walking or running, by varying the amount of pressure exerted by the outer and inner toe alternately, thus helping to maintain balance.

Discomfort and many minor foot problems, such as ingrown nails, calluses, blisters, and muscle cramps, are caused by ill-fitting shoes. Shoes that are too tight, too short, or too wide in the heels can easily be recognized and thus easily avoided; however, even shoes that are of good quality and seem to be the correct size may be ill-fitting, for the simple reason that many shoes have little relation to the shape and function of feet. Most shoes are manufactured in pairs, on standard blocks (called lasts) with identical right and left feet, whereas a person's right foot may differ markedly from his left foot in shape, size, and width.

More important, even, is the question of heels. Almost nobody distributes his weight *evenly* on his feet: depending on body type, some people use the heel more; others, the ball of the foot. Some use the left more, some the right. Increasing the height of the heel tends to throw the weight forward on the ball of the foot, but it also relieves strain on the long arch. Conversely, a low heel reduces the weight on the forward part of the foot but increases the strain on the arch. Thus, it cannot be said

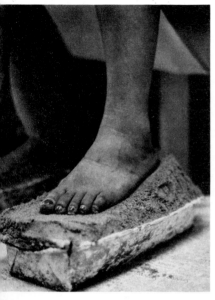 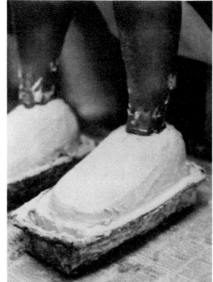 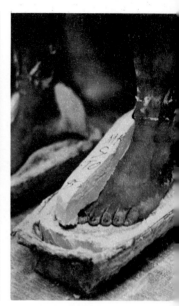

Above left: A client of T. O. Dey in New York City, ready to have a plaster cast impression taken of her feet—the first stage of the manufacture of custom-made shoes. The woman is sitting comfortably with her feet resting on a platform of moist sand, on which the exact contour of her soles will be impressed.

Above center: Plaster of Paris is then poured all around and over each foot and allowed to harden.

Above right: Before it is entirely dry, the plaster mold is cut lengthwise in order to free the foot. Subsequently, the parts are reassembled. This is the negative cast.

Below left: Positive casts are made from the negative ones, by filling the latter with liquid plaster. After this has set, the negative casts are removed, leaving behind the exact model of each foot.

Below right: the positive casts thus record the characteristics of each foot: its roundness, depth, length, width, ankle and leg alignment, balance. Any foot peculiarity— even deformity—can be camouflaged by T. O. Dey's skillful patterns. Unlike ordinary molded shoes, these custom-made shoes keep the "secrets" inside, allowing the outside appearance to follow the current fashion.

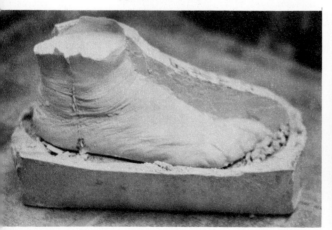 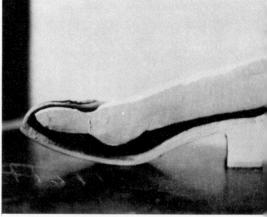

146

that either high heels or low heels are bad for the foot: heels should be of a height best suited to a person's specific weight distribution. For example, some women with very pronounced arches literally cannot walk with low-heel shoes without feeling pain. Others whose weight is already carried mostly by the ball of their feet look (and feel) off-balance once they wear shoes with heels that are too high for them.

In practice, however, many women (and men, too) wear shoes according more to fashion or personal taste than to their specific needs, and almost stoically prepare themselves for foot discomfort. At the other extreme are the foot-molded shoes, which are custom-made over a plaster-of-Paris cast of a person's feet. The end product takes on the shape of the foot both inside and outside, thus allowing the body weight to be transferred over the entire sole of the foot instead of concentrated at certain pressure points. The problem with foot-molded shoes is aesthetic: invariably they are extraordinarily unattractive.

At least one manufacturer of custom shoes—T. O. Dey of New York City—has found a solution for people who cannot wear ready-made shoes because their feet either are misshapen by such ailments as BUNIONS or ARTHRITIS, have too-pronounced or collapsed arches, or are too delicate or of markedly different size. This manufacturer builds shoes on a plaster replica of each foot, but manages to conceal all corrections *within* the shoe. Dey-Mould® shoes have a sculptured base that exactly matches the bottom of each foot, giving contact and support where needed. But on the outside the shoes are smooth, retaining a person's preferred style. In fact, customers can have favorite shoes, sandals, and boots reshaped inside or even entirely reconstructed in different, more suitable shapes. A top mold is made when additional depth is required to protect defects on the top of the foot; and special paddings can be added inside the top of a boot to conceal a polio defect, for instance.

T. O. Dey keeps customers' initial casts as a permanent record (which allows reorders to be placed by mail) together with a comfortable old pair of shoes as a guide.

FRAGRANCES

The following perfume oils may be used as they are, in small quantities, or diluted with a special diluent to make one's own favorite PERFUME or toilet water. Both the oils and the diluent are available at fancy drugstores such as Caswell-Massey in New York.

For toilet water, use twenty parts of diluent to one part of oil.

For perfume, use four parts of diluent to one part of oil.

FRAGRANCES

Almond, bitter
Amber
Anise
Basil
Bayberry
Bay leaf
Bergamot
Camellia
Caraway
Carnation
Cedarleaf
Cedarwood
Celery seed
Chypre
Cinnamon
Clove
Coriander
Cyclamen
Dill
Eucalyptus
Fennel seed
Fern
Frangipani
Frankincense

Freesia
Gardenia
Heliotrope
Honeysuckle
Hyacinth
Iris
Jasmine
Juniper
Lavender
Lemon
Lilac
Lily of the valley
Lime
Lotus
Magnolia
Mignonette
Mimosa
Narcissus
Nutmeg
Oak moss
Oleander
Orange
Orange blossom
Parsley

Patchouli
Peppermint
Pine balsam
Potpourri
Rose
Rose geranium
Rosemary
Russian leather
Sage
Sandalwood
Spearmint
Strawberry
Styrax
Sweet pea
Tangerine
Thyme
Tuberose
Verbena
Vetiver bourbon
Violet
White rose
Wintergreen
Wisteria
Ylang-ylang

G

GINSENG TEA

Ginseng is the common Asiatic name for the plants of the genus *Panax* of the Araliaceae family, which are found in Korea, China, Japan and part of Russia. Ginseng tea has a reputation as a general tonic, a "cure-all," and an aphrodisiac, partly based on the fact that its roots occasionally resemble human figures.

Ginseng is available now at most Chinese food stores and some "organic" food shops. Instant and "freeze-dried" preparations are also available there, all at quite high prices. Ginseng roots that closely resemble a human form have been sold for as much as $1000. Some "head shops" also sell ginseng—allegedly an aphrodisiac.

The major constituents of the plant are a mixture of chemicals called saponins and a variety of amino acids, CARBOHYDRATES and VITAMINS. Ginseng has the ability to help maintain an individual's HOMEOSTASIS under stress, to act as a muscle-stimulator, and to promote cellular growth after an operation and during healing. It also has several cardiovascular effects.

GIRDLES

Girdles are close-fitting undergarments, sometimes boned, sometimes partly or fully elasticized, extending from the waist, or just above, to just below the hips. They are meant to control the figure and, with garters or ribbons of gripping fabric attached, to support stockings.

A modern version of the girdle is the panty, designed in various lengths for the purpose of slimming heavy thighs. Once an indispensable part of women's clothes, girdles are still relatively popular, although in the last several years, according to a Warner Lingerie booklet, "the use . . . of PANTYHOSE took its toll by luring customers away from the slimwear department."

Like BRASSIERES, girdles are manufactured in a variety of sizes and styles, not all of which are appropriate for every woman. To facilitate the choice of the right girdle for her kind of body, a woman should first establish her own hip ratio, that is, the relationship between her hips and her waist. In practice, the hip ratio is the difference between hip and waist measurements. For instance:

A *straight-hip* figure—27″ waist, 35″ hips = 8 hip ratio;
An *average* figure—27″ waist, 37″ hips = 10 hip ratio;
A *full-hip* figure—27″ waist, 40″ hips = 13 hip ratio.

Some women may think that the tighter the girdle the better it will control the figure. In reality, if the girdle is too tight, the skin will bulge at the waistline or at the thighs.

The length of the girdle is also important. A girdle that is too long will interfere with normal walking; one that is too short will ride up and cut into the upper thighs, which is not only unattractive and uncomfortable but also unhealthy, especially for women who are prone to VARICOSE VEINS, as the girdle exerts pressure on the superficial veins of the legs.

A combination of brassiere and girdle is called a corselette, a body suit, or an all-in-one. The measurements for a corselette are usually the same as those of the bra, as the fabric used for it is generally stretchable enough to fit most figures. The corselette's shoulder straps are often detachable, so that the regular bra can be converted into a halter when the style of a particular dress requires naked shoulders.

The heat-molding techniques used for preshaped brassieres can also be applied to girdles, and in 1974 the first molded girdles were introduced on the market. The fabrics used are polyester and spandex.

GLUCOSE

Glucose (also called dextrose) is a sugar, found in animal and plant tissue, which provides the human body with fuel for energy. When food is digested, the CARBOHYDRATES (such as simple sugar and starch) in it are converted to glucose, which is the only form in which carbohydrates can be utilized by the body. Glucose is then carried throughout the body by the bloodstream. From the blood, with the help of insulin and other HORMONES, glucose enters the cells of the muscles, adipose tissue, and liver. When these cells have ingested sufficient glucose, most of the excess is stored in the liver as glycogen, in amounts so small that the stores are depleted within twenty-four hours—faster in cold weather or when a person is exercising. This storage system ensures the normal functioning of the body, for the liver releases just enough glucose to meet the requirements of the cells. In case new fat tissue is needed, for instance, glucose is broken down to produce glycerol, which reacts with fatty acids to form a new fat molecule.

Glucose utilization (combustion) is hampered when, because of a disease such as diabetes, either not enough insulin is available or it is present in a form that cannot be used. If a body lacks insulin, glucose cannot enter and be stored in the muscles and the fat cells; as a result, the glucose accumulates in the blood. Thus, blood-sugar level depends on a delicately balanced equilibrium between glucose supply from the liver and its utilization by the system. Incidentally, intravenous feeding nearly always contains glucose.

Indeed, glucose plays a central role in the functioning of the body, because its availability determines the rate at which fat and protein are utilized.

When glucose utilization is low, the stomach begins to contract in *hunger;* conversely, a high utilization corresponds to *satiety.*

GONADS

Gonads is a general term for primary, partially developed sex glands in the embryo that will later develop into either male sex glands—testicles —or female glands—ovaries.

GONOCOCCUS

Gonococcus, also called *Neisseria gonorrhoeae,* is the bacterium that causes GONORRHEA. Gonococci are found only in humans.

GONORRHEA

Gonorrhea is a venereal disease, i.e., one that is transmitted by sexual intercourse. Most contraceptive preparations immobilize or destroy bacteria of gonorrhea (and of SYPHILIS, too) within ten minutes; but when neither spermicides nor condoms are used, a man or a woman who has gonorrhea can infect his or her sexual partner.

Apart from today's supposedly increased promiscuity and sexual permissiveness, which are partly responsible for the spreading of gonorrhea, control of the disease is a problem because: 1) there are no vaccines available yet; and 2) it is difficult to find and treat asymptomatic carriers, i.e., people who have gonorrhea and who spread it unknowingly because they have no symptoms; 3) gonorrhea has an extraordinarily short incubation period; only a few days elapse between exposure to infection and appearance of the first symptoms.

Indeed, 80 percent of women with gonorrhea are asymptomatic, while men usually have distinct burning sensations and discharges that alert them of their condition. Recently, however, an increasing number of men have also been discovered to be asymptomatic carriers. One of the most serious consequences of gonorrhea in women is that the infection can spread from the cervix into the FALLOPIAN TUBES, thus causing permanent sterility.

For the moment, the immediate hope for control of gonorrhea is *early treatment,* which recently has been facilitated by a new blood test, GONOSTICON DRI-DOT®. However, until vaccines are available, prophylaxis will have to depend exclusively on vast and long-range programs of education and massive advertising campaigns encouraging routine checkups.

Treatment of gonorrhea is relatively easy: penicillin, either injected (two intramuscular injections) or administered orally (one single dose), has been the preferred drug for twenty-five years, and penicillin is still one of the most effective and inexpensive antibiotics available. Moreover, the doses used for gonorrhea can cure a coexisting incubatory syphilis. Tetracycline, another antibiotic, and sulfonamide, the most famous of the synthetic organic compounds better known as sulfa drugs, which were used against infections before the discovery of antibiotics, are also used in case the penicillin therapy fails or the patient is allergic to penicillin.

Unfortunately, in the last ten years the infective organisms (gonococci) have developed an antibiotic resistance that has made it necessary gradually to alter treatment. In the 1950s, 300,000 units of penicillin was very effective; in the 1970s, the recommended dosage is 4.8 million units—about eight times the amount originally required.

Apparently some doctors are still unaware that the old doses are no longer effective. Also, infected persons sometimes share their drug with sex partners who refuse to see a doctor. In either case, patients quite frequently receive an inadequate dose of penicillin and not only are *not* cured of gonorrhea but contribute to the breeding of more resistant strains of gonococci. Since most women who contract a gonococcal infection are totally unaware of their condition, it is important that they follow up after the treatment. The best and most reliable "test for cure" is a PAP SMEAR TEST of the cervix and the rectum seven to fourteen days after completion of the antibiotic treatment.

GONOSTICON DRI-DOT®

Gonosticon Dri-Dot® is a new, simple, inexpensive blood test for GONORRHEA that takes only two minutes and can be performed in a doctor's office. Though not yet officially approved by the Food and Drug Administration (as of 1975), Gonosticon Dri-Dot® is already considered much more practical than the standard gonorrhea test for women, which consists of a culture of vaginal secretions that must be processed by a laboratory and does not show results for twenty-four to forty-eight hours.

Gonosticon Dri-Dot® was developed by the pharmaceutical company Organon, Inc., in cooperation with the Massachusetts Division of Communicable Diseases. A drop of the patient's blood is combined with particles of latex rubber that are coated with a specific antigen for gonorrhea; if the particles visibly clump together, the test is *positive*, i.e., it indicates the presence of gonorrhea ANTIBODIES.

There is a drawback: if performed too soon after an infection is acquired, Gonosticon Dri-Dot® may be falsely *negative*, because antibodies have not yet begun to be produced. Also, the test may be falsely *positive* for a while after the infection has been cured, because, once established, antibody-forming systems tend to persist in the body slightly longer than the antigens. Consequently, Gonosticon Dri-Dot® should not be used as a "test for cure."

However, Gonosticon Dri-Dot® has many advantages; one of the most important is that, in cases of complications of gonorrhea, it can detect the presence of gonococci at sites *other* than the genitals.

H

HAIR COLORING

There are seven methods of hair coloring:

1) Permanent oxidation dyes
2) Temporary rinses
3) Semipermanent dyes
4) Bleachers and toners
5) Metallic dyes
6) Vegetable dyes
7) Crayons

Permanent oxidation dyes—These are preferred by professional hair colorists because they are applied cold, act quickly, have no adverse effect on hair, and can duplicate a variety of shades that are lasting, predictable, and remarkably natural-looking. For the moment, it is the best coloring method available, though in the near future it is quite possible that a process for actual repigmentation may be developed.

Permanent dyes consist of a pigment called *dye intermediate*, usually twenty-volume hydrogen peroxide and sodium hypochlorite, which are mixed together immediately before use. The mixture causes a physical and chemical reaction called oxidation within the hair. The peroxide changes the hair's structure by penetrating the keratin (hair protein), gradually lightening the melanin (the hair's natural pigment) and making the hair shaft more porous and receptive to a new color.

Permanent dyes are manufactured either as a cream formula, in which case they are applied with a brush or an applicator, one small section of hair at a time; or as a shampoo, which eliminates brushing and sectioning, making them easy to use at home. However, the shampoo is less effective and thorough than the cream.

Oxidation dyes are excellent for covering gray hair and for darkening or lightening hair two or three shades. (To change deep brown into very light brown, *bleaches and toners* must be used.)

After a first application, permanent dyes need to be applied only

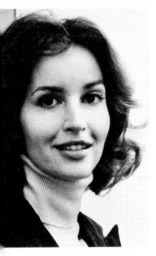 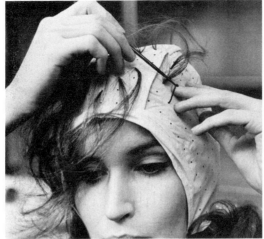 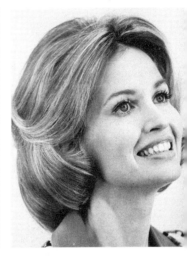

Top left: Although she was once a blond child, this New York model's hair has darkened to light brown. However, her complexion is still that of a blonde, so she decided to highlight her hair.

Top center: Following the instructions, she inserts the frosting needle through the cap holes and pulls out a number of hair strands to be frosted. The number of strands and their proximity determines how light the frosting will be.

Top right: The highlighting process is completed. The effect is that of sunlit natural blond hair, though no drastic bleaching has been used. *Courtesy of The Clairol Institute of Beauty, New York City.*

A Clairol brunette flanked by two Clairol moon blondes. No one, at this point, would care what their *real* hair color was.

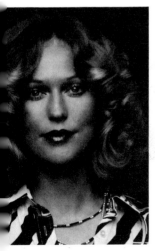 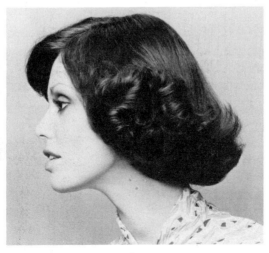 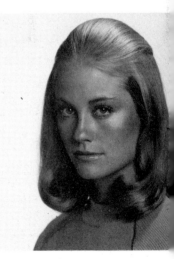

at three- or four-week intervals—the time it takes for hair to grow enough to reveal near the scalp the hair's original color.

Technically, before every application of permanent dye a person should undergo a PATCH TEST, which involves the application of a small amount of dye either to the skin behind the ear or to the inside of the arm at the elbow. The area should remain untouched for about twenty-four hours. If the reaction is *positive* (burning sensation, itching) the dye should not be used. A *negative* reaction, incidentally, means only that a person is not allergic to the dye at that particular time; it cannot predict whether he may become allergic later as a result of an acute condition such as a scalp irritation due to an illness, which may trigger an ALLERGY to hair dye. In practice, though, unless they already suspect the possibility of allergic reaction, very few hair colorists or their clients are willing to undergo the tedious and time-consuming procedure of a patch test.

Temporary rinses—These contain no oxidizing ingredients and affect only the hair's surface, which means that they cannot produce significant changes in color. They add highlights, tone down gray or yellow hair, brighten faded or sun-bleached hair, and darken reddishness. Some also act as a setting lotion.

Temporary rinses, which contain mild organic acids, were originally presented on the market mainly to help remove the dull film that might be left on the hair after a shampoo. Subsequently they became extremely popular because of the attractive highlights they added. These highlights can be removed from normal hair with a single shampoo. (Bleached or permanently waved hair is more porous, and the rinse lasts longer.)

Temporary rinses are available in either liquid or dry form. They usually consist of diluted solutions of the same acids used as additives (certified colors) in food and drugs and by the textile industry to dye wools and cellulose fibers. Others contain synthetic dyes other than certified colors, which produce stronger color effects but which can still be removed by several shampoos.

Semipermanent dyes—These are similar to temporary rinses in that they are organic acids requiring no developer—which means that they will not oxidize hair—but they produce more substantial color changes because, in addition to coating the hair surface, they slightly penetrate the shaft. Depending on the brand, they can be applied as shampoos or as rinses following shampooing, and can be gradually washed off by several ordinary shampoos. If the dye is left on the hair for about half an hour, the full color effect is immediate; if the dye is left on for only five to ten minutes, the color is less intense. Repeated weekly applications will gradually produce the effect that one long application accomplishes immediately.

Semipermanent dyes are best used to brighten drab shades of light hair and to neutralize the yellow tinge that gray hair sometimes has. However, to produce dark browns and black shades, the oxidation dyes are more successful.

Bleachers and toners—In order to lighten hair from dark brown to pale blond, a hair colorist must prebleach hair, that is, "strip" it of most of the existing color by a mixture of ammonia, hydrogen peroxide, and a hair lightener. After bleaching, a toner such as methylene blue is applied to give a small amount of natural-looking color to the bleached hair, which tends to be a lifeless yellow.

Bleaching increases considerably the porosity of hair, and frequent prebleaching sometimes weakens the hair, which may become extremely dry and brittle and finally break off near the scalp. An alternative to bleaching is frosting (or tipping, or streaking), a safer way for brown hair to acquire a blond look without actually being stripped of the entire color.

Metallic dyes—These are salts of copper, silver, and lead which react with the sulfur contained in the hair's keratin, thus forming a deposit of the corresponding sulfides. One drawback of these dyes is the limited range of available shades. Metallic dyes tend to produce harsh browns and blacks, while lighter shades fade or darken unpredictably. Also, since the coloring substance is deposited on the surface, the hair's natural luster is obscured.

Metallic dyes used to be advertised as "not dyes—just color restorers." Indeed, the color change happens gradually after several applications, a method that appeals to men self-conscious about changing the color of their hair suddenly. However, manufacturers are no longer allowed to use the term "restorer."

The advantage of metallic dyes is that they are almost totally harmless: they are not absorbed by intact skin, and they don't seem to provoke allergic reactions, as oxidation dyes sometimes do.

Vegetable dyes—Vegetable dyes, such as HENNA, indigo, camomile, logwood and walnut hull extracts, were used for centuries before being replaced by the permanent oxidation dyes. They are completely safe but they require elaborate applications and often produce colors that are limited, garish and uneven. With the exception of henna, vegetable dyes are no longer used today.

Crayons—These are temporary rinses that are manufactured in sticks and that are used for temporary retouching of newly grown gray hair between applications of permanent dyes. They can be rubbed wet directly onto hair or transferred to the hair from a wet brush.

HAIR FROSTING

Frosting is a technique of hair coloring that is obtained by bleaching tiny strands on a background of darker hair. When the frosting is limited to the front of the head, it is called highlighting.

There are two methods by which frosting can be performed. The first method is to place on the head a plastic cap dotted with small holes; selected hairs are then pulled through the holes and bleached. In the second method, a few strands of hair are placed on a small square of aluminum foil. The bleach is applied, starting half an inch from the scalp to the tip of each strand; the foil is then wrapped around the hair until the bleaching process is completed. After bleaching, a toner may be applied to obtain a more natural shade.

Frosting has certain advantages over total bleaching. For one thing, it does not have to be repeated so often as bleaching. Also, since the bleach does not touch the scalp, there is practically no danger of irritation or allergic reaction.

If frosting is done clumsily, it tends to have a salt-and-pepper look, rather like premature graying; and when the strands of lighter hair are too symmetrically bleached, they look unattractive and artificial—"spaghetti bleaching," as Marie McGrath, the famous New York colorist, called it. But if frosting is done skillfully, it can give to dark hair the illusion of blondness without having to strip it of all color. It can add golden highlights to plain brown hair and blend into blond hair youthful sunlike streaks.

A more recent variation of frosting that some beauty salons call naturalizing is to separate the hair in layers and give each series of layers a different strength of lightening, leaving some—close to the face or near a parting, for example—untouched so that there will be no revealing roots as the hair grows.

HAIR SPRAYS (OR LACQUERS)

Hair sprays are chemical preparations formulated to coat hair with a thin film to help keep the hairdo in place.

Hair sprays can be made of an almost unlimited combination of *synthetic* resins, which for this purpose are superior to *natural* resins because they are less susceptible to moisture and to flaking than the latter. This is important because when a woman brushes her hair too vigorously after repeated applications of spray, the film often sheds, forming flakes that give the appearance of DANDRUFF.

One of the natural resins, however, is still used in the preparation of certain hair sprays: shellac, a resinous secretion of *Tachardia lacca,* the lac insect. This raw material is a complex mixture of chemicals whose true composition is still difficult to analyze. Shellac is nonirritating to the scalp and makes a smooth, flexible film most suitable for a hair spray. Its major drawback is that it is difficult to preserve, as it is quite susceptible to bacterial attack.

Hair sprays have been available for many years; before the advent of the AEROSOL system, it was manufactured like a PERFUME atomizer (or an old-fashioned window spray), with a rubber bulb and a plunger.

Besides the resins, aerosol hair sprays contain alcohol and a propellant, which provides the force for the spray's self-dispensing.

The film formed by a hair spray is stronger than that of setting lotions; thus, hair sprays should be sprayed lightly, uniformly, and *only* on the surface. Quick drying—an essential quality of effective hair sprays—is obtained by adding to the preparation a small amount of plasticizer, a chemical that imparts flexibility to the preparation. Therefore, once it is sprayed, very little further styling or rearranging can be done to the hair.

HAIR STRAIGHTENERS

There are three methods of straightening naturally curly hair: 1) application of fixatives such as waxes, pomades, or film-depositing gums for a *temporary* straightening; 2) the use of a heated comb, a process called hot pressing, the effect of which lasts for about two or three weeks; 3) the use of chemical compounds which stretch hair *permanently*.

Applying waxes and pomades is the oldest method for temporarily straightening curly hair, yet it is not very satisfactory because the heavy oils and resins contained in the pomades simply glue the hair to the scalp, and hair regains its curliness as soon as the oils are washed off. Occasionally some people become hypersensitive to the PERFUME or to other ingredients used in the pomades and develop contact DERMATITIS.

In hot pressing, which has been in use for at least sixty years, a metal comb heated to about 400° or 500° F. is passed quickly through strands of hair that have been previously lubricated with a small amount of oil. The heat partially alters the molecular structure of the hair; when the comb is removed, the temperature drop causes the hair to stretch and temporarily retain its new position. However, once the hair is exposed to humidity—even just scalp PERSPIRATION—it tends to revert to its naturally curly state. Repeated use of hot pressing may cause some damage to the hair; an unskillful hairdresser may burn the scalp. A homemade variation of hot pressing is the practice, popular among teenagers, of ironing long hair to give it a perfectly straight look. Again, there is danger in this of burning either the hair or the scalp.

Unlike pomades and the heated comb, chemical straighteners are

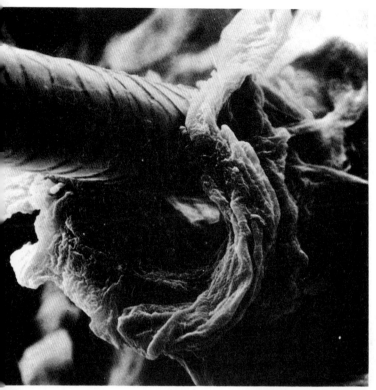

Photomicrograph, magnified 1,350 times, of a hair strand emerging from its follicle to the surface of the skin.

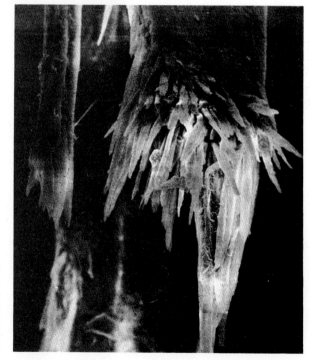

The fuzzy, ragged tip of a woman's hair that has not been trimmed in a long while. The outside layer—the cuticle—has broken away, and the cortex, the inner layer, is exposed to the drying effect of air. (Original magnification: 500 times.)

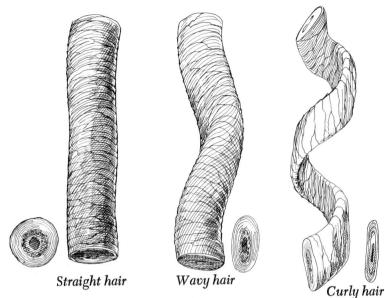

Straight hair   *Wavy hair*

Curly hair

Microscopic view of different kinds of human hair.

Above left: Straight hair, which forms naturally because of the even pattern of cell growth in the papilla, the essential part of the hair root. The cross-section of a straight hair shaft is usually round and symmetric.

Above center: Wavy hair, which is due to an *uneven* growth pattern in the papilla. The hair shaft cross-section is usually oval.

Above right: Very curly hair, a special form of hair, whose cross-section appears to be more or less flat. The flatter the hair shaft, the more it tends to turn upon itself and curl. The reason for curly hair is not well understood, but it probably is caused by an hereditary difference in the papilla.

Below left: Straight hair treated with a water set. Because the hair is merely wet with water and allowed to dry wound on curlers, its natural configuration is changed only for as long as the hair remains dry.

Below center: Straight hair treated with a permanent wave, which consists of first softening and breaking the chemical bonds of the hair, setting the hair in a new form, and finally rearranging the bond.

Below right: Curly hair straightened with the same ingredient—in slightly different concentrations—and on the same principle as permanent waving. The only difference between the two procedures concerns the way the hair is handled after the chemical bonds have been broken. In a permanent wave, the hair is wound on curlers while the internal bonds are being rearranged by a neutralizer; in straightening, the hair is combed flat before the neutralizer is applied.

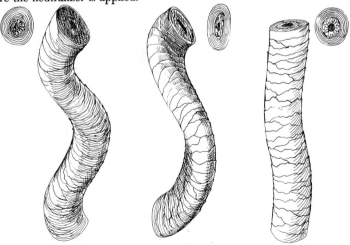

Water set   *Permanent*   *Straightened*   **161**

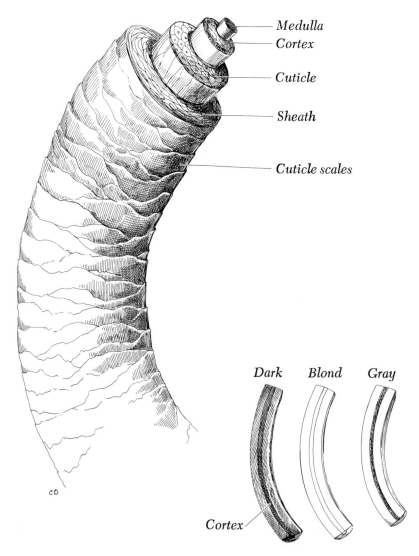

The visible part of the hair fiber is composed of three separate and distinct layers: the cuticle, the cortex and the medulla. Each of these layers has its own functions.

The cuticle is the outside layer. It consists of hard, flattened, horny scales that overlap one another in the direction of hair growth. The function of the cuticle is to protect the more delicate cortex.

The cortex is made of many millions of parallel fibers of hard keratin—the protein that forms the chemical basis of skin and hair—twisted around one another, ropelike. The natural color of hair is due to the pigment in the cortex, and the natural wave is due to physical changes in the cortex brought about in the follicle before the hair is mature.

The medulla is the inner layer of hair. It is made of a narrow column of cells. The medulla is often broken or even entirely absent from the hair shaft. Its function is not known.

At foot, left: Cross-section of a dark hair, with pigment in both its medulla and cortex.
At center: This hair is of the blond variety and has no medulla.
Right: Cross-section of a white hair. Although no pigment is present in its cortex, it has pigment in its medulla. This shows that it is the pigment in the cortex that gives color to hair.

162

permanent in their action, as they alter the chemical structure of the cortex—the hair shaft's middle layer. There are three types of permanent straighteners:

Sodium Hydroxide—Sodium hydroxide is an alkali that acts rapidly—in five to ten minutes—by swelling the hair and breaking the chemical bonds (the links between different atoms of a chemical compound) in the hair fibers, which in turn relax with combing. The chemical reaction stops when the hair is rinsed with abundant water.

Thioglycolate—Thioglycolate straighteners contain the same ingredients —in slightly different concentrations—as those used in permanent waving lotions; one such ingredient, thioglycolic acid, in this case is intended to reverse unattractive natural curliness rather than to curl the hair. Thioglycolate cream is applied to damp hair for a few minutes, and the hair is combed for about twenty minutes. Finally the hair is rinsed with water and treated with a special solution, which rebuilds new chemical bonds to produce straight hair. Thioglycolate straighteners are not always completely effective; however, they rarely cause damage to the hair or the scalp if used as directed.

Sodium Bisulfite—This type of straightener also produces changes in the chemical bonds in the hair. The lotion is applied to damp hair, which is then wrapped in a turban for about fifteen minutes and then combed for about twenty minutes. Finally the hair is rinsed with water, then with a stabilizer and a conditioner, which fixes the chemical bonds in the hair in their new straight configuration.

Bisulfite straighteners are considered by some to be more effective than the thioglycolates. If used according to directions, sodium bisulfite doesn't cause damage to either the hair or the scalp. Special care, however, should be observed when straightening bleached or tinted hair, whose structure has already been chemically modified. Some manufacturers supply specially formulated products for bleached or tinted hair, which apparently minimize any possible damage.

HAIR WAVING

There are several methods of waving hair. The simplest is, of course, the water set: the hair is merely wetted and allowed to dry under some sort of constraint, either straight or wound on a curler. Under these conditions, the natural configuration of the hair is changed to some extent. This type of set lasts only until the set is removed by excessive humidity or wetting.

The efficiency of the water set is much improved by drying the hair at high temperature (near the boiling point of water), a process similar to that used to press woolen pants. Depending on the temperature and the hair's pH—its degree of acidity and alkalinity—some very complex physical and chemical phenomena occur in the hair, and sometimes some minor damage is produced.

A more popular means of improving the efficiency of a water set involves the application of a setting lotion or a HAIR SPRAY, either before or after the hair has been wound on curlers. Many people believe that it is the resinous materials contained in these preparations that hold the hair in the desired configuration. "Actually, this is not the case," explained Dr. Martin M. Rieger, associate director of chemistry at the Warner-Lambert Company, in New Jersey. "The setting lotions applied to the hair produce spot welds, so that the adjacent or crossing hair fibers are in fact glued to each other and thereby maintain the set. The mechanical strength of hair fibers is too high, and no compound discovered to date is capable of restraining this fiber from assuming its natural configuration under ambient conditions of humidity. Theoretically, such compounds exist, or enough of a known compound can be applied to the hair to obtain a certain set by coating each fiber, thus changing the properties of each single hair. But this would produce a fibrous material that no longer feels like hair and which is aesthetically unacceptable."

Another method for setting hair is the permanent wave, which effects the change by chemically altering the hair fiber. Permanent waving can be: 1) *hot wave*, which depends on the action of steam in the presence of the appropriate chemicals; 2) *cold wave*, which uses chemicals at room temperature; 3) *tepid wave*, which operates at intermediate temperature, and which can utilize chemicals used in either the hot or the cold wave.

Hot waving is not practiced widely. Cold or tepid waving is achieved by treating the hair fiber with a softener, such as an alkaline solution of thioglycolic acid. Once it is softened, hair can be rearranged, bent, or stretched by the application of mechanical force. If the thioglycolate solution has a pH of less than eight, no permanent waves can be obtained; but if the pH is more than ten, i.e., at high alkalinity, the solution will act as a depilatory! Finally, the softness of the hair is reversed by the application of an oxidizing agent.

The softening agent breaks the bonds that cross-link the chains of keratin (hair PROTEIN) molecules in the hair fiber. The chains then can slip past each other and be rearranged, depending on the type of physical force exerted. In the case of straightening, the force comes from repeated combing while the hair is soft. In the case of waving, physical force is provided by the circular winding of the hair around curlers (one turn around the curler equals half a wave). The outer portion of the curled hair is stretched, while the interior portion is under a certain degree of compression. If a tight permanent wave is desired, the curlers are generally thin, and the processing time is relatively long. For a looser permanent wave, the rods are large, and the duration of the contact between the hair and the waving product is shorter. Since the curler often is held in place by a plastic bar or a rubber band, it should be kept in mind that these can exert additional stress on the side of the fiber. If this pressure is excessive, the fiber could be damaged.

After the curl has been formed, the hair must be restored by chemical oxidation. The most commonly used oxidizing agents are hydrogen peroxide (also used for hair bleaching) and sodium bromate. Incidentally, oxidation of the hair fibers could also be accomplished by air oxygen, but the process would be too slow, and the air may fail to eliminate completely the unpleasant odor of thioglycolic acid or other softeners.

Thioglycolic acid is generally safe, both for the operator, who is exposed frequently to its chemical action, and for the scalp of the person whose hair is being treated. Since the keratin portion of skin differs structurally and chemically from the keratin of hair, hair waving preparations do not affect the skin or penetrate too deeply, so that irritation or allergic reactions are unlikely. Nevertheless, since frequent exposure to the alkaline thioglycolates may remove some of the skin's protein constituents, thus making it more sensitive to the penetration of *any* noxious material, beauticians should always wear rubber gloves during the operations required for permanent waving.

HAND-LIFT

PLASTIC SURGERY, which can do wonders for the face, the nose, and the bosom, cannot do much to beautify hands. It cannot slenderize chubby fingers, mold thick wrists, or elongate square fingertips. And, except for toning down age wrinkles, dermatologists can do nothing either. There is, of course, a small group of super-specialized surgeons who combine the skill of plastic, orthopedic, and neurological surgeons and who are exclusively concerned with restoring the complicated functionality of the hands when it is impaired by injuries, ARTHRITIS, or congenital defects.

However, some plastic surgeons sometimes perform hand-lifts for women who, having undergone a FACE-LIFT, feel that their wrinkled hands reveal all the years the face-lift has subtracted from their faces.

The pioneer of this procedure is Dr. James Adamson, chief of the department of plastic surgery at Norfolk General Hospital in Norfolk, Virginia, though he credits a patient for inducing him several years ago to perform his first hand-lift.

A hand-lift is a relatively simple operation; it does not touch the fingers or probe beyond the skin of the back of the hand. It is, nevertheless, the work of a miniaturist, as no other area of the body is so closely fitted or made up of so many interdependent parts as the hand. A hand-lift requires general ANAESTHESIA and a tourniquet applied to the patient's arm in order to prevent blood from obscuring the hand's delicate structures during the operation. Then, an incision about 5 to 8 cm long is made between the wrist and the first crease of the little finger, where the skin of the top surface merges with that of the palm. Another incision, 1 cm long, is made horizontally, to coincide with one of the wrist's skin folds. The surgeon then proceeds delicately to undermine the skin of the back of the hand for approximately one-third of the surface—usually as far as the middle finger—carefully avoiding the nerves and the veins. The skin is gently pulled and draped back in place, exactly as in a face-lift. The excess skin is measured and sparingly cut off. The rest is closed neatly along the original L-shaped incision with a special paper tape which minimizes the scar by avoiding suture marks. The tourniquet is removed, and the hand is kept elevated for a few minutes as the blood flows back into it. The hand is then bandaged in the so-called position of function: fingers slightly curved, the thumb facing the other fingers, with a padded support fitted to the palm. Finally the hand is placed in a sling secured around the neck.

Bandages are removed in five days, and the paper tapes are replaced by a strip of gauze soaked in a special fluid that quickly evaporates, leaving a film that protects the fresh scar for a few more days. Convalescence lasts one more week, and the incisions, if they have been correctly made in the direction of the creases of the hand, leave scars that are hardly visible.

HANGNAILS

The ragged flaps and splits that sometimes affect nail cuticles are called hangnails. They are often due to excessive dryness of the skin in these areas or to inept MANICURES and may be worsened by a nervous habit of picking at the skin around the nail.

In order to avoid inflammation, hangnails should not be pulled, but removed at the base with sharp, clean scissors.

HEADACHES

Headache is a sensation somewhere in the head, face or neck, ranging from excruciating pain to a mere "strange feeling." Dull or sharp; steady, throbbing or stabbing; occasional, recurrent or chronic, headaches are known at one time or another to 90 percent of mankind, yet the word means something different to everyone, depending on an individual's PAIN threshold (the level at which the stimulation of nerve endings actually produces a sensation of pain), on his cultural background, and on his personal way of expressing feelings of pain.

Medically speaking, headaches are symptoms, that is, evidence of, and a warning for, some kind of physical disturbance. But in the case of headache, the distinction between *symptom* and actual *disease* is blurred. Headache is an extremely complex phenomenon, far from being understood, "truly a kaleidoscope of a disease, . . . confusing and even deadly in its effects," in the words of Arthur S. Freese, the author of *Headaches: The Kinds and the Cures.*

Interestingly, the brain itself does not feel pain; the only structures inside the skull that are sensitive to pain are the arteries and the veins, parts of the tissues protecting the brain, and a very few nerves. Outside the skull, however, almost everything is sensitive to pain: the scalp, the muscles of the neck and the face, the arteries and the veins.

Immediate headache pain may be caused by:

1) the pressure on sensitive tissues inside the skull, which may be caused, for example, by a brain tumor or abscess (often, though, the pain is "referred," that is, is felt in places other than where the tumor is, which of course makes it difficult to locate the source of the headache);

2) any swelling, inflammation or irritation of the arteries caused by fever, reactions to drugs, blood-pressure changes, etc.;

3) any prolonged contraction of the muscles in the neck, scalp and face because of poor POSTURE, anxiety, or an uneven bite.

The occasional headache obviously is not a problem: two ASPIRINS (or acetaminophen, an aspirin substitute) with a cup of coffee, a little rest, maybe a warm bath, a massage, or a walk in the fresh air, usually take care of it. Even the serious headaches that are diagnosed as being caused by a brain tumor, or which accompany MENSTRUATION or influenza, are resolved as soon as the cause is removed. The real headache victims are people who suffer from chronic, inexplicable and often unbearable pain. They are the ones who crowd the headache clinics and still puzzle teams of specialists—neurologists, endocrinologists, psychiatrists, pharmacologists—all over the world, for the cause of the vast majority of chronic headaches remains, to this day, obscure.

Also potentially dangerous are headaches that:

1) strike out of the blue;

2) are accompanied by convulsions or mental confusion;

3) are characterized by localized pain in the eye or ear, or in a specific area of the head;

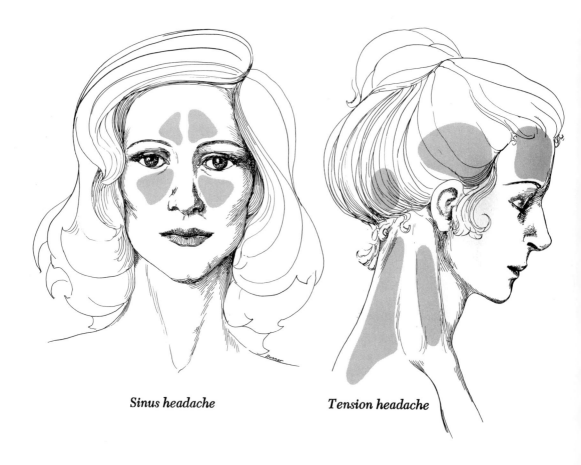

Sinus headache   *Tension headache*

4) follow a blow on the head;
5) are recurrent in children;
6) are daily or frequent;
7) are present for a long time and suddenly change pattern or character;
8) awaken a person from a deep sleep.

In 1962 The National Institute of Neurological Diseases and Stroke published the first comprehensive classification of headaches, which recognized the following fifteen major types of headaches:

1) *Migraine,* a syndrome of which vascular headaches (those caused by swollen blood vessels) are the most characteristic sign. Usually hereditary, recurrent, involving only one-half of the head (hemicrania), frequently preceded by nausea and loss of appetite, and by hypersensitivity to light, sound and smell. In its most severe form—the so-called "classic migraine"—it may cause hallucinations, distortion of vision, loss of consciousness and even temporary blindness.

2) *Cluster headache,* a recurrent and excruciating headache, sometimes

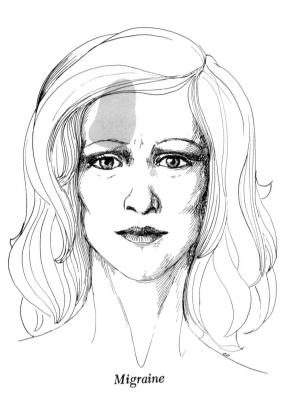

Migraine

Among the most common forms of headache are:

Left: Sinus headache, which may start with the swelling of the mucous membrane in the nose, due to a common cold. This blocks the openings of the sinuses and causes the secretion of the sinus lining to back up, which, in turn, causes a build-up of pressure and, ultimately, a headache in the areas marked in gray in the drawing.

Middle: Tension headache, usually long-lasting—weeks, months, even years—characterized by muscle contractions on the forehead, temples and neck, which are caused by stress and tension.

Right: Migraine, a syndrome whose most prominent sign is a vascular headache (swollen blood vessels). It is usually hereditary, recurrent, involving only one-half of the head (hemicrania). It is frequently preceded by nausea, loss of appetite, and hypersensitivity to light, sound, and smell.

called "suicide" headache. Strikes mostly men, usually awakening them from a deep sleep.

3) *Tension headache,* the most common of all headaches, usually long-lasting (weeks, months, even years); muscle-contracting usually caused by stress or tension.

4) *Combination headache,* a muscle-contracting headache that occurs as a reaction to the swollen blood vessels of an immediately preceding migraine attack.

5) *Nasal congestion headache,* involving the recurrent swelling of the mucous membranes in the nose, independent of ALLERGY, infection or nasal defects. Usually a reaction to pressure or stress.

6) *Psychogenic headache,* the result of a so-called "conversion reaction," in which emotional problems such as anxiety, depression, anger and frustration are converted into a physical symptom.

7) *Common vascular headache,* which, unlike migraine, is occasional, accompanying infections such as flu; carbon monoxide poisoning; lack of oxygen; reaction to certain drugs; brain concussion.

169

8) *Traction headache,* caused by the pulling exerted on sensitive tissues within the skull by tumors, abscesses, blood clots.

9) *Inflammation headache,* resulting from swelling of arteries and veins inside the skull, which in turn may be caused by meningitis or hemorrhages.

10-13) Headaches caused by any disturbance in the eyes, ears, nose, and sinuses; by allergy; by disturbances in the spine; and by tooth, gum, and jaw problems.

14) Headaches produced by *neuritis* (inflammation of a nerve).

15) *Neuralgias,* such as the so-called tic douloureux, a violent and unpredictable headache limited to a particular nerve—the trigeminal—which provides feeling in the face and forehead and is linked to other nerves in the nose, eyes, teeth, gums, upper lip, chin and tongue.

Following a trauma, a person may suffer from headaches that are combinations of several of those mentioned above.

Not all physicians agree with this classification; indeed, there are other types of headaches, based on different principles. At least one headache specialist—Dr. David R. Coddon, associate professor of neurology and the founder of the famous Headache Clinic at the Mount Sinai Medical Center in New York—does not classify headaches at all: considering their complexity and their overlapping characteristics, he feels that a description is all that is needed. Dr. Coddon also rejects the concept of the "migraine personality"—the traditional belief that people suffering from migraines are invariably meticulous, tense, insecure individuals who use migraine as a retreat from frustration and as a way to restore their reserves of energy. Migraine headache, Dr. Coddon believes, is a physiological problem, a series of biochemical changes involving hormones, blood vessels and the nervous system. What really matters is to pinpoint, whenever possible and as fast as possible, a headache's underlying cause. For this purpose, Dr. Coddon has recently compiled a questionnaire to be answered by each headache patient. Once computerized, the questionnaire will be of invaluable help to a specialist who has hundreds of possible clues to investigate before attempting a diagnosis.

In addition to a thorough history of his headache, a patient admitted to a headache clinic is asked to undergo:

1) X-rays of the skull, sinuses, cervical spine;

2) Blood count and other laboratory tests;

3) An ELECTROENCEPHALOGRAPH.

Prescription drugs for headaches that fail to respond to aspirin include antihistamines and minor tranquilizers. For migraine there is ergotamine tartrate, a derivative of a fungus called ergot, which is a powerful drug that is neither a sedative nor an analgesic but a vasoconstrictor—that is, it causes swollen blood vessels to return to normal. However, people suffering from high blood pressure, infections, or heart diseases cannot use ergotamine. For them, a doctor may prescribe inhalation of oxygen, or the application of cold packs (the most practical are made of a freezable gelatin encased in plastic, which can be kept in the freezer and which are easily applied to the head with a scarf or a bandage). To prevent a migraine attack, a drug called methysergide maleate (Sansert®) is sometimes prescribed. However, it often produces side effects such as nausea, cramps and swelling.

Among the experimental techniques that are currently being employed in treating or preventing severe, chronic headaches are ACUPUNCTURE, BIOFEEDBACK, HYPNOTHERAPY and the administration of certain PROSTAGLANDINS.

Clonidine, a drug used mainly for the treatment of high blood pressure, has recently been found to be effective in preventing migraine attacks in a limited number of cases. Propranolol, used to treat angina pectoris, seems to work in reducing the severity of a migraine attack.

However, the great hope for the future is a new, versatile, extraordinary drug called DIMETHYL SULFOXIDE (DMSO)—the aspirin of the twenty-first century, as it is sometimes referred to. As of 1974, DMSO has been turned over to the National Academy of Sciences for evaluation, which means that it may soon be available to the public, and perhaps do for headaches what ANTIBIOTICS did for infection.

HEARING AIDS

Deafness is not so rare as some people think, but it is not always easy to recognize. Except when it happens overnight, hearing loss can be so gradual as to be hardly noticed; having to strain to hear conversations, frequent need to have remarks repeated, or the conviction that "everybody is mumbling" may all be signs of deafness, yet many people may be unconsciously reluctant to relate these to deafness.

There are three major types of partial or total hearing loss:

Nerve loss—Resulting from damage to the inner ear caused, for example, by birth defects, aging, or a disease accompanied by high fever;

Conductive loss—Resulting from accumulation of EARWAX in the external canal; an infection in the middle ear; or a perforation of the eardrum;

Functional loss—Probably a result of psychological disturbance.

Conductive loss can usually be treated, but in many cases of nerve loss the only solution is a hearing aid, a device, basically comparable to a miniature telephone, that amplifies the sound reaching the ears.

Hearing aids won't help a person recover hearing, but they will help him to hear better. However, before considering a hearing aid, a person should first consult an otologist, for his hearing loss may be a type that can be treated. In case a hearing aid is needed, the otologist, together with a reputable hearing-aid dealer, will be able to choose the kind of aid that is best suited to a patient's specific degree and pattern of deafness, and to his daily activity and life-style.

A hearing aid consists of a tiny *microphone*, which picks up sound waves from the air and converts them into electrical impulses; an *amplifier*, which increases the strength of the electrical signals; a *battery*, which provides electrical energy to operate the aid; and a tiny loudspeaker, called the *receiver*, to which is connected a flexible wire from the amplifier, which converts the amplified signals back into sound waves and directs them into the ear through a plastic *ear mold*.

The ear mold is an essential part of the hearing aid system: it directs the amplified sound into the ear canal with great efficiency. If it doesn't fit properly, however, it may cause irritation and soreness, and produce whistles and squeals. Ready-made ear molds are available, but sometimes

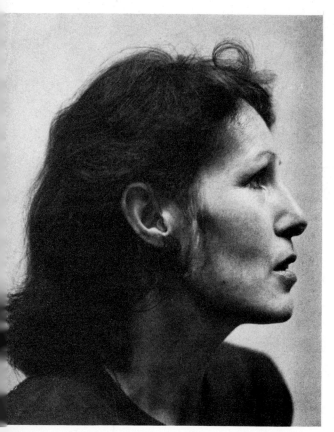

A forty-year-old woman with a mild hearing loss, shown here wearing a custom-made hearing aid in her right ear.

Though not completely invisible, this hearing aid—which was fitted by Allen Raiten, a certified hearing aid dealer in New York City—is contained in a small flesh-colored case that is placed neatly and inconspicuously behind the ear and is connected to the ear mold by a short transparent plastic tubule.

it is worth having an ear mold custom-made to the exact shape of a person's ear.

Good-quality hearing aids are usually equipped with adjustable *volume* and *tone* controls, which regulate the amplification of sounds so that they are neither too loud nor too soft, neither too high-pitched nor too low-pitched.

Modern hearing aids—quite different from the cumbersome units that were still in use only a few years ago—are powered by minuscule electronic devices such as transistors. They are not completely invisible—some parts of a hearing aid must show—but they are so small and light that any hairdo, with the exception of a crewcut, can easily hide them.

At present, hearing aids are manufactured in the following models:

In-the-ear—Fitted directly into the ear canal and supported by the ear shell itself. It is extremely light and has no external wires or tubes. Equipped with volume control but may not have tone control. Recommended for mild hearing loss.

Behind-the-ear—Contained in a small, curved, skin-colored case that fits neatly behind the ear. It is connected to the ear mold by a short plastic tube. Some models have both volume and tone controls. Recommended for mild to severe hearing loss.

Eyeglass—Similar to the behind-the-ear model, except that the device is built into an eyeglass frame.

"Cross-over"—Also built into an eyeglass frame; however, this system has a microphone beside the poorer ear, while the amplifier and the receiver are placed near the better ear. This system apparently prevents the head from blocking off sounds from the better ear.

On-the-body—This model has a larger microphone, amplifier, and power supply contained in a case that can be carried in a pocket or attached to clothes. This model is more powerful than the others, and the controls may be easier to adjust. Recommended for severe loss of hearing.

Directional—Consists of two complete hearing aids—microphone, amplifier and receiver—one for each ear. For many people this double system helps to filter out unwanted background noise.

Humidity, PERSPIRATION, HAIR SPRAYS and hair dryers may corrode a hearing aid and interfere with its performance, as may extremely cold weather and direct sunlight.

Batteries should be replaced periodically, and the ear mold detached and washed to prevent earwax from clogging it. Before being replaced, the ear mold should be thoroughly dried—one drop of water could block the passage of sound or even damage the entire system.

HEATING PADS

Heating pads are flexible pads that are used for applying heat to the body for therapeutic treatment. When *dry* heat is recommended, the pads usually consist of electric heating elements embedded in insulating material. *Moist* heat, which may be prescribed for the relief of muscular PAIN, ARTHRITIS and certain skin disorders, is provided by various types of steam packs, most of which, in order to produce heat, have to be immersed in hot water for quite a while.

In 1974, however, a more convenient instant heating pad, called Thermolaxor®, was developed by the Chem-E-Watt Corporation of Long Island, New York.

Thermolaxor®, which is based on a new technological invention in the field of electrochemistry, is self-heating, disposable, odorless, weighs less than one ounce, and can be used as either a moist or a dry heating pad. It consists of a heating element sealed between two layers of soft, porous polyurethane foam laminated with a perforated polyethylene film. Unlike other steam packs, it is not affected by toxic chemicals.

Heat is generated by holding the pad under a faucet for a few seconds and then squeezing out the excess water, to avoid dripping. If the tap water is warm, Thermolaxor® will start generating heat in three minutes; if the water is cold, it will take four or five minutes. Within ten minutes, the pad will reach a temperature of 140° F., and in fifteen to thirty minutes it will reach a peak temperature of about 167° F. After forty-five minutes it begins to cool off.

Special cotton felt pads, which are part of the heating element, absorb the water through the porous polyurethane foam, and the moist heat subsequently escapes through the small holes in the polyethylene film.

If the pad is too warm for a particular person, a thin cloth can be wrapped around it. When dry heat is needed, the pad may be inserted into a special polyethylene bag. The pads are flexible and will adapt to any part of the body: the shoulder, the knee, the elbow, the hand. Standard pads measure 4 by 6 inches and are sold in sealed packages of four. If one pad is not large enough, a second may be attached to it with adhesive tape.

HENNA

Henna *(Lawsonia alba)* is the Persian name for a small shrub found in India, Iran and the Middle East, and along the African coast of the Mediterranean. Its leaves can be powdered and used as a dye, producing a whole range of reddish shades from orange to deep purple, depending on the original color of the leaves.

As far back as Egypt's Third Dynasty, henna was used for tinting women's hair and fingernails, men's beards, the manes and tails of horses, and Moroccan leathers. Rubbed on palms and soles, henna was believed to reduce perspiration. The West, however, forgot henna for centuries, until the 1800s, when it became popular again for a while; in 1859, Adelina Patti, the celebrated Italian singer, made her triumphant debut in New York, appearing on stage with flaming henna-red hair.

Today, henna is practically ignored by cosmetology schools, though it is sometimes used by people allergic to permanent oxidation dyes. Still, every few years henna makes its way to the beauty pages of fashion magazines and in some French or Italian beauty salons; more than one woman has been momentarily tempted by the idea of adding a "natural" hue to her hair. More recently (1971) the revival of henna may have been part of the general interest in ORGANIC FOOD, natural COSMETICS, and home remedies in general.

The procedure involves mixing the powdered henna with hot water in a double boiler and applying the warm poultice on dry hair for about forty-five minutes, by which time it cools off, thus stopping the coloring process.

Henna never damages the hair structure and is not known to cause allergic reactions. However, the truth is that the red of henna rarely looks natural on hair; rather, it gives hair a vegetablelike shade—tomato, beet, eggplant—even if the decoction is heated to the right temperature, skillfully applied and precisely timed. If used often enough on the whole head, henna will accumulate on the hair surface and eventually acquire a characteristic orange-red shade that can be only partially mitigated by adding indigo—the same formula, it is said, Mahomet used to dye his beard.

HERPES SIMPLEX (COLD SORE)

Herpes simplex is an acute infection of the skin and mucous membranes caused by *herpesvirus hominis*. The condition is marked by itchy, recurrent cold sores and watery blisters, usually appearing at the borders of the lips and nostrils, and on the mucous surface of the genitals.

A cold sore can be triggered by fever, stress, menstruation, sunlight, or friction of the lip; increased local temperature seems to be an important factor. As a genital infection, it is now the second most prevalent venereal disease among young Americans.

At the end of 1973, medical researchers announced that this rather common and apparently trivial disturbance is not just a simple cosmetic problem but a serious disease. It can cause, among other things, eye problems, cervical cancer in women, and a venereal disease—not necessarily transmitted only by sexual intercourse—in men.

At about the same time, a new treatment called photodynamic

inactivation was developed by Dr. Joseph L. Melnick, professor of virology and epidemiology at Houston's Baylor College of Medicine. The treatment consists of swabbing herpes simplex lesions with a dye called proflavine—used for years as an antiseptic—and then exposing them to ordinary fluorescent light. The dye-light procedure is simple and inexpensive and requires no special equipment; it not only heals lesions more rapidly (by breaking up herpesvirus) but, over a period of time, also may progressively decrease the incidence of herpes simplex in the population.

The ideal time to give the dye-light treatment is early in the cold-sore course—at the first symptoms of tightness, stinging, tingling or burning of the skin. If the sores have already reached the stage of small, clear blisters, these are delicately opened and proflavine applied liberally.

The sores should not be exposed to light for at least six to eight hours. An ordinary fluorescent light, such as a desk reading lamp, is put as close as possible to the lesion—3 or 4 inches—for thirty minutes. Twenty-four hours later the light treatment is repeated. The dye alone will not kill the virus—only the dye *plus* light.

A few months after this new treatment was announced, the photodynamic inactivation therapy not only had gained wide popularity but had come under attack as potentially cancer-producing. Dr. Fred Rapp, a virologist at the Milton S. Hershey Medical Center of Pennsylvania State University, feels that there is a possibility that the treatment might convert some normal cells into cancer cells. But defective particles of the virus, which are suspected to be the CARCINOGENS, are produced *whenever* the virus multiplies, whether it is treated or not. The only question would be whether the treatment *compounds* this rather remote risk. Even Dr. Rapp concedes that most people who carry herpes simplex viruses under latent conditions do not develop tumors.

As of 1974, Dr. Melnick and Dr. Rapp agreed that, in any case, the dye-light therapy should be used only under a doctor's supervision. And indeed, many doctors are successfully using it. Others prefer to treat cold sores with daubs of ether or chloroform; still others vaccinate the patient with the regular smallpox vaccine. And a Denver dermatologist, Dr. Henry M. Lewis, recently suggested a third, even simpler solution that does not require a physician: soaking-wet tea bags applied to the lesions overnight. Apparently this treatment provides fast relief and clears the lesions rapidly.

HIRSUTISM (SUPERFLUOUS HAIR)

Hirsutism, also called hypertrichosis, refers to excessive growth of coarse hair in areas of a woman's body—face, breasts, arms, legs, and lower abdomen—where women generally have a soft, fine, more or less pigmented down. Needless to say, hirsutism is considered unattractive, though evaluation of what is superfluous hair depends on race, social standards, and a woman's personal sense of beauty.

In this respect, the word hirsutism is used generically, as true female hirsutism actually refers to a hormonal disturbance of a particular type of hair. Both men and women have four types of hair on different areas of the body, and both produce androgens (male sex HORMONES) and estrogen and progesterone (female sex hormones). However, not *all* hormones influence all types of hair:

1) *eyebrows* and hair on the *back of the scalp* are not influenced at all by any hormone;

2) *pubic* and *axillary* hair may be stimulated to grow by either androgens or estrogen and progesterone;

3) the hair on the *front* and the *top of the scalp* may be merely retarded by androgens;

4) the hair around the *mouth*, on the *chin, arms, legs*, and *lower abdomen* are stimulated by androgens alone.

Since androgens, in a woman, are secreted by both the adrenal gland and the ovaries, an endocrine disorder or a tumor in the adrenal gland or in an ovary may cause a woman to produce excessive amounts of androgens, with a rapid growth of coarse hair on her face, breast, extremities and lower abdomen. The same happens if a woman is treated with too large doses of drugs containing synthetic androgens. A few months after the treatment is discontinued, however, hair growth will return to normal.

Certain cases of hirsutism are definitely not related to endocrine disorders, yet their origin remains obscure. Some endocrinologists suggest that they may be caused by some biochemical alterations in one or more of the hormones. Indeed, some studies have indicated that some of these cases have benefited from a treatment of cortisone or female hormone. But the matter is still controversial. Others feel that the recent discovery that skin is capable of extracting and metabolizing androgens from the circulation, independent of the adrenal gland and the ovaries, may one day indicate that some of these inexplicable cases of hirsutism are related to androgen metabolism in the skin.

For the moment, once endocrine disorders are either treated or ruled out, excessive hair can be eliminated only by mechanical means. Depending on the texture and quantity, and on the area in which it grows, hair can be removed according to a woman's preference either temporarily, by depilatory creams, EPILATING WAX, plucking, or SHAVING; or permanently, by ELECTROLYSIS.

HOMEOSTASIS

Homeostasis, a concept introduced in 1926 by Walter B. Cannon, the famous Harvard physiologist, refers to the maintenance of form and function in the organism—the body's tendency "to keep things as they are." This seemingly uniform state of body harmony is actually the result of a constant turnover of body substances, and of continuous adjustments under the control of the nervous system and the endocrine glands.

One example is the system that controls the intake of food in the normal (as opposed to obese) person. Independent of consciousness and will, this control system determines what and how much a person will eat and at what point he will stop. Homeostasis is maintained when the intake of food matches the energy expenditure, as modified by cold weather, exercise, growth, pregnancy, and so forth. This matching of CALORIES eaten and calories spent is in direct proportion to the nature of the diet; in other words, normal people tend to eat approximately as much as they need *and no more*, so that the weight and the body reserves, at any given time, are essentially in balance.

As the body cannot, and does not, function without the mind, and as neither dominates the other, either one can be the *primary* or the *secondary* cause of illness. For instance, the stomach, as instructed by the autonomic nervous system, responds to fear or anger, but while doing so it may not conduct digestion properly; a dysfunction has been created. Conversely, a single imperfection in the metabolism may be at the root of a psychosis. Whenever the body-mind network is no longer synchronized, homeostasis is disrupted.

HORMONES

A hormone is a chemical substance that is secreted into the body fluids by an endocrine (internally secreting) gland and which has a specific effect on the activity of other organs that are remote from its point of origin.

HUMECTANTS

Humectants refer to smooth substances such as glycerin which are added in small quantities to MOISTURIZERS and CLEANSERS to improve their consistency.

Humectants are lubricants; they make the skin feel soft and smooth. However, unlike moisturizers, large quantities of humectants will actually *dry up* the skin because they absorb and retain moisture themselves.

Humectants are particularly undesirable for delicate skin when the air is dry, for they tend to sponge up whatever moisture is available from the skin itself.

HUMIDIFIER

A room humidifier is a rather simple device meant to correct one of the problems of temperature and humidity extremes—the overly dry air provided by most indoor heating systems, which can be particularly deleterious to human skin.

The colder the air, the less moisture it can hold; thus, when cold air is heated, its ability to hold moisture increases. This means that, when air is heated, the RELATIVE HUMIDITY (the amount of moisture in the air as compared with the maximum amount that the air could hold at the same temperature) will decline unless moisture is added. Suppose that the outdoor temperature is 20° F. and the relative humidity approximately 80 percent; when this air enters a house where the temperature is 75° F., the relative humidity may fall to 10 percent simply because the air's capacity to hold moisture has increased enormously. It is the relative humidity, not just the amount of moisture present, that determines whether people feel either very dry or very clammy.

One of the most elaborate kinds of humidifiers is that installed near a furnace and tapped into the water supply. However, with a steam-heating system (which utilizes circulating hot water) or with rooms that are individually heated by electricity, a self-contained, portable humidifier may be more efficient. It can be plugged into a wall outlet and should be placed in the middle of the apartment or near a staircase. If it is placed near an outside wall, the moisture tends to migrate into the wall's insulation space, condense, and freeze on cold days, reducing the insulation's effectiveness. However, many apartments and recently built houses are equipped with a so-called vapor barrier—a continuous plastic film, metal foil, or asphalt sheet placed between the walls and the insulation.

Humidifiers are generally classified as *evaporative* and *atomizing* types. The evaporative type consists basically of a fan forcing air through a wetted pad, evaporating moisture from it. The pad is a spongy elastic belt that rides the rim of a large drum or follows a roller-driven course through a water reservoir, which has to be refilled once a day. The atomizing model consists of a centrifugal pump that sprays water on a fixed pad which circles the pump. The best are those that blow the moist air straight up or at a wide upward angle—a draft from the front is not pleasant. Both types are equipped with a humidistat that, after being set, will automatically turn the humidifier on and off, keeping the humidity in the room constant.

Some models specify their humidifying capacity in cubic feet, but of course the estimate is only approximate, since other factors such as climate, air-exchange rate and so forth would have to be considered for a more precise determination of humidifying capacity.

Humidifiers should be stored empty of water, and the pad and reservoir should be periodically cleaned, because they may become clogged by mineral residue in the water (especially in hard-water areas).

For a short while in the mid-1960s, humidifiers were believed to give relief to ASTHMA, as an alternative to vaporizers, but the claim is no longer made, not even by the manufacturers of humidifiers. However, humidifiers are indeed useful in replacing some of the moisture needed by the human skin.

HYDROGENATION

Hydrogenation is a process whereby hydrogen is chemically added to FAT or OIL, not only to prevent rancidity and chemical decomposition (oxygenation) but also to increase the degree of saturation (a fat may be described as saturated or unsaturated depending on the number of hydrogen atoms in the molecule).

Labels usually don't mention whether a fat or oil has been hydrogenated, although this information really is not important. What *is* important to know is the proportion of saturated and unsaturated fatty acids that are present in a product, because saturated fats tend to raise the level of CHOLESTEROL in the blood, whereas unsaturated fats apparently lower it.

There are millions of people who are now deliberately eating unusually large amounts of unsaturated fats in the hope of forestalling or preventing coronary heart disease. However, there is no concrete evidence that a high level of unsaturates in the diet is beneficial or even harmless. For one thing, body tissues utilize more saturated than unsaturated fats and maintain a ratio of about three to one in favor of the former. If cholesterol were really harmful, a physician said recently, nature would not have put so much of it in the human brain.

HYPEROPIA (FARSIGHTEDNESS)

Usually called farsightedness, hyperopia is the direct opposite of MYOPIA. In this condition, light rays are intercepted by the retina *before* they come into focus. The focused image of a near object will fall *behind* the retina.

Convex lenses add focusing power and relieve some of the strain on the eye, thus producing clear vision without effort.

HYPERSOMNIA

Hypersomnia is the opposite of INSOMNIA. It is characterized by too much sleep, difficulty waking up and a tendency to escape from tension, anxiety or any crisis at all by going to sleep.

Sometimes hypersomnia is a symptom of serious emotional trouble: deeply depressed people often sleep excessively. As is the case with insomnia, this sleep disturbance is often complicated by the use of drugs.

"This oversleeping may be a good deal more common than we know," write Gay Gaer Luce and Dr. Julius Segal in *Insomnia*, "for sleep is an escape, and insomnia is not. . . . Even an unrefreshing, sudden sleep may generate less complaint than the inability to retreat into oblivion."

HYPERTENSION

Hypertension means, literally, elevated blood pressure. It refers, not to a *temporary* rise in blood pressure—which may be caused by excitement, exercise, too much coffee or lack of rest, as well as by a meal or cold weather—but to blood pressure that is *consistently* too high.

The degree of the pressure of blood on the walls of the arteries depends on the energy of the heart's action, the elasticity of the vessels, and the volume and viscosity of the blood. The maximum pressure occurs during the contraction—systole—of the left ventricle of the heart; the minimum, during dilation—diastole—of the ventricle. It is the increase in the diastolic pressure that is the key to hypertension.

Blood pressure is checked by wrapping around a patient's arm a sphygmomanometer—a cloth cuff with a dial, a rubber bulb, and tubes. This instrument indicates the pressure required to raise a column of mercury in a tube marked in millimeters; if the mercury in the sphygmomanometer rises to 120 mm, it means that the patient's blood pressure is 120.

Since recording blood pressure is painless and takes less than a minute, in theory the diagnosis of hypertension should be easy. In practice, however, 50 percent of the more than twenty-three million people in the United States who suffer from hypertension don't know they have it, and less than 10 percent are being effectively treated. The reasons are several: first, not all physicians check blood pressure routinely; second, the blood pressure of healthy people varies considerably with their age and, to some extent, with the time of day, which makes it difficult to define who is "normal" and who should be considered "hypertensive." In older people, for instance, higher levels of blood pressure are acceptable, even necessary to ensure an adequate blood flow in the aging body. And finally, many people are reluctant to consult a physician, or are unable to relate their HEADACHE, NAUSEA, anxiety, INSOMNIA, irritability, tendency to weep, PAINS in the arms, legs or back to hypertension—or worse, have no symptoms at all.

Blood pressure may rise abnormally essentially because of an increased resistance of the arteries to blood flow as a result of the thickening of the arterial walls. (The thickening consists of deposits containing CHOLESTEROL, which reduces the elasticity in the walls, which, in turn, increases the diastolic pressure.) Hypertension is called *essential* when the problem doesn't seem to have a direct cause and may simply have existed at birth, as part of a person's genetic makeup. Even people who seem to develop hypertension late in life almost always have shown a normal-to-high blood pressure in their youth. Hypertension is called *secondary* when the problem can be traced to some specific cause, such as a malfunctioning kidney or a tumor. Ninety-five percent of all cases of hypertension are essential; only 5 percent are secondary. The latter can often be corrected by surgery, but there is no easy solution yet for essential hypertension, other than drug therapy and life-long control. Untreated hypertension may be the cause, in part, of stroke, heart or kidney failure, and heart attack.

Many theories have been advanced in the last fifty years about the causes of hypertension, but to this day very little is known for sure. Essentially, scientists agree that hypertension is inherited; that men and women suffer it approximately in the same proportion, though women seem to tolerate it better; and that blacks are affected twice as much as Caucasians. Also, they agree that heavy smoking, high cholesterol levels in the blood, OBESITY, diabetes, lack of exercise, chronic anxiety and, in general, the strain of life today may worsen hypertension, though none of these can raise blood pressure to hypertensive levels.

For two decades it has been known that drug treatment of severe hypertension is very beneficial. Until a few years ago, however, it was believed that the preferable drugs were those which reduced the resistance in the arteries. In the early 1970s physicians discovered that the most effective hypertension drugs are those which primarily influence the heart's output of blood. Experiments with rats have shown that when the heart's output is reduced, the arteries' thickness is eventually reversed and hypertension cured. But it is still uncertain whether this is also true for human hypertension.

At present, antihypertension drugs have improved enough so that practically all cases of essential hypertension can be controlled; patients can lead lives of normal length and intensity with relatively small inconveniences. Even side effects such as feelings of depression, muscular cramps, upset stomach, dry mouth, and weakness usually can be corrected by lowering the dosage or using a different drug.

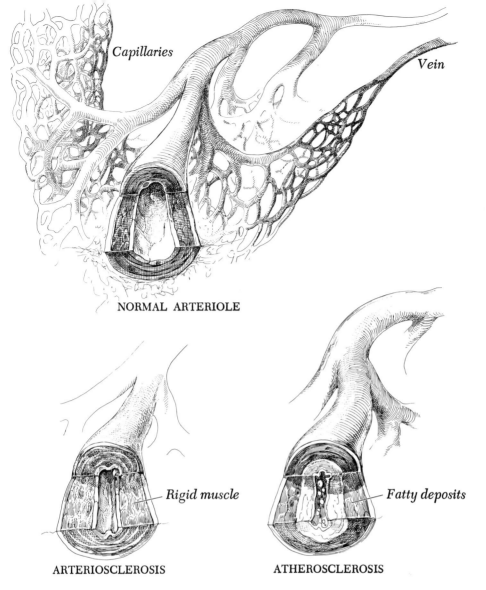

Capillaries

Vein

NORMAL ARTERIOLE

Rigid muscle

Fatty deposits

ARTERIOSCLEROSIS

ATHEROSCLEROSIS

Above: Arteries are tubular vessels into which blood is delivered from the heart to the various parts and organs of the body. Arteries branch out into arterioles, in which the outer coating is increasingly reduced, and ultimately into capillaries, which possess only the innermost endothelial layer.

Arteries and arterioles have thick, muscular, and elastic walls which, by expanding and contracting, constantly adjust to the blood pressure generated in the heart and transmitted into them, thus allowing for the smooth flow of blood throughout the body.

From the capillaries, the blood is carried back to the heart by the veins, which are thinner and much less elastic than the arteries, and are therefore provided with valves, to prevent the reflux of blood.

Left: An arteriole showing a reduced elasticity, hardening and thickening of its walls, a condition called arteriosclerosis.

Right: An arteriole with deposits in its inner lining of yellowish plaques containing cholesterol, a condition called atherosclerosis.

Arteriosclerosis and atherosclerosis are primary causes of hypertension: respectively, the loss of elasticity and the narrowing of the vessel channel limit the free flow of blood, thus giving rise to a pressure build-up.

183

Mild hypertension is easily controlled with a diuretic, which lowers the SODIUM content in the blood, and a small dose either of reserpine, a potent alkaloid obtained from the root of rauwolfia, a tropical shrub, or of methyldopa when depression or peptic ulcer contraindicate the use of reserpine.

Moderate hypertension often improves with the diuretic/reserpine (or methyldopa) combination. If this fails, hydralazine or guanethidine can be added to the diuretic and reserpine.

Severe hypertension requires higher doses of reserpine or guanethidine combined with a diuretic.

Accelerated hypertension is a medical emergency requiring immediate therapy, such as intravenous injections of diazoxone and other drugs administered under a physician's strict supervision.

Whatever the choice of drugs, physicians also advise the hypertensive patient to exercise, eat moderately, and, in order to avoid the vicious circle of worrying about hypertension and thus aggravating it, to be calm if at all possible.

HYPNOTHERAPY

Hypnotherapy has been a successful form of medical treatment for many centuries, yet only recently has it begun to be taught adequately in schools of medicine and to gain popularity as a legitimate addition to conventional therapy. The reason is that for a long time hypnosis had an aura of magic or of quackery; even today, some people still associate it with *stage* hypnosis, which brings to mind a Mephistophelian hypnotist calling a shill (or is it an innocent spectator, after all?) out of his seat in the audience.

Indeed, there is no accepted explanation of hypnosis—is it a state of altered susceptibility? Of super-concentration? A different state of consciousness similar to yoga or meditation? We still don't know, but we *do* know that hypnotherapy is *not* a form of sleep or an evil means of imposing thought control. We know what it can do and how to use it in reducing the pain of setting fractures, of changing a wound dressing. Hypnotherapy helps soothe anxiety and tension. It is used in the treatment of MIGRAINE, INSOMNIA, OBESITY, impotence, frigidity and motion sickness, and to help people overcome such psychologically oriented problems as heavy drinking, smoking, stuttering and nail biting.

However, in certain cases, such as CHILDBIRTH or PSYCHOSOMATIC DISEASES, hypnotherapy doesn't always work. Also, incompetent utilization of the trance state may bring superficial relief but ultimate harm by blocking out important symptoms. Finally, some feel that patients might develop an "addiction" to hypnotherapy. And although it is easier to

184

teach a person to hypnotize another than, say, to teach a policeman to deliver a baby, many doctors are reluctant to use hypnotherapy: they fear that it spoils the physician-patient relationship should the latter not respond to the trance!

Hypnotherapy works best with subjects who are intelligent, alert, psychologically healthy, and accustomed to a certain degree of discipline and concentration.

A successfully hypnotized person undergoes three basic states of mind: 1) compulsive compliance with the therapist's suggestions; 2) amnesia of the hypnotic experience; and 3) rationalization of his altered behavior. And since hypnosis is a multilevel phenomenon—it can be *light, medium* or *deep*—the more the subject moves into the trance, the more striking the modification of his behavior. Conversely, a *light* trance "is hardly more than a state of greatly increased physical and psychological relaxation, with an increased tendency to respond to suggestions of the therapist," in the words of Dr. James R. Hodge, head of the psychiatry section of Akron City Hospital, in Akron, Ohio.

There are many techniques to induce a trance, but usually it involves eye fixation; concentration on some object or event; elimination of external stimuli; and repetitive, soothing instructions by the therapist. Trance induction itself is the easiest step; the difficult stage of hypnotherapy comes once the patient has moved, smoothly and cooperatively, into the trance. It is at that point that the hypnotherapist functions successfully *as a therapist*—as long as he keeps the patient's clinical history well in mind.

HYPOCHONDRIASIS

Hypochondriasis refers to a morbid preoccupation with one's body and an exaggerated concern over physical health. A hypochondriac is usually obsessively aware of the functions of a specific organ or body process, and is convinced that he is incurably ill, though no organic sickness can be demonstrated. And even if the patient has a physical disorder, his worries are excessive, because the hypochondriacal symptoms play a major role in his life.

Hypochondriacs are more numerous than people usually think: every physician is familiar with this kind of patient, for although many of these need psychiatric help, they usually won't admit it.

The term hypochondriasis has many meanings. It can be: 1) a *symptom* of a variety of illnesses, such as depression or anxiety; 2) a *trait* of a childish personality; 3) or itself an *illness*, in which case hypochondriacal symptoms are a major feature of the patient's personality, literally incorporated into his way of talking and living.

Hypochondriasis is *not* a PSYCHOSOMATIC DISEASE, because, unlike HYPERTENSION, peptic ulcer, and ARTHRITIS, it does not have a somatic (physical) component. Hypochondriasis, therefore, is not always easy to recognize; inexperienced doctors especially may find it difficult to resist the patient's demand for examination and may tend to search for an organic disease. What a hypochondriac is looking for is a doctor who will understand him, not cure him of symptoms he is literally in love with. Reassurance and understanding for the patient's problems is practically all a physician can do, unless he has knowledge of PSYCHOACTIVE DRUGS and has experience in the prescription of antidepressants and tranquilizers, with which he can ease a hypochondriac's underlying depression or anxiety.

HYPODERMIC NEEDLE

This is a form of hollow needle used to inject liquid medication beneath the skin. It can also be used to inject liquid SILICONE during PLASTIC SURGERY and to aspirate fluid from CYSTS, or blood from a VARICOSE VEIN before treating it with a SCLEROSING SOLUTION.

HYSTERECTOMY

Hysterectomy means the removal of the uterus. This is a major operation that can be performed either through an incision in the abdominal wall or through the vagina. After she has undergone a hysterectomy, a woman can no longer menstruate or become pregnant.

Most frequently, hysterectomy is done because of the presence of fibroids, benign tumors of the womb. Less frequently, hysterectomy is necessary because of malignant tumors of the uterus, of the ovaries, or of the FALLOPIAN TUBES. If the benign tumors do not grow rapidly or to a large size, and if they do not cause other problems, most gynecologists feel that nothing need be done about them. In some cases—young women or women desirous of having more children—a more conservative approach may be indicated, i.e., removal of the fibroids alone with preservation of the uterus. This procedure, called myomectomy, cannot always be done, for it has a higher postoperative complication rate than hysterectomy, and the anticipated final result is frequently not achieved.

There are three kinds of hysterectomy: 1) *subtotal hysterectomy*, in which the body of the uterus, the fundus, is removed but the cervix is preserved; 2) *total hysterectomy*, in which the entire uterus (fundus *and* cervix) is removed; and 3) subtotal or total hysterectomy and *unilateral or bilateral salpingo-oophorectomy*, in which the uterus *and* one or both tubes and ovaries are removed.

If only a hysterectomy is done (without removal of the ovaries), no physiological, endocrine, or physical changes will take place, since the ovaries—the sources of the female sex hormones—are still in place. In some unusual situations, however, hysterectomy may have a psychological effect, that is, the woman may view the loss of her womb as a loss of femininity.

If the tubes and the ovaries are removed, a woman will no longer ovulate and will undergo those changes that occur with MENOPAUSE. During hysterectomy in women under forty, in whom the ovaries appear to be normal, the surgeon usually will choose to preserve the tubes and the ovaries. In this way, he tries to avoid castration and its effects. If the ovaries are removed, the beneficial effects of the female hormones can still be achieved by injectable or oral medications.

Most gynecologists do not perform hysterectomy for the sole purpose of sterilization, since the operation is a major one, not without risk or side effects. A hysterectomy may be suggested if other uterine pathology is present or if other contraceptive methods cannot be used or are inappropriate.

Occasionally hysterectomy may be done as a prophylaxis against future cancers of the uterus or cervix in "high-risk" patients, i.e., women who have repeatedly abnormal pap smears; women with abnormal bleeding problems, especially those who are also diabetic, obese, or hypertensive; women who have borne many children; women who have had multiple sexual partners, etc. At any rate, hysterectomy is a major surgical procedure that should never be undertaken lightly by patient or by surgeon.

I

ICHTHYOSIS (FISH-SCALE SKIN)

Ichthyosis is a rather common hereditary skin condition characterized by a dry scaling and thickness of the skin that resembles fish scales.

Ichthyosis ranges from mild to severe and usually appears shortly after birth. It often improves during puberty, a time when oil glands are very active, and is accentuated with aging, when even normal skin becomes drier.

There is no cure for ichthyosis, but a good dermatologist has the means of improving the excessive dryness and scaling of the skin.

IDIOPATHIC DISEASES

An idiopathic disease is, literally, a sickness peculiar to the individual, which, translated into lay language, means that the physician is not sure what the cause is.

IMMUNOLOGY

Immunology is a relatively new science that deals with the phenomena and causes of immunity. The existence of a natural defense mechanism in the human body—the immune system—has been known since the 1890s, when two German chemists, on the basis of the already known concept of vaccination, discovered the presence in the blood of ANTIBODIES that chemically fight invading antigens.

During the past twenty years, immunology has been linked with almost every branch of medicine and has brought extraordinary new insight into medical research in general. The immune system is now known to be crucially involved in fighting a vast number of diseases ranging from microbial infections to ALLERGIES, rheumatism, cancer and many other degenerative disorders of aging.

The immune system is dispersed throughout most of the tissues of the human body. It consists of millions of cells called lymphocytes—a type of white blood cell—and of antibodies, which are molecules made of blood PROTEINS called gamma globulin. Both lymphocytes and antibodies decay and renew themselves continuously.

The immune system "patrols" the body by identifying and destroying any foreign cells that invade the organism. The lymphocytes recognize these cells by the antigens on their surfaces. In other words, among the millions of various immune-system units (lymphocytes and antibodies) there is usually a set that "matches" a distinct antigen, mingles with it, and eventually destroys it.

Not only does the immune system identify antigens produced by any of the millions of species of animals, plants and microorganisms, but it also can distinguish foreign antigens from those belonging to the molecules of its own body. This discrimination between *self* and *nonself* is called self-tolerance. Incidentally, self-tolerance is not innate; the healthy immune system "learns" it during embryonic life, at which time it either eliminates or paralyzes all lymphocytes that could result in self-destruction. If a lymphocyte, after identifying an antigen, cannot become stimulated into producing antibodies (either because of the antigens' too high or too low concentration, or because the antibodies do not fit exactly with the antigen), it becomes paralyzed, or "suppressed."

Scientists feel that once they know more about the mechanism of lymphocyte paralysis, they will understand not only how the immune system learns to tolerate the antigens of its own body but also how the system is able sometimes to induce the organism to tolerate organ transplants.

Some lymphocytes have their origin before birth in the bone marrow and are called B-cells, while others are found in the thymus and are known as T-cells. The B-cells ultimately give rise to the antibodies, while the T-cells act on their own to attack foreign antigens. These cells are beneficial in attacking foreign bacteria, viruses and cancer cells, but unfortunately they are harmful when they attempt to destroy transplants of organs.

Lymphocytes and antibodies reach most tissues through the bloodstream, entering the tissues through the walls of the capillaries. After moving about in the tissues, they make their way back through a system of their own—the lymphatic system—whose vessels collect them (along with the lymphatic fluid and other cells and molecules) and pour them back into the bloodstream.

The immune system is comparable in the complexity of its functions to the nervous system. Both are diffuse organs, and both are unique in their ability to respond to an enormous variety of external signals. Their cells can both *receive* and *transmit* signals, and these can be either stimulating or inhibiting. The two systems penetrate most of the other tissues in the body, but they seem to avoid each other—lymphocytes *never* come into contact with nerve cells. Both systems adapt to the outside world and learn from experience, so to speak, building up a memory that is sustained by reinforcement but cannot be transmitted to the next generation.

The immune system can be mobilized and a person rendered immune to a disease by the injection of a VACCINE, a substance that contains a small amount of the germs of the disease that are dead, weakened, or else altered in such a way that they are unable to cause serious illness. The body reacts to these harmless germs by stimulating the specialized lymphocytes to produce a great number of T-cells and antibodies. Later, should the person come in contact with the disease, the body will have the antibodies to fight it.

INJECTABLE CONTRACEPTIVE
(MEDROXY PROGESTERONE ACETATE)

In the winter of 1973–74, the limited use of an injectable contraceptive was approved by the Food and Drug Administration. The drug is called medroxy progesterone acetate; its brand name is Depo-Provera.® For women who dislike CONTRACEPTIVE PILLS or suffer from their side effects, an injectable contraceptive may be more pleasant and still provide long-term protection against pregnancy.

The FDA has required that Depo-Provera® be labeled in such a way as to advise unequivocally both physicians and patients that, while the drug is clearly effective in preventing pregnancy, when its use is discontinued, it may either present the risk of infertility or allow a woman to become pregnant only after an interval of many months.

Before 1973, medroxy progesterone acetate already was marketed for treating cancer of the uterus; and physicians have known for a while that, if given at intervals of about three months, this drug could also act as a contraceptive.

As of 1975, however, Depo-Provera® has become controversial, and the FDA has reversed its approval, after reports of an increased incidence of cervical cancer in connection with the use of this contraceptive. The drug is currently being reanalyzed.

INSECT STINGS

Every year many persons are stung by insects of the class *Hymenoptera*, which includes bees, wasps, hornets and yellow jackets. Some people feel just a simple discomfort; others, especially if stung by many insects at the same time, react to the toxic properties of the insect's venom the way they would to a snakebite; still others have allergic reactions to the sting, which in extreme cases may result in shock and death.

There are two main kinds of bees: the social, such as the honey and bumble bees; and the solitary, such as the carpenters, the miners, and the mason bees. Of these, only the honey bee loses its life when it stings; therefore, it never stings in self-defense but only in defense of the hive. Wasps (which include hornets and yellow jackets) and all other bees sting not only in defense of the hive but also if they are merely disturbed.

The mechanism of allergic reactions to insect stings is not completely understood, but apparently the venom injected into the body by the sting acts as an allergen. After one or more stings, the allergen causes sensitizing ANTIBODIES to be produced in the body, which are then deposited in the tissue cells or remain in the blood. Each stinging insect contains its specific proteins, but all contain some that are similar, which means that if a person is sensitive to one insect he may be sensitive to others.

Reactions to insect stings vary. Apart from the extreme shock, moderately allergic people may react with large swellings, faintness, cramps, shortness of breath, wheezing, or a stuffed nose. The *emergency* treatment for an acute allergic reaction to insect stings is an immediate injection of adrenalin, the only drug that will prevent shock. Cortisone and antihistamine tablets are useful but act too slowly in an emergency situation.

There are *preventive* treatments available for people who are already aware of their sensitivity to insect stings. One such treatment is desensitization, a series of immunizing injections that often consist of a mixture of the venom of four insect species, since the insect causing the allergic reaction may not be known.

Desensitization, however, is recommended mostly for people who have serious reactions involving areas of the body distant from the sting. If the reactions are limited to the site of the sting, the physician's prescription at the time of the sting is sufficient.

INSOMNIA

Insomnia means inability to sleep. When it is transitory, there is no real problem—everybody experiences occasional sleep disturbances and is able, eventually, to adjust to a new environment, a different work shift or an uncomfortable bed, or to recover from an illness, fear, grief or voluntary sleep loss.

For some, however, insomnia may be a chronic symptom of physical or emotional trouble. Itching, chronic cough, powerful drugs prescribed for other ailments—each may contribute to poor sleep. Insomnia may also be an early sign of depression or severe anxiety, or may accompany the euphoric cycle in manic depression. And sleep loss alone produces its *own* physiological and psychological symptoms; prolonged insomnia can produce FATIGUE, hallucinations, and some of the manifestations of psychosis.

Still, insomnia is a misnomer, for *total* lack of sleep does not exist, except for people with rare diseases or injuries to the nervous system. And even though a person may claim he cannot sleep at all, he actually does sleep for a good part of his "sleepless nights." This does not mean that he is lying but rather that the series of repeated cycles of brain and body activity occurring during NORMAL SLEEP has been disrupted, for any of a variety of reasons. This is particularly true in the case of an elderly person because of the altered activity of the central nervous system and the changes in metabolism that occur in old age.

Sometimes insomnia can be treated simply by improving a person's sleep environment. A physician may recommend sleeping alone in a ventilated, dark, quiet room; making a conscious attempt to slow down mental activities toward evening; taking a warm bath; having a light meal with a light alcoholic drink, while avoiding drinks containing caffeine. He may also suggest that the patient spend his sleepless hours doing something fruitful or pleasant, rather than anxiously awaiting sleep. Above all, the doctor may recommend that, rather than trying to conform to other people's sleeping styles, the patient respond to his own internal cycles of alertness and torpor.

Indeed, people have individual sleeping styles and pre-sleep rituals that are almost as distinctive and just as unconscious as handwriting. Some people have to check all faucets and locks, for instance, before they can "surrender" to sleep; others need to be naked or warmly clothed, or lie in the exact center of the bed, with a night light or in complete darkness. Still others must wash their feet, have a last cigarette, drink a glass of milk, exorcise their fear of sleep/death by concentrating on elaborate images, etc. More important, people differ in the amount and depth of sleep they need: some regularly sleep eight to ten hours, others require only five or six; some sleep only at night, others prefer frequent naps throughout the day. There are light sleepers and heavy sleepers; selective sleepers, who are awakened only by certain sounds; early risers, whose body temperature climbs swiftly in the morning; and "owls," who are physiologically timed to perform best in late afternoon.

People vary, too, in the types of sleep disturbances they experience. A person may have one or more of these symptoms: inability to fall asleep or stay asleep; frequent nighttime or early-morning awakenings, or awakenings in the middle of a dream; lack of satisfaction with sleep; constant feeling of fatigue. If a physician decides to prescribe sleeping pills (not all forms of insomnia improve with drugs, and some worsen), these have to be selected specifically for the particular kind of sleep problem. For example, a fast-acting, short-lasting drug is suitable for a person who has trouble falling asleep but useless for someone who awakens often during the night. Conversely, a drug with a delayed but prolonged action is right for a person who awakens too early.

Hypnotic drugs—sometimes loosely called sedatives, since high doses of certain sedatives might put a person to sleep (incidentally, still higher doses might act as ANAESTHETICS)—function by reducing, in various degrees, the activity of the nervous system. Hypnotic drugs include:

1) *Barbiturates*, such as secobarbital, pentobarbital, amobarbital and dozens of others—all members of the same chemical family, but with different qualities and marketed under different brand names;

2) *Nonbarbiturates*, such as chloral hydrate, glutethimide, ethchlorvynol, methyprylon, methaqualone;

3) *Major tranquilizers*, such as chlorpromazine, whose primary use is as an antipsychotic drug;

4) *Minor tranquilizers*, such as chlordiazepoxide and diazepam, which are primarily antianxiety drugs;

5) The so-called *monoamine oxidase inhibitors (MAO)*, which are antidepressant drugs;

6) *Antihistamines*, which are chiefly used in treating allergy but which may also produce drowsiness and sometimes sleep;

7) Nonprescription hypnotics, compounds which usually consist of an antihistamine, a mild sedative such as scopolamine, potassium bromide or passion flower extract, and, for no apparent reason, VITAMINS.

These are all valuable chemical compounds when they are expertly used, but the ideal hypnotic—one that would provide quick action and sufficient duration of sleep, with no habituation, withdrawal, hangover or disruption in the pattern of normal sleep—has yet to be formulated.

Besides sleeping pills, insomnia can be treated with HYPNOTHERAPY, electrosleep and relaxation EXERCISES.

In hypnotherapy, a suggestion is planted in the mind of an insomniac that will help him to dissociate himself from the anxiety, stress or whatever it is that causes his wakefulness, allowing him later to fall asleep. Incidentally, many people, without realizing it, often use some form of autohypnosis to put themselves to sleep—concentrating on the rhythmic hum of a jet's engines, for instance, which allows them to sleep even on the uncomfortable seat of a noisy plane.

Electrosleep is an instrument developed about twenty-five years ago by Russian scientists, equipped to direct a very mild electrical stimulation at the lower region of the brain. Electrosleep does not produce sleep at the time of the electrical stimulation but apparently induces patients to relax and fall asleep *after* the treatment.

Relaxation exercises consist of teaching anxious insomniacs to become aware, one by one, of the muscles of their feet, legs, abdomen, shoulders, and face, and to contract and relax each one separately and progressively (in a manner not unlike that used for women undergoing PREPARED CHILDBIRTH), so that they can differentiate between tenseness and relaxation and consciously decide to relax. This in turn slows down the kind of frantic mental activity that keeps anxious people awake.

Much of the insomnia that people suffer from, then, is *voluntary*, especially for those who rely on drugs to make up for the excessive and disorderly use of their energy resources, thereby establishing a vicious circle of sleeping pills and stimulants. In the near future, doctors may treat insomniacs, not by prescribing hypnotics, but by teaching them—perhaps with such techniques as BIOFEEDBACK—what the good sleeper instinctively knows that he should do: tune into his own physiological cycles and respond to his body's own periods of activity and repose.

INTERFERON

Interferon is one of the many substances produced by the body. It acts like a natural antivirus and is now being produced in the laboratory as a remedy against the COMMON COLD and influenza.

Interferon is an ideal antiviral substance: it is nontoxic, does not stimulate the production of antibodies and seems to be effective against a wide range of viruses.

Interferon acts, not directly on viruses, but on cells, making them resistant to viruses. There are two ways in which interferon could be utilized in the treatment of disease: 1) by administering an "inducer" that would stimulate natural interferon production in the body (under appropriate stimuli, all cells can be made to produce interferon for a few hours); or 2) by directly administering synthetic interferon. For the moment, however, a nontoxic and effective inducer has not been found; as for synthetic interferon, it has thus far been difficult to produce enough of it for commercial use.

INTERTRIGO

Derived from the Latin verb *terere* (to rub), intertrigo refers to the area of skin in obese people that is chafed by friction of adjacent surfaces, such as under the breasts, in the groin, or between the thighs.

INTRAUTERINE DEVICE (IUD)

The IUD is a tiny, flexible object, usually made of plastic or metal, which is placed inside the uterus to prevent pregnancy. An IUD is usually inserted by a gynecologist. This can be done at any time, but it is easier when the cervical opening is slightly dilated—after childbirth or ABORTION, for instance, or during MENSTRUATION, which, incidentally, excludes the possibility of pregnancy at the time of insertion.

The device is compressed into a thin tube inserted into the uterus. A plunger pushes the device out of the tube and it springs back into its original shape.

Some IUDs have a small thread attached that projects from the uterus into the vagina far enough to be felt by the patient, to verify whether the IUD is still in the uterus. However, some physicians feel that the thread may be an irritant and/or may increase the risk of infection, because it connects the sterile uterine cavity with the vagina, which is contaminated by external bacteria.

The ancestors of the IUD comprise such heterogeneous materials as cork, wood, ivory, glass and pewter, as well as pebbles (for female Arabian camels), twisted pieces of paper (for ninth-century Persian women) and gold and silver pessaries (for sixteenth-century French

Left: Photomicrograph (original magnification: 80 times) of a cross-sectioned string from an old model of the Dalkon Shield®, made up of a bundle of fibers enclosed loosely within a plastic sheath.

Right: Photomicrograph (original magnification: 21,000 times) of a space between three fibers within an old model of the Dalkon Shield®. Visible are the bacteria that this type of string allowed to proliferate and invade the uterine cavity of women who had been fitted with it.

As of 1975, the design of the Dalkon Shield® has been modified to a single-fiber string. *Courtesy of Dr. Howard J. Tatum, The Rockefeller University, New York City.*

women). Finally, in the 1930s, a German gynecologist devised a silkworm gut knotted into the shape of a ring. By now it had a modern shape, but the insertion of a foreign substance into the uterus still provoked all sorts of side effects and, ultimately, expulsion.

The modern IUD did not appear until the 1950s, when a group of Japanese physicians successfully began to use a ring made of biologically inert substances such as nylon and polyethylene. No one knows exactly how or why the IUD works. One of the current theories is that the device causes the EGG CELL to move down the FALLOPIAN TUBES so rapidly that when it arrives in the uterus it is not yet ready for implantation. Another theory is that the IUD provokes a mild, nonbacterial inflammation of the endometrium (the lining of the uterus), resulting in the production of an unknown substance with a spermicidal action. For some women, the IUD is the ideal contraceptive: its use is removed from the sex act; it is almost as efficient as the CONTRACEPTIVE PILL; it requires practically no effort to use, unlike the Pill, which a woman must remember to take every day; and it does not interfere with menstruation or fertility. In fact, once inserted, it can be forgotten until the following yearly check-up.

There are some disadvantages: about 35 percent of the women who try an IUD cannot tolerate it. Either the body rejects it, or it simply makes a woman uncomfortable. Worse, it sometimes causes a pelvic infection, vaginal infection, and, in rare cases, perforation of the uterus. However, these problems are in most instances quickly detected, and the IUD can be removed by simple surgery. Almost everybody complains of cramps after the IUD is first inserted, and heavy bleeding between menstrual periods lasts a few months. Often, all that is needed is to switch to another shape (or size) of IUD.

Among the IUDs currently in use are the fin-shaped Dalkon Shield®, the Lippes Loop®, and the Safe-T-Coil®. Recently perfected and apparently safer and more effective are the Copper-T 200®, the Copper-7®, the Y-shaped Ypsilon®, and the Progesterone-T®. Still being studied is a fluid-filled IUD. The Majzlin Spring®, which used to be quite popular some years ago, was seized in the spring of 1973 at the recommendation of the Food and Drug Administration because it was determined to be unsafe.

In 1974 the FDA also required that the sale and distribution of the Dalkon Shield® be suspended, following reports of 209 cases of septic (infectious) abortions and eleven maternal deaths in women using this IUD. However, the FDA did not recommend removing the Dalkon Shield® from women who reported no trouble with it.

Subsequently, Dr. Howard J. Tatum, associate director of the biomedical division at Rockefeller University in New York City, conducted a study that showed that all IUDs' strings—except that of Dalkon Shield®—"consisted of either a single or a double segment of monofila-

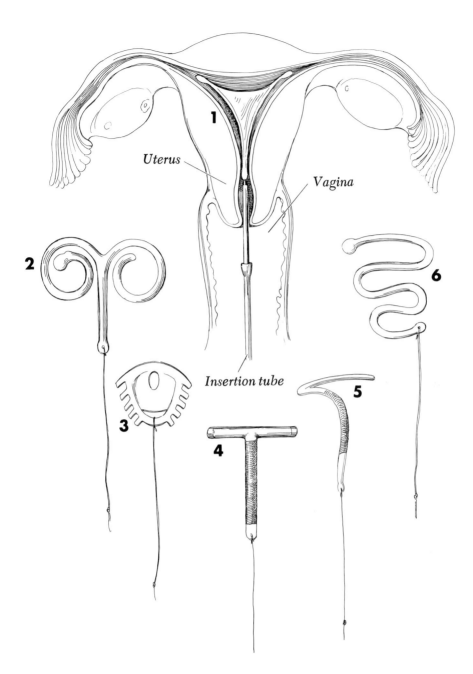

Uterus

Vagina

Insertion tube

1) YPSILON®
2) SAFE-T-COIL®
3) DALKON SHIELD®
4) COPPER-T®
5) COPPER-7®
6) LIPPES LOOP®

ment plastic thread." The Dalkon Shield® utilizes a single string consisting of a bundle of monofilaments enclosed freely within a thin plastic sheath. Both ends of this string are open.

The structure of this string immediately suggested to Dr. Tatum that it might function as a wick for fluid containing infectious bacteria. In 1975 it was announced that the string of the Dalkon Shield® would be modified to the monofilament type of other IUDs.

Copper-T 200® is a T-shaped device made of polyethylene impregnated with barium sulfate. A spiral of pure copper wire is attached to the vertical arm of the plastic. The horizontal arms of the T serve to anchor it high in the uterus wall, the fundus, so that the insert can be pulled out without further pressure. Since the Copper-T® is small, it can be inserted easily, without dilating the cervix, which reduces the bleeding and pain often accompanying insertion of an IUD.

The copper apparently alters ENZYMES in the secretion of the endometrium, making it "inimical to sperm," as they say in medical papers. Moreover, the copper, which experts are sure will be used in most IUDs of the future, may offer some indirect prophylaxis against GONORRHEA, unlike inert IUDs such as the Lippes Loop®, which offers no protection against venereal diseases. Body rejection is rare, but a few perforations have been reported. The Copper-T® must be replaced approximately every two years because the copper dissolves with time. Most of it is lost in menstrual blood.

A new, long-acting variation of the Copper-T® is being studied, the TCU 220®. It has copper sleeves instead of wire, which should slow down the rate of copper dissolution.

Copper-7® is similar to the Copper-T®; it, too, is made of plastic and has a copper wire wound around it. Only the shape is different: a 7 instead of a T.

Ypsilon® has been developed by Dr. Samuel Soichet, professor of obstetrics and gynecology at Cornell Medical College of New York. This is a Y-shaped IUD made of inert, medical-grade SILICONE rubber, capable of reaching from the cornua (the opening of either side of the uterus, leading to the FALLOPIAN TUBES) to the cervical canal. The stem of the Y is made of soft silicone; the arms have tiny beaded ends large enough to fit the cornua. A fine web connects the arms, allowing the device to adapt to any uterus, regardless of its tilt, barely touching the walls, thus avoiding any excess pressure.

The silicone causes minimal or no inflammatory reaction of the tissue.

The contraceptive mechanism of the Ypsilon®, too, is a mystery. Dr. Soichet theorizes that the Y's gentle pressure against the endometrium somehow promotes the production of a substance that, in turn, stimulates certain changes in the uterus and the tubes, thus preventing pregnancy.

Two different sizes of the Ypsilon® are now available: the smaller is for women who have never borne children; the larger, for women who have an unusually large uterus or who have recently experienced childbirth. The Ypsilon® has an extremely low rate of expulsion and *not one single perforation*. A few pregnancies occurred when too small a size was used. If a woman wishes to remove the Y, she can be instructed to do it herself, by pulling gently on the device's slender silicone tail.

Progesterone-T® was designed by Dr. Antonio Scommegna, of the Michael Reese Medical Center in Chicago. The device is T-shaped and is designed to continuously release minute quantities of progesterone. Based on the observation that, after an egg cell is fertilized, natural progesterone is cyclically released to transform the lining of the uterus into the so-called decidua—tissue suitable for the egg's growth—the synthetic progesterone released by this device causes premature development of the decidua, thus disrupting the cycle and either preventing implantation of the egg cell or expelling the already implanted cell.

Women continue to ovulate normally, with no alteration in the menstrual pattern. Body rejection is rare; bleeding and pain are minimal. Progesterone-T® can be left in place approximately one year; after that it must be replaced, since the amount of progesterone it can contain is limited.

A fluid-filled IUD is being studied by Dr. Jack M. Futoran of San Francisco. It is a nonrigid IUD filled with a saline solution after insertion to "custom fit" the uterus. The pouch, made of silicone rubber reinforced with Dacron mesh, is in the shape of an inverted isosceles triangle, measuring 28 mm along its base and 35 mm along each leg. A thin silicone tube runs out from the point and is used to inject the saline solution, up to a maximum of 0.6 cc.

After insertion, the saline solution is injected until the device fills the uterine cavity. After filling, a knot is tied in the tube.

IRON

Iron is one of the minerals essential to human health, even though the amount required each day is relatively small. Iron was the first among the so-called micronutrients (another is VITAMINS) for which a specific need was recognized. In fact, the metabolism of iron was generally understood before the discovery of many currently known vitamins (for more than one hundred fifty years, iron salts have been successfully used to treat patients with ANEMIA due to iron deficiency), yet even now gaps remain in the knowledge of iron metabolism and the exact nature of iron deficiency.

Iron is needed by the body to produce hemoglobin—a PROTEIN

substance that constitutes the pigment of red blood corpuscles—which has the function of transporting oxygen to the muscles throughout the body. Iron is stored mostly in the bone marrow, the liver and the spleen in two forms, ferritin and hemosiderin. Conservation is one of the most important characteristics of iron metabolism: within the body, there is a constant exchange of iron between bone marrow, red blood cells, and other tissues. One percent of red blood cells is destroyed every day, releasing about 20 mg of iron, 90 percent of which is reutilized to make more hemoglobin.

Iron is widely distributed in nature and is found in some amount in most foods. Since the average diet in the United States contains ten to twenty times the minimal daily requirement of iron (about 1 mg for men, but 2 mg for women because they lose iron during MENSTRUATION), deficiency should never be a problem. However, 1) only 10 percent of the iron in food is actually absorbed, because iron tends to form bonds with various food substances and cannot be absorbed in the bonded form; 2) the stored reserve of iron is 800 mg for men and 300 mg for women; 3) 1 mg is lost daily in the feces, urine, sweat, and bile, with women losing an additional 1 mg a day; 4) iron absorption is influenced by, among other things, the rate of red-blood-cell production, *independent of* the body's iron content. Incidentally, the amount of iron lost through menstruation is nearly *doubled* when an INTRAUTERINE DEVICE is in use, compared to the amount lost by women using oral CONTRACEPTIVES.

Thus, some doctors feel that simple nutritional deficiency—not enough of the food rich in iron—is almost never the cause of anemia in adults, and are opposed, for instance, to adding iron to enriched flour as unnecessary and perhaps dangerous: the *more* iron present in the blood, the *less* it can be absorbed; conversely, iron deficiency (during pregnancy, for instance) causes increased absorption and is the only case in which an iron supplement should be prescribed.

J K

JEJUNOILEOSTOMY

Jejunoileostomy, also called intestinal bypass, is an operation that attempts to reduce the efficiency of the intestines of pathologically obese people so that a considerable portion of the food eaten will be wasted.

At the University of Southern California, the University of Minnesota, and Vanderbilt University, medical researchers have for the last ten years conducted elaborate studies in the cautious selection of the appropriate patients for intestinal bypass, the evaluation of the surgical procedure, the investigation of the metabolic results, and the possible complications.

I say *appropriate* patients because intestinal bypass is not a miracle cure for all overweight people who wish to lose weight without having to go through the torture of dieting. Surgery may be advisable only for a few severely obese people who cannot adhere to DIETS or establish new eating habits, and whose health is in danger because of the almost inevitable risks of diabetes, HYPERTENSION, coronary artery disease, and a shortened lifespan.

Each of the three research teams has developed its own procedure, but all three agree on the operation's basic principle: reduction of the small intestine's length in order to diminish the *surface* of the intestine and the *time* for absorption of food. They also agree that the reduction should be performed in the jejunum (the first two-fifths of the small intestine) and in the ileum (the last section of the small intestine), and that the ileocecal valve (the one-way valve at the junction of the small and the large intestine) should be preserved.

Intestinal continuity is restored either by uniting the shortened jejunum to an appropriate point of the ileum, or by first connecting the two segments of the jejunum and the ileum with a procedure called anastomosis, and then connecting it directly to the colon in the large intestine.

In either case, the bypassed segment is not cut off, in order to make possible the reestablishment of normal bowel anatomy should it become necessary. The original concept was that a patient would lose weight steadily and continuously and that in time the normal continuity of the bowel could be reestablished. But all researchers at the three centers agree that this is not necessary, since the functioning segment of the jejunum eventually assumes the absorbing capacities of the bypassed segment. Restoration is performed only in those cases in which side effects become intolerable to the patient.

The major side effect is diarrhea, which usually lasts a few months and can cause an excessive fluid loss and a depletion of potassium and calcium. Also, certain patients are disappointed to discover that they will never become really slender. However, the loss of weight is always dramatic—sometimes hundreds of pounds! Not all surgeons are yet capable of performing this still experimental surgery; but, as often happens with certain daring medical discoveries, it is the enthusiasm of lay people that provides the incentive to scientists to perfect their techniques. However, in the case of intestinal bypass, a tempting operation for people who are physically grotesque, surgical techniques and understanding of the enormous metabolic risks still have a long way to go.

JET LAG

Most people who travel by air across large time zones suffer—often for several days—from jet lag, a SYNDROME which may include a slight sense of unreality, memory lapses, depression, constipation, wakefulness and hunger at unusual hours, as well as brittle nails, roughened and greasy skin, and oily hair.

"Jet lag," a *Medical Tribune* editor once wrote, "is like leaving your endocrine glands at home asleep while you try to cope with a wakeful world thousands of miles away."

For people who frequently travel by jet, such as pilots, stewardesses, businessmen and politicians, jet lag may worsen into jet fatigue—a gradual progression of HEADACHES, burning or unfocusing eyes, gastrointestinal problems, loss of appetite, shortness of breath, INSOMNIA and, occasionally, nightmares, and, for women, menstrual irregularities. All symptoms usually disappear when these people take a respite from flying.

In general, although individuals vary widely in how well they adapt to jet travel, the body's susceptibility to jet lag is greater than most people think. Scientists and airlines have been concerned with jet lag for many years, but only in 1969 was a controlled study of jet passengers' physical and psychological reactions first attempted. In this study, which was organized by Trans World Airlines and Syntex Laboratories, Inc., a pharmaceutical company, eight men and six women were flown from London to San Francisco; samples of their blood and urine were taken around the clock, their blood pressure and heart rates monitored, their alertness tested, and their sleep patterns recorded on an EEG.

The physical and chemical findings for the nine-hour time shift these volunteers had undergone indicated that all body systems are disturbed by major time-zone changes; that it takes at least seven to ten days for temperature, pulse, and breathing rate to resume their normal patterns in the twenty-four-hour day; and finally, that disturbances of sleep are a major cause of distress in most travelers.

Psychological tests showed, too, that most jet travelers' manual dexterity, coordination and speed of reaction time, judgment and reasoning power, and quickness of decision are affected to some degree.

Finally, the study showed that there is a clear difference in the duration of jet lag depending on whether one flies east or west. The period of adjustment to a time-zone change is at least five days when traveling east to west; seven days or more, west to east. One possible explanation is that, since many of the body's physiological functions follow a pronounced circadian rhythm—a daily rhythm of activity and rest—the whole biological clock mechanism is upset when the light-dark cycle is interrupted. For the same reason, jetting down the lines of longitude seems to be less disruptive than along lines of latitude, because the sun rises and sets at the same time, no matter how long the trip.

KELOIDS

Keloids are benign tumors that sometimes develop along the edges of healing wounds, burns, surgical incisions, infections, or even INSECT STINGS.

Normal fibrous tissue grows to form new COLLAGEN and to unite the edges of a wound, but in the keloid it continues to grow abnormally. The resulting scar is thick, tough, sometimes painful and with whitish ridges.

Keloids develop most frequently on the chest, face and neck. They are very rare on eyelids, arms, or legs, and they are more common among blacks and dark-skinned Caucasians; for some reason, blond people almost never suffer from keloids.

When keloids are just slightly raised, a cortisone cream is enough to control them. When keloids have been present in an area for some time, injections of cortisone are more effective; but when they are very large, excision combined with cortisone therapy is the best solution.

KOHL

Kohl is a cosmetic that has been used from the earliest times in the East by women to darken the eyelids, in order to add to the eyes' brilliance. It is usually made of finely powdered antimony, but soot obtained from burnt almond shells or frankincense is also used.

Like HENNA and other exotic preparations, kohl is periodically revived as a "natural" COSMETIC. In general, however, it can be used to good effect only by women with black hair and eyelashes. For all others, the subtler shades of modern cosmetics are usually preferable.

L

LACTATION (BREAST-FEEDING)

For centuries, all over the world, nursing a baby has been a phase of every mother's life. But in the last thirty years, proper refrigeration, pasteurization of cow's milk, and nutritionally sound formulas have given mothers a choice between breast- and bottle-feeding their babies.

In the late 1960s, however, the trend of bottle-feeding—which in this country apparently still appealed to lower-middle-class and immigrant women as one of the advantages of a technologically advanced society—began to lose appeal among middle- and upper-class women.

For some women, breast-feeding is not only natural but a pleasure; others are reluctant, apprehensive, or simply eager to learn about its "technique," which for a long time few had the authority to explain. This lack of information accounts for the extraordinary success in the last several years of La Leche League, the organization that began in 1956 with a conversation between two mothers at a picnic in Franklin Park, Illinois. These women, having happily nursed their own babies, decided to help other mothers through publications, telephone conversations, and personal correspondence. At present, La Leche ("leche" is Spanish for "milk") comprises more than one thousand groups throughout the United States and other countries.

In flawless sanitary conditions and temperate climates, there seems to be little difference between breast-fed and bottle-fed babies. However, human milk seems to have several physiological advantages: it can never be contaminated by bacteria and it is always ready, always the right temperature, always of the same consistency. It is more digestible than cow's milk and less likely to provoke allergylike reactions in the baby. More important, human milk may well have immunological significance, i.e., it may contribute to the formation in the baby of ANTIBODIES from the mother's system, preventing such illnesses as polio and influenza. Also, as a baby needs much more energy to extract milk from his mother's nipple than from a bottle's rubber nipple, from which milk usually flows a little too freely, his jaws and gums develop better; he learns proper swallowing habits, and he will have less chance of teeth problems in adult life.

Breast-feeding is generally better psychologically, too: for one thing, the baby gains a lasting sense of security from the warmth and closeness of the mother's body while suckling her milk. But if a woman truly resents nursing, she will communicate her nervousness to the baby, in which case, naturally, a bottle formula is preferable.

As for the mother, though lactation is not a guarantee against pregnancy, she is less likely to become pregnant while nursing, because the baby's continuous suckling maintains in her body high levels of prolactin, the hormone released by the pituitary gland immediately after childbirth. Prolactin causes the breasts to produce milk for as long as they are suckled and tends to suppress ovulation.

Also, lactation acts on a woman as a kind of sexual stimulation. Some of the responses are the same as those occurring during intercourse: erection of the nipples and discharge of oxytocin, another pituitary hormone that, besides facilitating the flow of the milk from the ducts to the milk pool beneath the nipple, causes the uterus to contract and therefore to return more rapidly to its prepregnant size.

The most common reasons why women hesitate to breast-feed are fear of not being able to nurse (i.e., fear of not having enough milk for the baby's diet, or of not being able to produce rich enough milk); fear of developing sagging breasts; fear of being relegated to the home twenty-four hours a day for months; fear of developing sores on the nipples because of the baby's too-vigorous suckling or biting, and embarrassment at having occasionally to expose the breast in public.

But the well-informed mother knows that her milk is always right for her baby (even if it looks thinner than cow's milk), that the baby's suckling will stimulate the production of enough milk for his needs, and that anxiety about nursing may interfere with her let-down reflex, the hormone-regulated mechanism that starts the production of milk. She knows, too, that breast changes occur with pregnancy, regardless of nursing; that breast sores, if treated properly, heal quickly; and that babies can be taught not to bite. "Sioux Indian mothers," notes Sally Wendkos Olds in *The Complete Book of Breastfeeding*, "still thump their babies when they bite the breast. The babies turn blue in the face with rage—but they learn not to bite." The mother may prepare an occasional "relief" bottle in case she has to leave the house for more than three hours; this bottle may contain either a ready-to-feed formula or a small amount of her own milk that she has previously pressed out, either by hand or with a little electric pump, and refrigerated. And finally, a button-front BRASSIERE, a loose-fitting cardigan unbuttoned from the bottom, and a strategically placed scarf make decorous nursing clothes.

For about two days after delivery, before starting to produce true milk, a woman's breast releases colostrum, a thick, yellowish fluid that contains more PROTEIN, MINERALS, VITAMIN A and nitrogen and less FAT and sugar than milk, and which usually contains antibodies as well—the ideal first food for a newborn baby.

During the first few days after delivery, some women may experience an engorged breast, which means that one or more milk ducts are blocked and the milk cannot pass through. This is usually caused by swelling of tissue, increased blood circulation in the breasts, and the pressure of newly produced milk. The engorged breast improves as soon as the baby begins to suckle vigorously and often. In addition, a woman can press the milk out after each feeding so as to empty the breast more thoroughly. In more severe cases, in order to avoid mastitis (breast infection), the doctor may prescribe synthetic oxytocin to facilitate the flow of milk through the ducts, or diethylbestrol, an estrogen compound, to inhibit milk production temporarily. Because of this property of estrogen, CONTRACEPTIVE PILLS are never prescribed for a nursing woman.

There is no definite time for weaning; a mother and her baby know instinctively when it is time to stop nursing. But whenever weaning seems advisable—after seven or eight months, one year, or sometimes even two years—it should be done gradually and gently over a period of several weeks. In this way, neither the baby nor the mother will feel discomfort: the baby slowly becomes used to being spoon-fed, and the milk pressure in the mother's breasts gradually diminishes until it stops.

LANOLIN

Lanolin is a fatlike substance that adheres to wool fibers and is secreted by the oil glands of sheep. It has been used for years as a base for creams, ointments, hand lotions, shaving creams, SHAMPOOS and various other cosmetics because of its emollient and emulsifying qualities, i.e., it promotes softness of the skin and facilitates the mixing of ingredients that do not mix readily. In other words, when used in the proper concentration, lanolin makes creams spread and adhere more perfectly.

A few people have been found to be allergic to lanolin, and some dermatologists claim that the recent trend toward "glossy" types of eye and lip cosmetics (which contain a more refined type of lanolin oil rather than ordinary lanolin, which usually contains a certain amount of WAX) is responsible for increasing incidence of DERMATITIS. However, most dermatologists and chemists dispute this claim, and while they concede that some people may be allergic to certain types of lanolin (and the cause of the allergy may be related to something as remote as the breed of sheep the lanolin was extracted from!), they feel that the instances of allergic reaction are too infrequent to cause concern.

LAXATIVES

Laxatives, the remedy for constipation, are a very popular medicine in the United States. Most of them are available without prescription. They are sometimes abused by people who attribute excessive importance to punctual, regular daily bowel movements and who mistakenly think that a small upsetting of this routine is a sign of constipation. In reality, constipation is a medical problem caused by different disturbances that bring about an inability to move the bowel.

Strong laxatives are called cathartics. The most common are saline mixtures—magnesium sulfate, milk of magnesia, sodium phosphate, potassium phosphate—which attract fluid into the bowel by osmosis and cause a fluid evacuation.

Milder laxatives such as cascara, castor oil, and phenolphthalein act by increasing intestinal motility, whereas mineral oil and dioctyl sodium sulfosuccinate soften the stool; however, finely emulsified mineral oil can traverse the bowel wall so as to interfere with the absorption of fat-soluble VITAMINS.

Psyllium seed and certain foods such as bran and prunes are natural laxatives that act by increasing the bulk of the stool, thus compensating for a lack of an adequate amount of bulky food in the diet, a requirement for normal bowel activity.

One must take care in using laxatives. If food is hurried through the digestive tract with a laxative before it can be fully digested, the body not only loses water, sodium and potassium salts but may become dependent on the laxative. Constipation should be treated by first finding the underlying cause; this may be something as serious as appendicitis, in which case laxatives are dangerous. But irregularity often is simply a consequence of eating improperly, not drinking enough water, leading a too-sedentary life, or not heeding the so-called gastrocolic reflex (the contractions in the colon induced by the entrance of a large quantity of food in the empty stomach). In these cases, too, laxatives are superfluous.

LECITHIN

Lecithin is one of the phospholipids, fatlike substances containing nitrogen, fatty acids and phosphorus that are found in animal tissue (especially nerve tissue), semen, egg yolk and, in smaller amounts, bile and blood.

One of lecithin's properties is that of a natural emulsifier—it helps FAT mix with WATER in the body—and as such it is active in the metabolism of fat in the liver.

The commercial form of lecithin is extracted mostly from SOYBEANS. It is used as an emulsifier and an emollient in COSMETICS—COLD CREAM, SOAPS, lipsticks—and in foods such as margarine, mayonnaise, and chocolate candies to maintain the stability of the oil ingredients. It is also added to fish oils that have been enriched with VITAMINS A and D.

Lecithin has been, and still is, a favorite among health-food enthusiasts, who recommend it as a food supplement (either by itself or mixed with vitamins and other supplements) because it supposedly breaks up and disperses CHOLESTEROL in the blood, thus preventing the cholesterol from accumulating in the arteries (atherosclerosis). There have also been claims that lecithin can be effective in the treatment of ARTHRITIS and HYPERTENSION, and in improving brain power.

However, many doctors and nutritionists do not believe that supplements of lecithin in the diet have any effect in lowering the cholesterol level in the blood. For one thing, the exact mechanism by which cholesterol is deposited in the arteries is not fully understood; also, there is no evidence that lecithin can prevent atherosclerosis. However, neither is there any evidence that lecithin is harmful to health.

LIFESPAN

Every living being has a duration of existence that is characteristic of the species to which it belongs—a few minutes for a bacterium; a few days for an insect in its winged phase; a few months for an annual plant; a few score years for man; a few centuries for a sequoia tree.

LIPECTOMY

Lipectomy generally means excision of fat tissue. Most commonly, it refers to a number of PLASTIC SURGERY procedures for the removal of excessive fat in the chin, the abdomen, or the thighs and buttocks.

Excision of fat from the chin is usually called SUBMANDIBULAR LIPECTOMY, while excision from the thighs and buttocks is often referred to informally as the "RIDING BREECHES" OPERATION.

Abdominal lipectomy is indicated when the abdomen, as a result of frequent pregnancies, old scars, sudden weight loss or predisposition, has become so flaccid that no amount of MASSAGE or EXERCISE can ever correct it. In this operation the surgeon draws, with surgical ink, a vertical guideline from the pubic hairline through the navel up to the ribcage, dividing the abdomen exactly in the middle. The incision line is drawn horizontally along the pubic hairline, continuing on either side across the inguinal fold and curving slightly downward. The surgeon then undermines the skin all the way up to the ribs in order to prevent later tension on the suture line. The skin around the navel is split and the navel circumcised and left solidly attached to the deeper tissue so that it will receive a good blood supply. If the abdominal muscles, too, are very flabby, the surgeon must reinforce them by opening and then vertically suturing the membranes covering them (the aponeurosis) in order to tighten and realign the outspread muscle fibers. This procedure will slim the waist and give the abdomen a graceful contour. The skin is then pulled downward, and the amount of skin and fat to be excised is calculated.

After a temporary suture has been placed in the midline, the new, higher position of the navel is calculated and a small incision made to mark the location. The navel is then surfaced through the incision and sutured delicately into place.

A padded dressing, topped by well-balanced weights (which should not hamper respiration), is applied to help the skin adhere evenly to its bed in order to prevent swellings. The dressing is removed after one or two days.

As for the "riding breeches" operation, here, too, general ANAESTHESIA is required. However, convalescence is shorter: only three or four days in the hospital. Sutures are removed after about ten days, but the patient should not exert herself or carry heavy objects for at least four weeks.

LITHIUM CARBONATE

Lithium is a ubiquitous, highly reactive, silvery-white alkaline metal used in nuclear technology. It is present in countless mineral springs—from Montecatini, Italy, to Lithium Springs, Georgia—where it still takes the credit, as it has for decades, for curing such conditions as gout, renal calculi, and rheumatism.

Lithium carbonate is the most widely used of the lithium salts, as it contains the most lithium. It is an extraordinary PSYCHOACTIVE DRUG, currently used in the treatment of manic depression, the enigmatic, cyclical mental disturbance in which a person seems to go through a periodic transformation of character—from a state of ebullience (the *manic cycle*, marked by compulsive speech, dangerous elation, overactivity, no need to sleep) to one of apathy and desperation (the *depressive cycle*) and back again, relentlessly.

Dr. Ronald R. Fieve, chief of psychiatric research at the New York State Psychiatric Institute at Columbia Presbyterian Medical Center, is a pioneer in lithium research. In 1970, under the aegis of the New York State Department of Mental Hygiene, Dr. Fieve became head of the first lithium clinic in the United States, where, together with an interdisciplinary team, he has been conducting a series of metabolic and genetic studies. Some of these studies have already dramatically demonstrated what had been merely supposed: at least one form of manic depression is genetically transmitted by an anomalous gene on the female CHROMOSOME.

As a treatment for manic depression, lithium carbonate is unique in that, unlike other psychoactive drugs that either calm anxiety or uplift depression, it reduces the duration and the intensity of *both* the manic cycle and the depressive cycle. Thus, lithium acts as a prophylactic, i.e., it prevents the recurrence of the disease.

Lithium does not cure mood disorders the way an antibiotic cures an infection; a single dose has no effect. The drug's therapeutic properties depend on its continuous presence at a certain minimum level in certain tissues of the body. At present, the rules for using lithium are empirical, based mainly on the experience gained in clinical practice and on findings of animal studies.

Lithium is given orally in the form of a tablet or capsule. From the stomach, it enters the bloodstream rapidly and almost completely: less than 1 percent is eliminated in the feces. From the bloodstream, lithium is carried easily around the body into various tissues, at different rates for different tissues—quickly into the kidney, more slowly into the liver, very slowly into the brain.

Lithium also differs from other psychoactive drugs in that it rarely produces any undesirable effects on emotional or intellectual functioning. However, lithium may at first cause some temporary physical side effects such as NAUSEA, diarrhea, thirst, FATIGUE and sleepiness.

Manic depressive people are often highly successful, energetic and creative. In the mild form of the disorder, many of these patients refuse to continue with lithium carbonate therapy because they feel that this drug—which so effectively normalizes a person's mood, putting him on a more even keel—acts as a "brake," preventing their productivity and interfering with their careers. Others feel that the manic phase is often so enjoyable that, rather than eliminate or limit it, they prefer to take their chances and hope that a depression will not occur afterward. Still others are loath to accept lithium therapy as a lifetime need, since the mere idea suggests permanent commitment to a drug, periodic blood tests, and the stigma of an incurable illness, which they attempt to deny by discontinuing therapy after several months of use.

For the most part, though, manic depressive patients accept lithium and are cooperative, both in taking the drug and in permitting control of the lithium level in the blood at regular intervals.

LOOFAH

Loofah is the fibrous part of the pod of a tropical gourd. It is used as a slightly abrasive sponge to rub away the dead cells of the skin surface.

Loofah is thin and flat but swells up like a sponge when wet. It is available in its elongated, slightly irregular natural shape; as a strap with two handles; or in the form of a bath mitten, sometimes with the rough, natural loofah on one side and terrycloth on the other.

Loofah is most pleasant when used with soap in a warm bath. Occasionally, though, it should just be rubbed delicately—without using soap—over the entire body, including the face, to make the skin smooth without depleting it of its natural oils.

M

MALE CONTRACEPTIVE PILL

In 1974 Dr. C. Alvin Paulsen of the University of Washington developed a sperm-reducing (from a normal one hundred million to two hundred million to less than fifty million per ejaculation) drug compound that produces a temporary infertility in men *without* causing side effects—including any diminishing of the sex drive.

This male oral contraceptive, which is expected to be ready for the general public around 1980, will probably consist of a daily pill containing a *small* dose of androgen, the male hormone. Supplementing the pill will be a monthly injection of a *large* dose of androgen.

MAMMOGRAPHY

Mammography, one of the methods for early detection of BREAST CANCER, is simply the projection of an X-ray image of the breast's soft tissue on photographic film. It does not have total accuracy in determining the difference between benign and malignant tumors—sometimes, for instance, the tumor may not show sufficient density to be visible on X-ray film, especially in premenopausal patients—but with good technique and interpretation, it can be about 85 percent accurate. Mammographies are particularly accurate in detecting cancer in older patients and progressively less so the younger the patient is.

In the detection of tiny lesions, several projections from different angles are necessary. The accuracy of mammography has been improved in the last few years by the use of an apparatus called Senograph®, which was designed specifically for mammography.

As far as X-ray exposure is concerned—one of the reasons why many gynecologists still hesitate to recommend mammography as a routine breast cancer check-up—new units are being devised that reduce the amount of radiation. But even now, in the words of Dr. Henry P. Leis, Jr., clinical professor of surgery and chief of the breast surgery service at New York Medical College, "a yearly mammogram for twenty-five years would only give about the same amount of radiation as is used in treating bursitis of the shoulder."

Recently a new technique has been developed by Dr. Gilbert Baum, director of the ultrasound laboratory at New York City's Albert Einstein College of Medicine. It is called ultrasound mammography, and it apparently can identify breast masses with less danger to the patient and provide more information than the X-ray mammogram. The ultrasound mammogram is made by flashing to the breast a beam of high-frequency sound waves such as those used in sonar devices. The returning echoes

This is a mammogram, i.e., an X-ray image of a breast's soft tissue on photographic film. It is that of a sixty-year-old patient of Dr. Herman C. Zuckerman, a well-known New York radiologist.

Although mammography is one of the methods for early detection of breast cancer, in this case the patient came to Dr. Zuckerman when she already had a large carcinoma in her right breast (clearly visible in the X-ray), which required an immediate radical mastectomy.

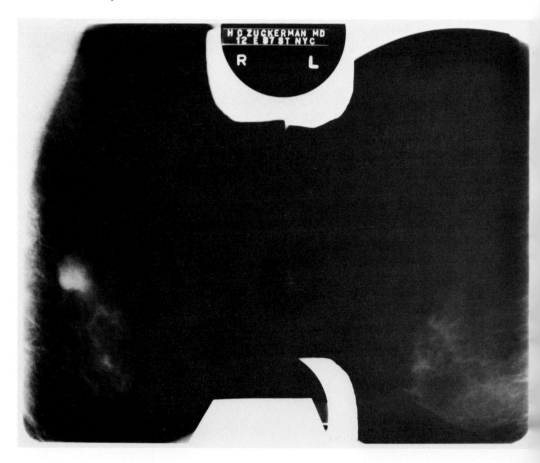

are then converted into images, which are displayed on a television screen and which represent a three-dimensional cross-section through the breast skin to the chest wall. Computerized equipment supplies a gray scale to give a smooth image similar to a black-and-white photograph (the X-ray provides only a silhouette), with the denser regions of the breast appearing darker on the screen. Because the difference among the shades of gray used are difficult to perceive, the picture is then converted to color, also by computer, with each color representing a specific echo intensity. The result is an extraordinarily clear picture of the breast's internal structure. Weaker echoes show up at the blue end of the spectrum; strong echoes are at the red end.

Tumors give a weaker echo than healthy tissue and are immediately apparent on the color-coded mammogram as unnatural yellow areas with shadows behind them. Different kinds of breast masses give different ultrasound pictures. CYSTS, for example, are characteristically round and have a tail.

At present ultrasound mammography has not been developed enough to permit the sound to be transmitted into the breast through the air. The breast must be immersed in a tank of saline solution through which the sound is beamed.

MANICURE

Manicure is the cleaning, shaping and polishing of the nails and the moisturizing and massaging of the hands.

Hands, much like hair and skin, reflect the body's health. When a person suffers from some disease, infection, or deficiency, the growth and appearance of nails can change. And nails can have conditions of their own: bacteria and fungi, for instance, may invade nailbeds and the soft tissue that surrounds them.

Hands reveal a person's age and give a good clue to his daily occupation and to the kind of manicure he receives—every stage from total neglect to frequent, professional care. Overmanicured hands are just as unattractive as neglected ones, not to speak of the infections, HANGNAILS, and uneven growth that a too vigorous manicure can cause to the delicate structure of the nails.

In the last several years, the scientific understanding of the nail structure has advanced considerably, as have nail preparations such as CONDITIONERS, mending preparations, polishes and removers, which are now on a par with many other COSMETICS. But the rules for a good manicure have remained the same for ages. The tools—clippers, curved scissors, files, buffers, cuticle scrapers—also have changed little over the years, both in shape and in function.

A modern professional manicurist still displays in front of a client a little table with a strong lamp attached to it, a small pillow covered with a clean towel, a bowl with lukewarm water and a mild soap—the same accoutrements listed in a once-popular turn-of-the-century booklet of instructions for the perfect manicurist. As a postscript, the author wrote: "Temperature of the hand is a matter to be noted by the manicurist, especially that of her own, since a cold or damp hand is unpleasant to a patron and might suffice to drive some away after one sitting."

As reasonable and well known as the rules for a good manicure are, people still need to be cautioned about the proper way to care for their nails. Periodically, women's magazines publish in their columns lists of "Dos and Don'ts" about nail care, without fear of being repetitive. For example:

Don't cut nails; *do* always file them with an emery board.

Don't cut cuticles; *do* push them back with an orangewood stick.

Don't use fingernails as tools; *do* use a pencil to dial a telephone.

Don't file nails back and forth; *do* file them toward the center and underneath the edge.

Don't immerse hands in too hot or too cold water.

Don't use polish remover too often.

Do soak nails in warm oil once a week.

Do use rubber gloves whenever handling chemicals or detergents, or when cleaning vegetables or dusty objects.

All of this is easy to do but tedious to remember. "Thank God there are very few perfect nails," noted, half-seriously, Elba Tamburino, one of the most sought-after manicurists in Manhattan. "To have perfect nails, a woman would have to wear gloves all the time and sit all day without doing anything with her hands. Real women, women who are alive, *never* have perfect nails!"

Most of these rules apply also to the care of feet and toenails—pedicure. Naturally, feet are more subject than hands to calluses, fungi and ingrown nails, and to conditions that are related exclusively to shoes or to walking habits. For this reason, the distinction between a pedicurist and a podiatrist—a foot specialist—is sometimes blurred. Though podiatrists usually frown on it, expert pedicurists are often perfectly capable of taking care of minor problems of the feet.

MASSAGE

The word massage refers to the pressing of the skin and the muscular parts of the body and exercising traction on the joints with the hands or with instruments such as a vibrator for therapeutic or hygienic purposes. Massage is essentially a *passive* exercise and is most effective and pleasant when performed by an experienced masseur on a body in repose. (There are, too, some *active* movements of massage, which consist of a special form of gymnastics, designed to exercise particular muscles or groups of muscles.)

Massage was extensively practiced by Arabian physicians, from whom it was probably adopted by the French, who are generally supposed to have revived this method of treatment, which has been practiced since time immemorial but has from time to time fallen into disuse in Western countries; in some places, it has even fallen into disrepute on account of its association, in the words of *The Encyclopaedia Britannica*, Eleventh Edition, "with vicious abuses." To this day, the basic massage strokes are usually referred to by their French names: *effleurage* (stroking); *pétrissage* (kneading); *friction* (rubbing); and *tapotement* (tapping).

Among the Greeks, Romans, Egyptians and, later, the Turks, massage came to be part of the ordinary procedure of the bath without any special therapeutic intention, and the usage has survived until today, when skillful masseurs are found not only in the physiotherapy department of large hospitals but at BEAUTY SPAS, salons and gyms, and are appreciated almost exclusively for the sense of well-being, relaxation and luxury that they can give to people through massage.

Many kinds of massage are practiced today—from the use of high-pressure hoses for massaging bodies submerged in water to the spinal manipulations of CHIROPRACTIC. In the United States, however, most masseurs use the so-called Swedish massage, based on a system developed in the early 1800s by Per Henrik Ling, a Swedish medical-gymnastic practitioner.

Each masseur usually works out his own technique and develops a very personal style. However, no matter what variation is used, the principle of the Swedish massage is essentially the same: the masseur moves the limbs while the patient resists, thus bringing the opposing muscles into play.

Effleurage—This is performed by stroking the body in the direction of the blood course in the veins, i.e., toward the heart. It can be done with any part of the hand—heel or palm, balls of thumbs or knuckles. The pressure exerted is as heavy as possible.

Pétrissage—"Kneading" or "rolling" in English, this stroke is executed by slightly lifting the large muscles of the back, arms, and legs from the bones, holding them between the fingers, and then allowing small portions of the muscle to slip through the fingers back to the bone. The pressure can vary from light to heavy, depending on the area and the effect desired. Kneading is often used to relieve spasms in the legs, arms and shoulders.

Friction—This stroke involves deep rubbing over large areas of the body. The pressure is heavy and exerted by palms flat on the skin with circular motions that increase in radius as the massage progresses. *Friction* is sometimes done with fingertips. It stimulates the flow of blood through the capillaries, and is beneficial for minor pains in nerves and muscles.

Tapotement—This is usually done toward the end of a massage session, because it is too energetic for a body that has not yet been manipulated. The masseur holds his hands rigid, with fingers close together and extended as far as possible. Holding his hands parallel, he strikes the skin with rapid, judo-choplike movements. The blows should be firm but not excessively so: the patient should never recoil. *Tapotement* is often used for the muscles of the abdomen, with the patient lying on his back with feet lifted just enough to tense the stomach muscles. The face, head, Adam's apple, collarbone, breasts, and genitals should never be tapped. Various techniques include consecutive fingertip, fingernail, and circular vibrating movements.

A skillful massage has a consistent, rhythmic pattern. The speed varies with each stage: slow for *effleurage;* consistent and moderate for *pétrissage;* optional for *friction;* and rapid for *tapotement.*

As a rule, OILS and other lubricants are not used, but several masseurs favor unscented oils, COLD CREAM or talcum powder, in order to smooth the skin and prevent irritation. Alcohol is also used for rubs to relieve PAIN in overexerted muscles.

A person should never receive a massage after a meal: the blood rushes to the stomach during the digestive process and should not be diverted and made to circulate faster in other parts of the body. Nor is a massage recommended for a person who is hungry and anticipating a meal. Immediately after strenuous exercise, it is always best to take a lukewarm shower first before a massage.

Despite the tendency on the part of some masseurs to exalt massage as a cure-all, there are conditions for which it is of no use at all. Torn ligaments, fractured bones, and dislocations do not improve with massage, though it may speed recovery once these conditions have been medically treated. Massage will not replace DIETS and EXERCISE in weight control; and there is little evidence that it strengthens or tones muscles, since it does not force them to contract. Massage of the scalp cannot restore hair, and there is no reason to believe it will "melt" away CELLULITE or help reduce frigidity or impotence.

A truly relaxing and pleasant massage is best received in a cool, quiet, well-ventilated room, at a time of day when a person has no pressing engagements on his mind. The masseur should be strong enough to do the work without obvious exhaustion—which may make a poor impression on the patient—and have a fine sense of touch and resistance so as to know exactly how much pressure to exert: too much will hurt and too little is ineffective. The masseur's presence should be pleasant but never overwhelming: his personality, at least during the massage, should be almost entirely concentrated on his massaging technique. An experienced masseur, for instance, never wears a distinctive PERFUME or after-shave lotion.

"When you find one [massage] you really like," *Vogue* magazine wisely suggested recently, "treasure the person who gives it, as it's all a matter of personal choice."

MASTECTOMY

Mastectomy, also called mammectomy, refers to the surgical removal of a breast because of cancer or painful, recurrent CYSTS.

Surgical procedures for patients with potentially curable breast lesions include:

Radical mastectomy—For nearly a century, this has been the accepted treatment of breast cancer throughout the world. It consists of the complete removal of the breast and of part, or all, of the three levels of lymph glands (or nodes) in the armpit, the chest, and behind the collarbone. The modern version of this surgical procedure is the so-called *modified radical mastectomy*, which preserves most or all of the chest muscles. Very few surgeons nowadays use the *extended radical mastectomy*, in which the chest muscles also are removed.

Simple mastectomy—This procedure involves the removal of the entire breast, but it preserves the lymphatic glands when these have not been infiltrated by malignant cells. However, it is not always simple for the pathologist to determine whether the lymph glands have been tainted.

Subcutaneous mastectomy—This is a procedure that has become popular only recently. It consists of removing only the breast tissue while preserving the skin and the nipple. Subcutaneous mastectomy is recommended for patients with so-called *premalignant* lesions, such as fibrocystic disease (also called cystic mastitis), fibroadenoma, and intraductal papilloma—three types of benign tumors that could eventually become malignant. The cosmetic defect can be easily corrected later with a SILICONE prosthesis, the same as is used for augmentation mammaplasty.

Partial mastectomy—This procedure, also called *lumpectomy*, is a local excision of the tumor with about one-third of the breast tissue. It is recommended only for a very few women with small, peripheral lesions. Lumpectomy was first presented in 1970 by Dr. George Crile,

Jr., emeritus consultant at the department of general surgery, Cleveland Clinic Foundation in Cleveland, Ohio, to the American College of Surgeons, as a less drastic alternative to radical mastectomy.

Lumpectomy became instantly famous (and controversial) among doctors and women throughout the country following an article by Dr. William A. Nolen in *McCall's* magazine. Dr. Nolen, the author of *The Making of a Surgeon*, reported Dr. Crile's innovation in such enthusiastic terms (without mentioning, for instance, that only *very* few cases of breast cancer qualify for lumpectomy) that many women began to believe that radical mastectomy was just a barbaric practice of the past.

Some of the most conservative surgeons are currently blaming lay magazines for endangering women's lives by urging them to become involved in decisions relating to their cancer treatment, rather than leaving the decisions entirely to the surgeon as in the past. But it is not entirely the magazines' fault: they have merely brought to public attention a controversy over treatment of breast cancer that has been going on since 1948 between the advocates of the traditional radical mastectomy and those who believe that partial mastectomy is less disfiguring and disabling and shows the same rate of survival as radical mastectomy.

Dr. Crile, one of the leaders of the second group, argues, for instance, that death from breast cancer is due to distant METASTASES and that in most cases the factors that regulate the spreading of a cancer seem to be beyond the control of either the surgeon or the radiologist. More important, Crile says, "in some kinds of cancer, lymph nodes act more as an immunological barrier to spread than as a source of dissemination."

A successful mastectomy means that a patient can expect to be alive and well at least five years after the operation. Five years is the somewhat unofficial line at which cancer specialists declare a "cure," although breast cancer is one kind of malignancy that can recur later. However, it is quite common for a breast-cancer patient to live for twenty to thirty years after her mastectomy.

MEDICAL KIT FOR TRAVELERS

The following basic items will provide most of the medical needs for one person on a two-week trip. Some people, of course, may want to substitute or add some drugs, depending on their individual prescriptions, their health history or their itinerary. For example, patients who wear glasses or contact lenses should have not only an extra pair but also the exact prescription of the correction needed. And the cardiac patient should have digitalis available in the handbag as well as in the medical kit in case luggage is lost.

For *aches and pains*	Codeine®		No more than once every 6 hours.
For *constipation*	Dulcolax® suppositories or milk of magnesia tablets		Use as directed.
For *diarrhea*	Kaopectate®		1½ tbls. followed by 1 tsp. after each bowel movement until diarrhea ceases.
For *gastrointestinal upset*	Donnatal®	30 tablets	1 tablet 4 times a day.
For *motion sickness*	Dramamine®	15 tablets	1 or 2 tablets 4 times a day.
For *respiratory infection* (cold, sinusitis, allergy, or other signs of respiratory congestion)—	Chlor-Trimeton®	14-16 tablets	1 tablet every 3 to 6 hours for minor symptoms.
	or Coricidin® decongestant	14-16 tablets	1 tablet every 4 hours (not to exceed 4 a day).
	or Benadryl®	10 tablets	50 mg tablet 2 or 3 times a day for more severe allergic symptoms.

The tropical traveler should add to these drugs the following items: disposable needles and syringes; salt tablets; insect repellents; a mosquito net; an antimalarial such as chloroquine; water-purifying tablets such as halazone.

And finally, a medical kit for travelers should contain adhesive tape, antiseptic, aspirin, sleeping pills, a thermometer, scissors, tweezers, bandages, gauze, sunburn lotion, a Red Cross first-aid book, and, when possible, a Blue Cross–Blue Shield membership card, together with information about the traveler's blood group and Rh type.

For women only: tampons, especially when traveling abroad; and, if the traveler takes CONTRACEPTIVE PILLS, an additional supply of her prescription—abroad, her brand of pills may not be available—in case her return home is delayed.

MENARCHE

A young girl's first menstrual period is called menarche. The age of onset varies widely—from ten to sixteen years of age, though it usually occurs between the ages of twelve and fourteen. If menarche has not occurred by eighteen, it is called "delayed menarche" and often implies some endocrine or psychogenic disorder. However, a physiological delay is relatively common, and it is up to the gynecologist to evaluate its exact causes before hastily administering hormone therapy.

The first sign of puberty is usually breast development—thelarche—and usually begins from nine to eleven years of age. As the first clinical sign indicating release of estrogen by the ovaries, breast development indirectly signifies that the link between the pituitary gland and the ovaries is intact and beginning to function.

Soon after thelarche, between eleven and twelve, the adolescent girl notes the appearance of pubic hair. Underarm hair does not appear until the growth of pubic hair is complete. At about the age of twelve, a sudden spurt of growth occurs in the girl's body, culminating in the onset of her first menstrual period. Menarche is therefore the last stage in a sequence of events, "a late status symbol of adolescence," in the words of a noted gynecologist.

After menarche, menstruation may begin at regular intervals of approximately four weeks, but only a small percentage of young girls start menstruation with such punctuality: usually it takes a minimum of a few months and a maximum of two years for regular menstruation to set in.

During the last century, the age of menarche onset has apparently dropped in western Europe and North America at the rate of about three or four months every decade. According to the Harvard Center for the Study of Population Growth, better nutrition makes women reach a crucial weight sooner. Once this weight is achieved—regardless of other nutrition-related factors such as height—a series of biochemical changes takes place that triggers the hypothalamus and the pituitary gland into starting the regulation of the reproductive cycle.

Pakistani researchers have an entirely different explanation. Investigating the old gynecology textbooks' observation that menarche occurs sooner in tropical climates, where daylight lasts longer, they demonstrated that young female mice kept under prolonged illumination have an earlier onset of puberty than those living in ordinary light.

On the other hand, there have been studies that have concluded that adolescents in northern Europe reach menarche more frequently in wintertime, and that blind girls reach it earlier than girls with sight.

These studies are contradictory only on the surface, for there is no doubt that light (or darkness) is a synchronizer of hormonal rhythms, and that the intensity, duration and quality of light have an influence on the menstrual cycle and the reproductive system in general.

MENOPAUSE

The term menopause refers to the end of a woman's MENSTRUATION, namely, the end of her reproductive years. Usually it occurs after forty, but it occasionally happens as early as twenty-five. In menopause, the ovaries stop releasing eggs and the body curtails production of female hormones, notably estrogen. These events may occur abruptly or over a period of time called climacteric.

Estrogen deficiency causes the skin to lose its elasticity and the vaginal mucosa to become dry and much thinner, which makes it more susceptible to infections. Though sexual energy remains the same, intercourse may become unpleasant.

Some women never experience premenopausal and menopausal symptoms—for them it literally means nothing more than the end of menstruation and, in certain cases, a pleasant relief from the fear of pregnancy. But many others have severe symptoms that can be traced to the nervous system and to metabolic or psychogenic causes. The adjustment period may last for years.

The main symptom of the climacteric is hot flashes: blood vessels dilate, sweat glands become overactive, and waves of heat sweep up from the breast to the face. Other symptoms are INSOMNIA, nervousness, palpitations occurring at rest, and an often irrational feeling of irritation, which may be a sign of estrogen deficiency. Some women become depressed, too, but some doctors believe that depression is not a symptom of hormonal deficiency: it is a psychosomatic effect that may be associated with the awareness of growing older. Others suggest that depression, too, may be connected with the decrease of estrogen activity.

There are four schools of thought on how to treat these symptoms:

1) One point of view is that menopause is a natural physiological event, and that no treatment should be given because of the side effects of the so-called hormone-replacement therapy.

2) There are those who consider menopause an endocrine-deficiency syndrome and believe that *every* woman over forty should be treated as a preventive measure, because estrogen in particular may prevent some of the manifestations of aging, especially postmenopausal skin atrophy, arteriosclerosis, and osteoporosis—deterioration of the bones, making them porous and dangerously fragile.

3) Another group maintains that menopausal symptoms should be treated for only a short period of time, i.e., as long as it takes to control them.

4) Gynecologists in general believe in treating most women who have symptoms and even women who have undergone HYSTERECTOMY (with the exception of women with a family history of BREAST CANCER or uterine cancer, with neurotic fear of HORMONES or with liver or circulatory problems). Hormone-replacement therapy, they feel, should be carefully dosed for the individual needs of the patient, should be frequently monitored, and should be sustained for as long as treatment is needed in the postmenopausal stage.

These doctors point out 1) that there is no evidence of any adverse effects from estrogen therapy, even if administered for years, as long as it is *cyclic*—three weeks on, one week off; 2) that there is no really good evidence that synthetic estrogen has prophylactic qualities (for one thing, it cannot restore lost bone, though it may prevent some of the excessive bone deterioration); 3) that it makes no sense to use estrogen therapy for a short period of time, because symptoms will reappear as soon as treatment is discontinued.

Estrogen is not the only hormone used in the hormone-replacement therapy; progesterone is sometimes added, especially when estrogen causes fluid retention in certain women. Moreover, the withdrawal of the progesterone during the one-week-off phase promotes the shedding of the uterine lining, just as happens when production of natural progesterone is slowed down to allow normal menstrual bleeding. Also used are small doses of methyltestosterone (a synthetic male hormone), which attenuates depression, increases the sense of well-being, and prevents overstimulation of the breasts by the other hormones.

Estrogen treatment, as mentioned previously, is best administered on a cyclic basis, as with certain CONTRACEPTIVE PILLS. Some doctors prescribe estrogen in tablets for twenty-one days, with estrogen and progesterone combined during the last seven days.

Like the oral-contraceptive users, menopausal and postmenopausal women may have changes in VITAMIN and mineral needs, though opinions vary here. Controversial, too, is whether hormone-replacement therapy could promote any form of cancer. Some doctors believe that it could, especially if estrogen is administered *continuously* rather than cyclically. Others feel that there is absolutely no such evidence; on the contrary, they point out the possibility that estrogen may act as a protection against at least some forms of cancer.

MENSTRUAL EXTRACTION

Menstrual extraction, also called mini-abortion, is a safe and effective early abortion technique that has to be performed no later than the seventh week of gestation. In fact, it can be performed a few days after a menstrual period is missed, *before* the development of a positive PREGNANCY TEST.

In this procedure, a flexible plastic tube 5 mm in diameter called a cannula (which was developed by Harvey Karman, a Los Angeles psychologist) is inserted through the cervix into the uterus. Most of the uterine lining is then removed by suction with a small, specially designed syringe.

Since the tube is thin, it usually can be used without dilating the cervix; and since it is flexible, it eliminates the danger of perforation.

The operation can be done with local anaesthesia in a doctor's office and takes about five minutes. Pain and bleeding are minimal, and after relaxing half an hour in the waiting room a patient can leave the office unaided.

Since pregnancy tests available to the public are usually not accurate for some time after a missed menstrual period, some of the women seeking this technique may not be pregnant. But if a fertilized EGG is present in the uterus, it will be sucked out along with the rest of the uterine shedding. Technically then (and probably also legally), menstrual extraction cannot be considered an abortion but rather a method of birth control—and as such it may sometimes be performed unnecessarily. On the other hand, there are women—many of them Catholic—who prefer not to know whether they are pregnant. Also, a menstrual extraction can spare a great deal of anxiety for a woman who fears pregnancy and who normally would have to wait weeks for a reliable PREGNANCY TEST.

MENSTRUATION

Despite decades of laboratory experiments and clinical investigation, physiologists are still baffled by the complexities of menstruation—the most dramatic influence in a woman's life.

There have been, and still are, many taboos about menstruation and the potency of menstrual blood. To most ancient cultures, menstruation was profoundly relevant to rites of passage into the adult role; and the correlation, made by primitive men, between lunar changes and menstruation persisted in one form or another for centuries. Recently, scientists have reconsidered the possibility that lunar rhythms may be pertinent to understanding human ovulation cycles.

The menstrual cycle consists of several hormonal stages. It begins in one of the most important glands in the human body, the pituitary gland, which lies under the brain near the middle of the head and is controlled, through the hypothalamus, by the higher brain centers. The pituitary gland secretes the *first* HORMONE of the cycle, the FSH (Follicle-stimulating hormone), into the bloodstream and alternately to the right ovary and to the left ovary. The target of FSH is one of the FOLLICLES, the tiny cavities contained in each ovary. (Each follicle holds thousands of immature egg cells). The FSH carries a double "message" to the follicle: to start maturing one of the unripe egg cells, and to start producing the *second* hormone of the cycle, estrogen.

Estrogen's main purpose at this stage is to stimulate the endometrium (the mucous membrane that lines the uterus) to thicken with small blood vessels, which are meant to provide nourishment for the developing egg cell in case it becomes fertilized by a male sperm cell. While the estrogen level rises in the bloodstream, the pituitary gland releases the *third* hormone, LH (luteinizing hormone), which instructs the follicle to release the egg cell that has been maturing in it. The mature egg is swept into the oviduct, the tube that will lead it into the uterus, where it may become fertilized.

If the egg cell is fertilized, it will attach itself to the uterine wall and continue to develop for nine months. Meanwhile, the follicle continues to produce estrogen, which continues to thicken the uterine walls and also increases its supply of LH. At the same time, a *fourth* hormone, LTH (luteotrophic hormone), is activated, causing a dramatic change in the follicle. It becomes bright yellow and is now known as *corpus luteum,* yellow body. This dramatic change in color means that progesterone, the *fifth* hormone, is now being produced and sent into the uterus. Progesterone is essential to maintain pregnancy, since it continues to enrich the wall of the uterus, preventing it from being shed. Progesterone also signals the pituitary gland not to stimulate other follicles to start producing mature eggs.

If the egg cell is *not* fertilized, a decreased supply of progesterone signals the pituitary gland to stop releasing LH. In turn, the production of estrogen and progesterone is slowed down, and the endometrium begins to shed its built-up lining of tiny blood vessels. This shedding process is what happens when a woman menstruates. Menstrual blood does not coagulate; to be precise, it clots at first but then undergoes liquefaction in the uterus because of certain ENZYMES. Why this happens is still a mystery.

As soon as the uterus's old lining has been sloughed off and the blood vessels have regressed, the new lining is ready for a new growth. The pituitary gland starts the cycle again, signaling the ovary to develop another mature egg.

The human menstrual cycle is characteristically irregular, both in overall length and in variation of the hormonal level and pattern in their various stages of activity. An average menstruation occurs every twenty-one to thirty-five days (from day one to day one) and lasts two to seven days. But even women who are most regular can experience a great fluctuation in cycle length—for instance, a twenty-six-day cycle one month and a thirty-three-day cycle the following month. Also, many women are either occasionally or permanently anovulatory, that is, their ovaries fail to produce and release a mature egg.

The basal body temperature is *lower* during the first part of a cycle than during the last two weeks. At ovulation the temperature drops a few tenths of a degree; twenty-four hours later, it abruptly rises several tenths of a degree above the base line. Absence of menstrual flow is called amenorrhea. (This symptom is often present in young girls who go on low-calorie crash DIETS.)

Painful menstruation is called dysmenorrhea. Cramps, excessive or absent menstruation, even anovulation may signal emotional problems: after all, emotions and ovulation are sparked in the same areas of the

This chart illustrates the normal variations in basal body temperature and hormone levels of a woman during her menstrual cycle.

Since the body temperature always drops abruptly just before ovulation and rises to a peak within twenty-four hours, a woman who monitors her daily temperature for several months may establish with a certain amount of accuracy her ovulating rhythm. This calculation is often used to facilitate or avoid pregnancy, as conception can occur only during ovulation.

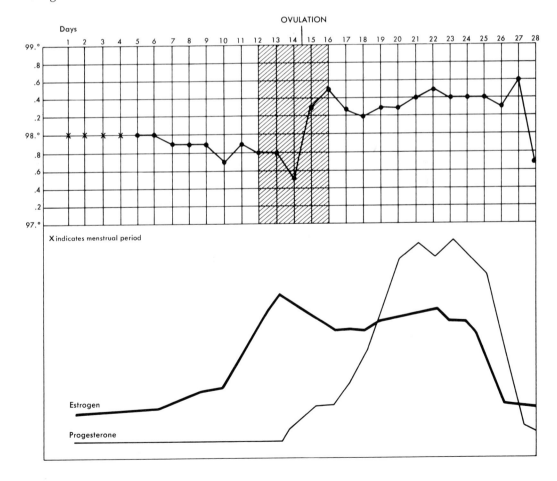

brain, the pituitary gland and the hypothalamus. It is more than possible that emotions and menstruation affect each other. Incidentally, the menstrual cycle probably has its subtle counterpart in men, for in at least one study there have been signs of monthly hormonal rhythms and monthly mood cycles in men.

A heavy menstrual flow is called hypermenorrhea, not a real problem but often a nuisance. Hypermenorrhea can be corrected with a special preparation that has a low-estrogen, high-progesterone content (much like a CONTRACEPTIVE PILL), which reduces the buildup of the uterine lining and therefore its shedding.

It would be impossible to enumerate here all the important biochemical changes that occur—echoed in the premenstrual symptoms—as a result of the chain of hormones in the phase just before each menstrual cycle. Clearly, the slightest variations in the level and activities of such important hormones as estrogen and progesterone reverberate throughout the nervous system and the metabolism. Since at least 60 percent of all women have premenstrual and menstrual symptoms, these symptoms must be considered normal, except when they become so severe as to alter a woman's life. "When one considers how many functions, chemistries, and intermeshed cycles must cooperate to produce an ovum each month," writes Gay Gaer Luce in *Body Time*, "it is astonishing that the cycle proceeds as smoothly as it does."

METASTASIS

Metastasis is the transfer of disease-producing cells or bacteria from an original site of disease to another part of the body, with development of a similar lesion (such as a malignant tumor) in the new location.

MIDWIFERY

The midwife, according to Webster (Third Edition), is a woman not qualified as a physician who assists other women in childbirth.

In Europe midwifery has been a respected profession for centuries, and to this day midwives in Holland, France and England perform countless normal deliveries, often without the help of a physician. In the United States the midwife has been traditionally associated with extremely poor, isolated rural communities where "real" doctors are not available. In the last few years, however, the rank of midwife in this country has begun to rise again. The modern version of the old-style, empirically trained "granny" is the nurse-midwife, an integral part of the specialized obstetric team who receives extensive training in every aspect of maternal care.

In 1970 the American College of Obstetricians and Gynecologists made the midwife's position official, stating in part that in "medically directed teams, qualified nurse-midwives may assume responsibility for complete care and management of uncomplicated maternity patients." The Maternity Center Association, a national health agency that founded the first nurse-midwifery school in the United States in 1931, and its director, Ruth Lubic, are credited with much of midwives' recently improved status.

It is now agreed that the special skills of an obstetrician are not needed for most normal deliveries. Spontaneous labor in a normal woman is a sequence of processes so complicated and so perfectly attuned to one another that any interference would only disturb their rhythm. There is no need for a specialist to sit for hours, watching a normal process taking

A nurse-midwife lifts a newly born baby after managing his normal birth. *Courtesy of The American College of Nurse-Midwives, Washington, D.C.*

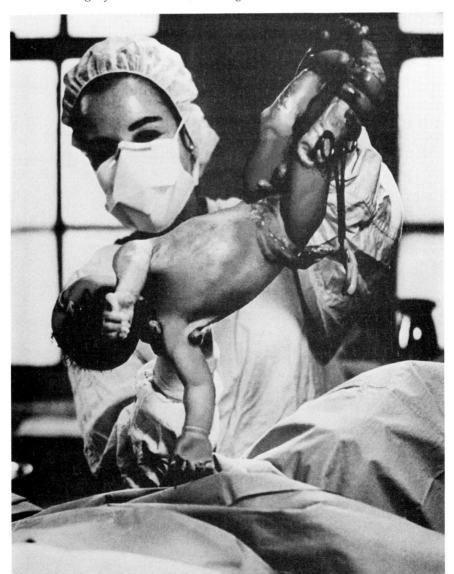

place; a healthy woman in labor mainly needs comfort, a friendly person wiping her forehead, offering a few drops to drink, and reinforcing confidence in her own strength. "If I had to do this [a normal delivery] . . . often," said a Dutch obstetrician recently interviewed by *Contemporary Ob/Gyn* magazine, "I am sure that I would yield to the temptation to shorten labor without real indications, to drug the parturient without trying . . . to give her moral support and without trying to coach her during the last hours of labor."

But, of course, nurse-midwives are trained to do much more than comfort a woman in labor. They can examine pregnant women, feel the position of the baby, administer drugs, help women during labor until delivery, help physicians with difficult deliveries, and assist the family after the baby's birth. A midwife is also trained to recognize immediately any complication and to alert the physician while setting the hospital machinery into motion at the earliest stage.

Some feminists have proposed that nurse-midwives in this country be authorized to perform deliveries on their own and that normal childbirth be handled entirely at home. This attitude is shared to a degree by a number of young women, especially in California and New York, who in the last few years have created almost a trend of delivering babies at home.

However, between the two extremes of unassisted childbirth at home and a delivery in the impersonal, almost frightening atmosphere of a big hospital, where pregnancy is often dealt with as a sickness rather than as a natural event, the nurse-midwife can offer the ideal compromise: the link between human feelings and scientific knowledge.

MILIARIA (PRICKLY HEAT)

Miliaria, better known as prickly heat, is a disorder of the sweat glands caused by temporary blockage of the sweat duct openings on the skin surface.

Especially during hot weather, when a person perspires more readily, if the sweat cannot reach the skin's surface it may break through the walls of its ducts and create an inflammation in the skin.

Miliaria is characterized by patches of small red blisters, accompanied by intense burning and itching. It is especially common in areas where two skin surfaces touch each other, as in the skin folds of overweight people.

Treatment consists mainly of keeping the skin cool and dry with air-conditioning; engaging in only limited physical activity; wearing light, loose-fitting clothes; and taking cool showers or plain-water baths, followed by dusting with talcum powder.

MINERALS

Like VITAMINS, minerals are essential for good health and for growth. The body requires just the right amount of minerals from the diet.

Minerals have two general body functions: *building* and *regulating*. Their building function affects the skeleton and all soft tissue. Their regulating function includes a variety of systems, such as heart beat, blood clotting, nerve responses, and transport of oxygen from the lungs to the tissues.

Some minerals (called macrominerals) are present in relatively large amounts in the body and are needed in relatively large amounts in the diet. The other minerals—which occur in living tissues in such small amounts that until recently their precise concentration could not be measured—are called trace elements.

Macrominerals

CALCIUM—Present in the body in greater amounts than any other mineral: two or three pounds, almost all concentrated in the bones and the teeth. Good sources of calcium are milk and milk products; green, leafy vegetables; citrus fruits, and dried beans.

CHLORIDE—Part of hydrochloric acid, which is found in high concentration in the gastric juice and is very important for digestion of food in the stomach.

MAGNESIUM—Found in all body tissues, but mainly in the bones. It is an essential part of many ENZYME systems responsible for energy conversions in the body.

PHOSPHORUS—Present in large quantities in the bones and teeth, and an important part of every tissue in the body. Good sources of phosphorus are meat, poultry, fish, eggs and whole-grain foods.

POTASSIUM—Found mainly in the fluid inside body cells. Potassium is abundant in almost all foods, both vegetable and animal.

SODIUM—Found mainly in blood plasma and in the fluids outside the body cells. Combined with chlorine, it becomes sodium chloride—table salt. Good sources of sodium are meat, fish, eggs and milk. Many processed foods such as ham, bacon, and bread have a high sodium content because salt or sodium compounds are added in the processing.

SULFUR—Present in all body tissues and related to PROTEIN nutrition because it is a component of several important amino acids. It is also part of two vitamins—thiamine and biotin.

Trace Elements

CHROMIUM—Acts with insulin and is needed for GLUCOSE utilization. Good sources of chromium are liver and whole-grain cereals.

COBALT—Not essential in itself, cobalt is a part of VITAMIN B$_{12}$.

COPPER—Involved in the storage and release of IRON to form hemoglobin for red blood cells. Good sources of copper are shellfish, nuts, dried legumes and most unprocessed foods.

FLUORINE—Found in small and varying amounts in water, soil, plants, and animals. As fluoride, it contributes to solid tooth formation and results in a decrease of dental caries, especially in children.

IODINE—Required in extremely small amounts, but the normal functioning of the thyroid gland depends on its adequate supply. For this reason, in 1924 iodized salt was introduced and, later, noniodized salt required to be labeled with the statement: "This salt does not supply iodine, a necessary nutrient."

IRON—Widely distributed in the body, mostly in the blood, with relatively large amounts in the liver, spleen, and bone marrow. Iron is an important part of compounds necessary for transporting oxygen to the cells and making use of the oxygen when it arrives. Good sources of iron are liver, egg yolk, fish, beans, peas, dried fruits, and foods prepared from iron-enriched cereal products.

MANGANESE—Needed for normal tendon and bone structure, and a part of some enzymes. Good sources of manganese are coffee, tea, nuts, peas and beans.

SELENIUM—Acts on VITAMIN E. Its content in foods depends on the amount available to the growing plant or animal.

ZINC—An important part of the enzymes that, among other functions, move carbon dioxide from the tissues through red blood cells to the lungs, where it can be exhaled. Good sources of zinc are meat, fish, egg yolk and milk.

Because of the changes in the environment due to scientific and technological progress, man's intake of trace elements may be changing, scientists say; yet the nature of these changes and their significance to human health are still poorly understood. What *is* known is that even infinitesimal amounts of various chemical substances such as nickel, SILICONE and tin play an important role in the human body.

MOISTURIZERS

The ultimate moisturizer is water—water is all the skin surface needs to feel soft and smooth. But what we usually call moisturizers (EMOLLIENTS or VANISHING CREAMS) do not themselves enter the skin to moisturize it—as so many labels emphatically promise—but rather provide a film that seals in the available water, thus slowing down water's inevitable evaporation.

Normal moisture is supplied by the inner layer of the skin to the outer layer; however, moisture is quickly depleted when the skin is exposed to the dry air of an overheated room, or to cold, windy air, or simply when it is unprotected from intense sunlight.

Also, SOAPS and CLEANSERS remove not only dirt but also most of the skin's natural moisturizer: the film of oil secreted by the sebaceous glands that rises to the skin surface through the pores.

Older skin needs a more frequent and more consistent use of moisturizers than young skin for several reasons. First, the cells produced by the older skin's outer layer build up instead of shedding easily as they used to, causing the skin to become coarse and dry. Second, the outer layer's ability to hold water decreases. Third, the oil glands' activity diminishes—all of which combine to worsen the lack of moisture. As Dr. Bedford Shelmire, Jr., points out in his book, *The Art of Looking Younger*, the buttock skin of a middle-aged woman, which has been protected by clothing for years (while her face has been exposed to all the dangers of her environment) is always astoundingly smooth and soft, like baby skin.

Indeed, some form of moisturizer should be used *all the time* by any woman (and any man, too) over eighteen. Even people with very oily skin should use moisturizers, combined with products that reduce oil without overdrying or irritating the skin. All OILS, whether of animal, vegetable or mineral origin, will moisturize skin to about the same degree: turtle oil, cocoa butter and mineral oil show no particular differences. The many types of available moisturizers differ only in their consistency—light or heavy—which is determined by the concentration of the ingredient. Therefore, Dr. Shelmire reasons, there seems to be no point in using exotic (and expensive) ingredients such as shark oil, avocado oil and mink oil when Vaseline®, for example, will do just as well.

Among the numerous apparently *useless* ingredients added to moisturizing products are HORMONES, VITAMINS, PROTEINS, royal jelly, seaweed and aloe vera, as well as cucumbers, strawberries and herbs.

Certainly, exotic creams and oils presented in exquisite containers are much lovelier and smell much better than simple mineral oil. However, it is important to realize that their high prices have little to do with their moisturizing action.

MOLDS

Molds play an important role in allergic diseases. Mold spores (minute reproductive bodies) are major causes of bronchial ASTHMA, ALLERGIC RHINITIS and eczema, and they often complicate the ALLERGY TO POLLEN, because most mold-sensitive people are sensitive to other allergens, too, especially to pollens; and if the symptoms occur during the pollination season, it may be difficult to establish what is causing them.

Molds that are involved in allergy are microscopic, superficial growths produced on living organisms—such as plants—and various organic substances, especially when damp and decaying, such as food, leather, wood and soil.

Allergy to molds was once considered uncommon, limited to people regularly exposed to large numbers of spores in the air, such as farmers in the Midwest. Recently, however, mold spores have been found, either seasonally or even the year round, in many more regions of the United States.

Summer cottages, resort hotels, motels and damp basements are fertile grounds for the growth of molds, which may lie dormant throughout the winter and flourish with the first rise in temperature.

Molds may contaminate many foods such as bread, cake, fruits and meats. In certain foods, however, molds are used intentionally to create a specific taste, such as in aged cheeses, beers and wines.

Treatment of mold allergy is basically the same as for most allergies: medications prescribed by the physician and avoidance of the allergen. Desensitization treatment is given in the same way as in pollen allergy: subcutaneous injections of mold extract administered once or twice weekly before the season of the allergen's emergence, and continued until the patient is completely free of symptoms.

MOUTHWASHES

A mouthwash is a liquid preparation for freshening the breath, and for cleansing the mouth and teeth by removing or destroying bacteria caused by the fermentation of food particles trapped inside the mouth.

Mouthwashes are manufactured either ready for use or to be diluted from a concentrated form such as tablets. The most recently developed form is an AEROSOL spray. They usually contain alcohol, a DEODORANT, a sweetener, and a flavoring such as cinnamon, clove, eucalyptus, thyme, peppermint, anise or wintergreen.

Some mouthwashes also contain an astringent, such as zinc or aluminum compounds, which shrinks and protects enflamed mucous surfaces in the mouth and reduces excessive salivary secretions by precipitating (rendering insoluble) the PROTEINS in the saliva, so that these can be flushed out. Astringents, however, should not be used too often, as they might irritate the tissues and be harmful to the calcified structure of the teeth.

Other mouthwashes, available by prescription, contain fluoride (as do certain TOOTHPASTES) for the general purpose of preventing caries. Still others are formulated for relieving infection or mitigating conditions of the teeth or throat, though halitosis—chronic bad breath—is often a symptom of tooth-and-gum disease or some gastrointestinal problem, neither of which can be cured by a mouthwash.

For people with healthy but hypersensitive teeth who are advised not to use a toothbrush too often, a mouthwash is a quick and extremely practical cleanser. After a spicy meal, a nap, or excessive smoking, a few drops of a mouthwash can be more pleasant and refreshing than any other cosmetic product.

MYOPIA (NEARSIGHTEDNESS)

An eye that can see near objects clearly but cannot focus well on distant ones is nearsighted, or myopic.

In myopia, parallel rays of light falling on the eye focus *in front* of the retina. To correct the condition, concave lenses are used to diverge the light just enough to focus a sharp image on the retina.

N

NAIL CONDITIONERS

Nail conditioners are PROTEIN-like substances that are painted on the bare nail for strengthening the nail plate. As with hair CONDITIONERS, such preparations serve to fill in tiny imperfections in the nail plate but do not influence the growth pattern or the character of the nail itself. Nail polish may be applied over these conditioners.

NAIL HARDENERS

PROTEIN, which is the basic component of nails, can be hardened by certain chemicals. One of the most effective is formaldehyde, a powerful disinfectant gas that, when dissolved in 40 percent solution in water, is widely used as a preservative, especially in laboratories, where it helps to maintain the form and cellular structure of tissues to be examined.

However, skin reactions after exposure to formaldehyde are not uncommon, and such reactions may become more frequent because of the public's greater contact with formaldehyde in various forms. For example, formaldehyde has been used in the manufacture of cosmetic products other than nail hardeners; also, certain fabrics with a permanent-press finish are treated with formaldehyde resins.

Yet, formaldehyde definitely hardens nails. If a nail hardener containing it is scrupulously applied *only* to the free edge of the nail, with care taken so that it does not touch the rest of the nail or come in contact with the cuticle, it can safely and successfully be applied to the bare nail or even over nail polish.

Another group of nail-hardening preparations merely function as temporary support for fragile, flaking and splitting nails by coating them with a strong film that resembles clear nail polish. In some products, nylon fibers are suspended in the thick liquid, and when the preparation dries, the enmeshed fibers provide the nail with additional strength.

These nail hardeners are meant to be worn alone or under nail polish. The only drawback to them is that, once they dry, they tend to have an irregular, streaked surface which many women find unattractive.

NAIL PATCHES (OR MENDERS)

Nail patches refer to kits containing a thick, clear polish, tiny squares of very fine fabric (or tissue paper), and a small stick, designed for mending partially torn nails, especially long ones.

The polish is applied both over and under the nail; the tissue is trimmed, stuck to the wet polish, pressed over the break, and folded under the nail. Finally one more coat of polish is painted over the mended nail.

The result is reasonably satisfactory and lasts several days. The patch is easily removed with nail polish remover.

NAIL WHITENER

A nail whitener is a white pigment, made of titanium dioxide or chalk added to wax or a water-soluble resin, that is intended to give a neater and more even look to the free edge of bare fingernails. It is applied *underneath* the nails with either an orangewood stick or a pencil.

For best results, fingertips should be soaked in lukewarm water and blotted lightly, and the undernail coated with the whitener in such a way that the nail bed is not damaged by the stick's (or pencil's) point. Care should also be taken not to smudge the pigment on the skin surrounding the nail.

NARCOTICS

Substances that have the physiological action, in a healthy organism, of producing lethargy or stupor (which may pass into a state of unconsciousness and ultimately result in death) are called narcotics.

Certain substances of this class are used in medicine for the relief of pain and are called anodynes, while others produce sleep and are known as hypnotic drugs. Technically, ANAESTHETICS too may be classified as narcotics, though they are usually volatile substances causing unconsciousness for a comparatively short time, and as such are conveniently separated from the *true* narcotics, the effects of which are much more lasting.

These distinctions are to a large extent artificial, as it is evident that a substance capable of producing sleep or partial insensibility to pain will *in large doses* inevitably cause profound coma ending in death. Therefore, the same substance may sometimes be classed as an anodyne and at other times as a hypnotic. For example, small doses of OPIUM or of one of its preparations relieve pain, whereas larger doses act as a hypnotic.

NAUSEA (MORNING SICKNESS)

About 50 percent of pregnant women suffer from some form of nausea in the first few months of pregnancy. An obnoxious odor or a repelling sight may cause nausea, or even vomiting, in any woman, whether pregnant or not; however, the hormonal status of pregnancy seems to create a heightened tendency to nausea, whose frequency and severity may be related to the amount of circulating levels of HORMONES in the blood. Sometimes nausea is psychic in origin—an emotional reaction to being pregnant.

The common name for nausea is morning sickness, which suggests that it usually starts first thing in the morning, when the stomach is empty. Eating breakfast doesn't always relieve the nausea, but most women find that it disappears by noon. For some women, however, it may persist all day, worsening in the afternoon. In general, though, nausea is unpredictable: it may last for weeks, perhaps as long as three months, and suddenly cease, whereas other women never experience it.

Except for VITAMIN B$_6$ (pyridoxine hydrochloride) and a mild sedative, few remedies seem to work for nausea; besides, physicians hesitate to prescribe medications during the first trimester of pregnancy for fear of producing congenital anomalies in the baby.

Some women eventually find their own way of avoiding or minimizing nausea: lying down after a light meal, keeping a few crackers near the bed and eating them before getting up in the morning, avoiding strong kitchen odors and tobacco smoke.

"There is one consolation that I can offer," recently wrote Dr. George Schaefer, a New York obstetrician, "and that is that women are more likely to carry full term when they have nausea. We think this is due to excessive secretion of one of the hormones that 'protect' against early delivery."

NERVOUS BREAKDOWN

"Nervous breakdown" is a colloquialism that can signify almost any kind of emotionally upsetting experience. The term is no longer popular and indeed is too vague to be useful. However, when the average person used to say nervous breakdown, he really meant an emotional illness serious enough to disrupt work and the continuity of living. In the sense of mental depression, Dr. Leonard Cammer, the author of *Up From*

Depression, believes that the image of the breakdown of a machine is still quite appropriate.

Our muscles produce caloric energy, which is obtained by a constant supply of food. But before this energy can be produced, the brain and the nervous system, in coordination with glandular secretions and other biochemical processes, must activate muscles with tensional energy. Every moment of the day we all spend a certain amount of tensional energy, without which we could not function. The question is, how much tensional energy do we generate? How well do we utilize it?

Some people distribute their daily quotas wisely and feel only moderately tired at the end of an average day. But some build up too much energy and never learn how to spend it profitably; others have to use enormous amounts of energy to cope with prolonged periods of stress. The former bottle up energy until it spills over in the form of physical ailments; the latter become exhausted and can no longer adapt to life's stresses—their tensional energy system has broken down.

NEVI

Nevi refers to pigmented spots on the skin that are composed chiefly of melanocytes, specialized cells in the skin (probably nerve cells) that produce melanin, the dark pigment of the skin and hair.

Most nevi appear a few years after birth as small spots that gradually enlarge as a person grows. Everybody has a number of nevi, either superficial, located in the epidermis, or deep, at the junction between epidermis and dermis or in the dermis itself.

Nevi vary greatly in size and in thickness, as well as in color, which ranges all the way from flesh color to blue-black, depending on the concentration of melanocytes. Small, flat, brown nevi are called freckles; large, raised, sometimes hairy ones are generally referred to as moles.

Nevi are not always easy to recognize, because not all pigmented spots on the skin are nevi. For example, WARTS, certain port-wine stains, and seborrheic keratoses—none of which has anything to do with melanocytes—are often mistaken for nevi.

Many people consult dermatologists about nevi, either because they wish to have them removed for aesthetic reasons or because they are concerned that a particular nevus might be malignant. Some nevi can indeed be removed without difficulty, either by excision or by ELECTRODESICCATION. A few of them, however, are potentially dangerous in that they can turn into melanomas, malignant tumors that often metastasize with great rapidity. A nevus may become a melanoma, for instance, following excessive exposure to sunlight. This form of SKIN CANCER, incidentally, is particularly frequent among fair-skinned women.

When a nevus suddenly begins to grow, to change in color, to itch and to bleed, one should consult a doctor immediately. But these changes are not necessarily a sign of malignancy, and a skillful dermatologist is usually able to recognize whether the changing nevus is indeed turning into a melanoma. In case it is, or even if a melanoma is only suspected, the nevus should never be electrodesiccated but should be promptly removed with a wide, deep incision and examined under a microscope.

NOISE POLLUTION

Dr. Vern O. Knudsen, a pioneer in acoustics, described noise as "one of the waste products of the twentieth century—as unwanted and unnecessary as smog and polluted water." The human ear, unlike the pupil of the eye, which automatically contracts when light intensity increases, is relatively helpless against constant or sudden noises in the environment, though it is able to adapt to a great variety of noisy situations; and hearing loss is directly related to the total amount of noise a person is exposed to over the years.

Noise is measured in units called decibels (db), which indicate the intensity of sound. Sound is also measured in relation to its pitch, or frequency. The frequency scale that approximates the frequency response of the human ear is called the "A" scale, so that when sound levels are measured, they are often expressed as dbA.

One db represents the weakest sound that can be detected by a keen human ear in quiet surroundings—approximately that of "a baby mouse urinating on a dry blotter three feet away," in the words of Dr. John E. Watson, chief of the Audiology-Speech Pathology Service at the Veterans Administration Hospital in Palo Alto, California.

The total range of sound levels from the threshold of hearing to the threshold of pain is 0 to 140 db. For the sake of convenience, the decibel scale is logarithmic rather than linear, which means that for an increase of 10 db, loudness increases *ten times*, not 10 percent. For instance, street traffic is measured at 70 db, ten times louder than ordinary speech, which is measured at 60 db. A pneumatic drill (80 db) corresponds to a hundredfold increase in the acoustic level of ordinary speech. Sounds at 140 db—the level of jet operations on a carrier deck—are one trillion times greater than at 1 db.

"Noise not only impairs hearing," wrote Dr. Watson. "It also can raise a person's blood pressure, increase heart rate, impede convalescence, hinder concentrated mental effort, interfere with relaxation and sleep, cause stress and nervousness and thereby increase the troubles associated with tension—irritability, INSOMNIA, accident-proneness, cardiovascular disease." More dramatically, the noise level in many large cities has been rising steadily at the rate of 1 db a year. As of 1974, we have a noise pollution whose increase goes hand in hand with that of air pollution. For instance, doctors believe that the past decade of extraordinarily amplified rock music may have affected the hearing of an entire generation. True, the difference between sound and noise is in part psychological—what *we* make is sound; noise is what *other* people make. Still, human nerves cannot distinguish between noise and sound, and even exciting music, when it is above 90 db, will produce damage as any other noise.

In 1972, the Federal Noise Control Act was signed into law; this act empowered the Environmental Protection Agency to establish standards for all noise sources that are a threat to public health. The standards were established in 1974, but until their effects are fully realized, all we have at our disposal are masking-sound machines, which produce a rhythmic or monotonous, so-called "white" sound that is meant to drown out other noises, and ear stopples. Needless to say, neither can be considered a practical antidote to noise. Ear stopples are generally inadequate and often annoying, and masking-sound machines, while being of some psychological help to insomniacs, are ineffective in the presence of loud noises.

NONBARBITURATE HYPNOTICS

The term nonbarbiturates refers loosely to a group of hypnotic drugs, such as glutethimide (whose trade name is Doriden®), methyprylon (Nodular®) and ethchlorvynol (Placidyl®), that were put on the market in the mid-1950s as mild, nonaddictive substitutes for BARBITURATES. Interestingly enough, chloral hydrate (Beta-chlor® and Triclos®), a derivative of alcohol and to this day considered a very mild nonbarbiturate hypnotic, has been available since 1832, even before the first barbiturate—barbituric acid—was synthetized.

Nonbarbiturates once enjoyed great popularity; unfortunately, it has turned out that they are just as habit-forming and intoxicating as barbiturates. One of the most publicized cases is that of methaqualone, marketed in the United States since 1966 under such trade names as Quaalude®, Somnafac®, Optimil®, and known among drug addicts and pushers as "ludes," "quacks" or "sopors." As of November 1973, methaqualone has been put into the same legal category as barbiturates and opium derivatives; physicians and pharmacists must maintain strict inventories and issue the drug only on nonrefillable prescriptions.

One of the problems of nonbarbiturates may well be their very *mildness:* sometimes a small dose will have no effect, and many people, having been assured that nonbarbiturates are harmless, may be inclined to escalate the dose until they experience the same abnormal sleep patterns, physical and mental disturbances, and withdrawal problems that occur with barbiturates.

NORMAL SLEEP

Whether during the day or during the night, approximately once every twenty-four hours human beings go to sleep for a variable length of time in order to refresh themselves and to recharge their bodies with energy.

Sleep represents one of the phases in a minutely regulated daily cycle of activity and rest called circadian rhythm (from the Latin *circa dies,* around a day), which is an important organizing principle in man's physiology.

Sleep is not a unitary condition: it is composed of many stages of detachment from the surrounding world, an orderly sequence of subtle changes constantly occurring throughout the body and the mind, intermeshed with each other and the rest of the organism. Sleep is normal when the sequence and the relative duration of each stage are constant. Any alteration of, or interference with, any of the stages may provoke a sleep disorder.

At the onset of sleep, the body relaxes, the eyes close, breathing becomes even, the pulse becomes steady, temperature gradually lowers, and the brain—when monitored by an ELECTROENCEPHALOGRAPH—shows an electrical activity of a frequency of about nine to thirteen waves per second, the so-called Alpha rhythm.

What follows is a sudden, faint spasm of the body, called the myoclonic jerk, which results from a tiny burst of activity in the brain.

At this time, the body crosses the threshold of wakefulness and enters into *Stage I* of sleep, from which a person still could easily awaken, convinced he has not been asleep.

After a few minutes, the body descends deeper, into *Stage II;* the brain shows a sudden burst of activity, and the eyes slowly roll from side to side.

Within thirty minutes, *Stage III* is reached. Brain waves slow down, muscles relax, breathing becomes even, body temperature and blood pressure fall slightly.

Stage III soon merges into *Stage IV,* the deepest level of sleep, called Delta sleep. Breathing and heart rate are even; the body temperature continues to fall. Delta sleep lasts about twenty minutes, after which the body climbs back toward the threshold of consciousness but without fully awakening.

Suddenly, the quality of sleep changes again and drifts into the REM (rapid-eye-movement) stage: the sleeper begins to dream, moving his eyes as if watching a movie. The heart beats irregularly and the blood pressure fluctuates; men have an erection. Yet the body remains relaxed, except for imperceptible twitchings of toes and fingers. The REM stage lasts about ten minutes, after which the body is ready to begin the cycle again, from *Stage II*. Ninety minutes later the sleeper will reach a new REM stage; and the entire cycle is repeated about four or five times during the night. Toward morning, the body no longer reaches the depth of Delta sleep, and its REM periods are longer. Sleep is lighter, body temperature begins to rise—the body will soon awake.

Human beings spend about twenty years of their lifetime sleeping, yet as long as sleep is normal, most people hardly seem concerned with that mysterious portion of their daily lives. Only when they experience INSOMNIA, the distressing symptom of a variety of illnesses and at times itself an illness, do people realize the importance of a good night's sleep. Keeping regular hours of sleep is one of the ways the body rewinds and resets the internal clock that regulates thousands of other body rhythms.

NUTRILITES

Nutrilites are substances such as VITAMINS, amino acids and fatty acids that are obtained by man from his food and that are required in small quantities for normal metabolism and growth.

OBESITY

Obesity is the common symptom of several dissimilar organic and emotional disturbances—all related to the ingestion of too much food—which can trigger this complex phenomenon at birth or in midlife, suddenly or over the years. Obesity is still imperfectly understood; opinions differ about the assessment and the treatment of it, and only recently have precise measurements and acceptable criteria for obesity—as opposed to overweight—been formulated.

Overweight refers to body weight in excess of a standard; it does not specify whether the excess is fat, bone, muscle or fluid. Obesity, on the other hand, refers to the condition of fatness; that is, an excessive amount of adipose tissue. Not all overweight people are obese, but most obese people are overweight.

There are several ways to measure adiposity; one of the simplest is the skinfold measurements. The triceps (the muscle along the back of the upper arm) skinfold is the easiest to measure and the most representative of total body fatness.

In theory, since excessive fat is the end result of an imbalance between the number of CALORIES ingested and the amount of energy expended, it should be easy to lose weight. Once a person realizes that one pound of fat has approximately the energy value of 3,500 calories, that a daily surplus of 500 calories means a gain of one pound of fat a week, and that a daily reduction of merely 250 calories—plus 250 calories' worth of exercise—can take off a pound of fat a week, one should have little problem reducing. In reality, there are so many different conditions and factors that affect the intake of food and output of energy that logic alone won't induce an obese person to lose weight.

Our present knowledge indicates that the ultimate cause of calorie/energy imbalance may be one or a combination of the following factors:

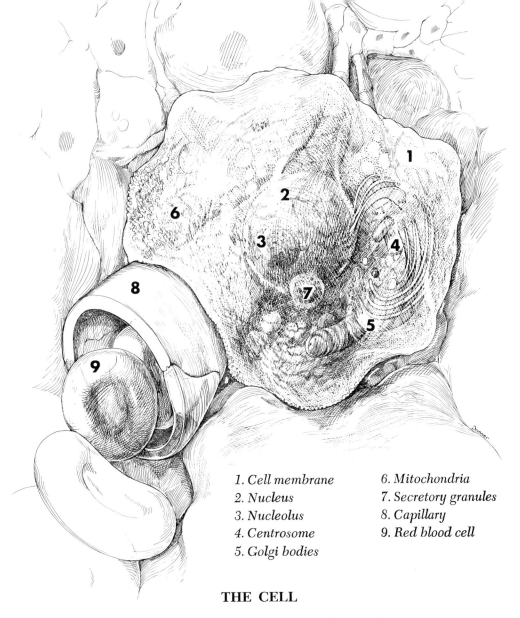

1. Cell membrane
2. Nucleus
3. Nucleolus
4. Centrosome
5. Golgi bodies

6. Mitochondria
7. Secretory granules
8. Capillary
9. Red blood cell

THE CELL

A typical cell is composed of two parts: the outer jellylike cytoplasm and the inner nucleus.

The cytoplasm is enveloped by a very thin membrane which controls the exchange of nutrients and wastes between the cell and its environment.

Within the cytoplasm are small bodies called mitochondria, responsible for storing energy within the cell. Other structures within the cytoplasm are: the lysosomes, which are rich in enzymes; the endoplasmic reticulum, which functions as a transportation system within the cell; the ribosomes, which help in the production of proteins; and the Golgi bodies, which parcel up the proteins.

The nucleus, which during periods of cell division undergoes a series of changes called mitosis, is a spherical body with a thin envelope and a translucent internal nucleoplasm containing one to several semi-solid bodies called nucleoli. Inside the nucleus are masses of material called chromatin. During cell division, the chromatin first aggregates into threads and then into bodies called chromosomes, which carry the factors for the genetic constitution of the individual. Close to the nucleus lies the centrosome, a structure essential to the process of cell division.

Genetic and constitutional predisposition. The evidence is absolute in animals, and is strongly persuasive in man, too, that some forms of obesity can be hereditary. With one fat parent, a person's chances of becoming fat are roughly thirty percent; with two fat parents, eighty percent.

Dr. Jules Hirsch, head of the Department of Human Behavior at Rockefeller University in New York City, not only demonstrated that it is possible to make an actual count of the number of fat cells in the human body but, by taking a count of human fat cells at various stages of growth development, concluded that the actual *number* of fat cells is determined in the first few months of life.

For people born with a predisposition to being fat, Dr. Hirsch believes, how much a baby is fed during his first year of life will determine whether he will end up with an increased number of fat cells. If the overfed baby grows into an adult who continues to eat more calories than he burns, the fat cells will be not only *more numerous* but also *larger*. However, if the baby is fed normally, he will have a normal number of fat cells as he grows and will become obese only if he overeats later in life.

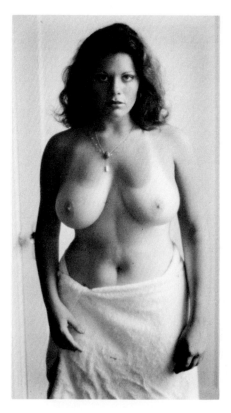

This nineteen-year-old girl, an almost perfect example of endomorphic body type at seventeen, is now clearly overweight. After each drastic diet she has tried, she happily could claim losses of as much as thirty pounds. Yet, the "after" picture we hoped to publish of her did not materialize: so far, each time, she has gained her weight back.

Dysfunction in metabolism. Metabolic obesities—as Dr. Jean Mayer, professor of nutrition at Harvard School of Public Health, calls this dysfunction—refer to an inborn or acquired error in the metabolism of tissue. Normally, the GLUCOSE level in the blood provides a signal to the "feeding center" in the hypothalamus, indicating whether one needs to eat. The hypothalamus responds directly to the glucose by generating signals felt as either appetite or satiety, depending on whether the glucose level in the blood is low or high.

Because we depend on glucose (stored in the liver as glycogen) as a reservoir of energy, when glucose is low, the rhythm of the liver may indirectly influence our desire to eat. Activated by an enzyme called glycerokinase, glucose turns into a glycerophosphate compound that reacts with fatty acids in the adipose tissue to form a fat molecule.

When a cell requires energy, its enzymes break up the bond holding the molecule of fat, releasing glycerol and WATER in a process called hydrolysis, during the course of which energy is discharged. The fat molecule is thus irreversibly split and the released glycerol cannot be reutilized to form new molecules of fat: a "repressor" neutralizes the enzyme's action.

In metabolic obesity, the "repressor" is absent, and the enzyme reincorporates the just released glycerol into fat. Glucose, no longer needed for fat synthesis, backs up in the blood. High blood glucose causes the pancreas to secrete a larger amount of insulin. The combination of higher levels of glucose and insulin causes the liver and other organs to produce more fat from sugar than normal.

To lose weight in this case is possible, but because of the faulty metabolism, what is lost is mostly muscle: the body tends to utilize for energy the proteins in the muscles *before* utilizing the fat reserves.

Impairment of the central food-regulation mechanism. This mechanism, as we have seen, is located in the hypothalamus, at the base of the brain, though people recognize hunger by an indirect set of signals: stomach contractions, feelings of emptiness, etc. Normal people eat every day approximately as much as they need for their metabolism and to balance the kind of activity they perform, *and no more.* In practice, of course, they sometimes eat a little more or a little less; however, the deficit or the excess is minimal and is compensated for during the next few days. Over a period of two weeks, a normal body's weight and its reserves are always essentially in balance.

People with "regulatory obesity," as Dr. Mayer calls it, cannot respond to hunger pangs, because the rhythmic signals from their bodies no longer serve as guides for eating—they are "out of touch" with their own sensation of hunger. In the laboratory, animals with a damaged hypothalamus may eat incessantly and become enormously fat, or they can stop eating altogether if the damage is in a slightly different location. However, after prolonged fasting, these animals' fat production rate can be brought back to normal levels, and their body composition returns to normal.

Psychosomatic factors. These factors operate through either the nervous system or the cerebral cortex. These conditions are responsible for only a small number of the obesities usually seen in our population. Most obesities are not associated with any known or proven organic deficit but are the result of a long-term caloric imbalance.

Physical inactivity. This not only is one of the most common causes of obesity but is almost always a component of psychological disturbances. Overeating is often a compensation for tension, a response to stress, frustration, and the social disapproval of fatness. Especially among adolescents, a sense of rejection and guilt follows, leading to social isolation, which diminishes the opportunities for exercise, which in turn accelerates the development of obesity. An early pattern of overeating may also develop in children growing up in families that have failed to respect them as individuals. These youngsters feel that they are not in control of their own sensations and actions—that they don't *own* their bodies.

Physical inactivity may also be a result of social and economic conditions which have eliminated the need for hard physical work *without* creating the means or the incentive for voluntary physical exercise.

ODOR VOCABULARY

Acacia	Citronella	Lavender	Pine
Aldehyde	Citrus	Leaf	Pineapple
Almond	Clove	Leather	Pistachio
Amaryllis	Clover	Lemon	Plum
Amber	Cocoa	Licorice	Potato
Animal	Coconut	Lilac	Primrose
Anise	Coffee	Lily of the Valley	Raspberry
Antiseptic	Cognac	Lime	Rhubarb
Apple	Corn	Magnolia	Rose
Apple blossom	Cucumber	Malt	Rubber
Apricot	Earth	Marigold	Rum
Arbutus	Elder flower	Melon	Sage
Azalea	Fat	Mimosa	Sandalwood
Bacon	Fern	Mint	Seed
Balsam	Fig	Moss	Smoke

Banana	Fish	Muguet	Spearmint
Basil	Gardenia	Mushroom	Strawberry
Berry	Garlic	Musk	Sweat
Bouvardia	Geranium	Mustard	Tea
Broken twig	Ginger	Narcissus	Thyme
Butter	Grape	Nut	Tobacco
Camellia	Grass	Nutmeg	Tuberose
Camomile	Green bean	Onion	Valerian
Camphor	Ham	Orange	Vanilla
Caramel	Hay	Orange flower	Verbena
Caraway	Heather	Orris root	Vermouth
Carnation	Heliotrope	Paprika	Vinegar
Carrot	Herb	Parsley	Violet
Cassia	Hickory smoke	Peach	Walnut
Cedar	Honey	Peach flower	Watercress
Celery	Honeysuckle	Pear	Watermelon
Cherry	Hyacinth	Peony	Wax
Cherry blossom	Iris	Pepper	Wine
Chocolate	Jasmine	Peppermint oil	Wisteria
Chrysanthemum	Jonquil	Phenol	Witch hazel
Cinnamon	Juniper	Pickle	Wood

ONYCHOLYSIS

Onycholysis is the medical term for a condition in which a nail separates from the nail bed, beginning at the free edge and proceeding to the root.

Onycholysis can be caused by many dermatological disorders, such as PSORIASIS, various fungal infections, and disturbances to the lunula, the crescent-shaped area at the base of the nail. Certain drugs, such as formaldehyde, an ingredient of NAIL HARDENERS, may also cause onycholysis.

As the nail becomes separated from the nail bed, white areas appear under the nail plate. This may happen suddenly, with only slight discomfort. If the nail bed becomes infected, the white areas may change to a greenish color or to black.

Minor white spots or streaks may also develop in the nails whenever the growth and hardening process—keratinization—of the cells in the nail plate originating in the nail root (the matrix) is incomplete or changed. White spots can also be caused by minor traumas, such as may occur during an inept MANICURE.

Despite its alarming appearance, onycholysis can be easily cured by a dermatologist. As for the minor white spots, these are rather common and usually do not require treatment.

OOPHORECTOMY (OVARIECTOMY)

Oophorectomy, commonly called ovariectomy, refers to the surgical removal of one or both of a woman's ovaries, a procedure that becomes necessary when certain types of CYSTS or tumors develop on or inside an ovary.

The removal of one ovary still allows a woman to become pregnant; however, the removal of both inevitably produces sterility, causes MENSTRUATION to cease and produces other changes typical of MENOPAUSE.

ORAL SURGERY

Doctors still are not sure why jawbones sometimes grow unevenly, asymmetrically, so that one side of a person's face becomes larger than the other, or why the lower jaw may stop growing halfway while the upper reaches normal maturity. But anyone who suffers from malocclusion (bad bite) or jaw misalignment; improper breathing, speaking, chewing, or swallowing; or osteomyelitis (infection of the bone marrow) should, if the orthodontist and the dentist cannot help, seek the aid of an oral surgeon.

There is no age limit to oral surgery: some doctors feel that the traditional theory of waiting for an adolescent to reach full growth before operating on his bones may no longer be valid when it concerns the jawbones. Even a child with incipient jaw defects may now be operated on, years before his jaw reaches its full growth.

Oral surgery is an ancient specialty mentioned in Egyptian hieroglyphics and discussed around 400 B.C. by Hippocrates, the legendary Greek physician, who described a system of leather straps and wiring to repair dislocated and fractured jaws. The modern oral surgeon has gone one step forward: he considers not only the functional but also the aesthetic impairment of an asymmetric face structure.

Whatever type of oral surgery is needed, the preparation is always exhaustive, the surgeon investing as much as thirty hours of research in each patient. First he takes impressions of the teeth and of the upper and lower jaws—the maxilla and the mandible—and casts several sets of a plaster model, since there is always more than one solution for every problem. Photographs of both profiles are made, as well as a cephalogram, a special X-ray of the skull in profile, over which the surgeon superimposes a transparent sheet of acetate. On it he draws lines to and from a number of fixed points of reference that give him the exact length of certain bones and the relationship of the jaws to the face, of the upper jaw to the lower, and of the teeth to the jaw.

With the two-dimensional cephalogram and the three-dimensional

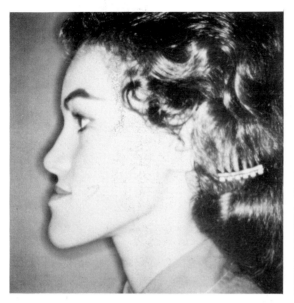
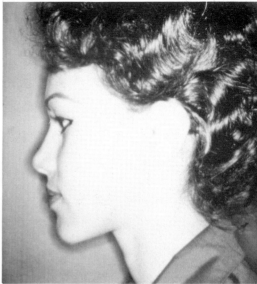

Left: A twenty-two-year-old patient of Dr. Stanley J. Behrman of New York City, with a severely protruding lower jaw.

Right: The same patient after oral surgery. The lower jaw has been shifted back with an operation performed from the outside, through a vertical incision in either side of the neck, coinciding with one of the skin's natural creases.

This operation, though extraordinarily successful, was performed several years ago. When presented with similar cases today, Dr. Behrman operates only inside the mouth, thus avoiding any visible scar at all.

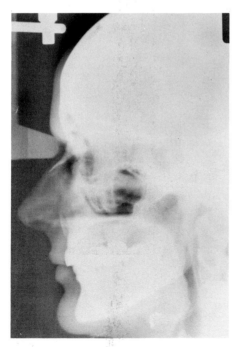

A cephalogram—a special X-ray of a woman's skull in profile, over which a transparent sheet of acetate has been superimposed. On it, several lines to and from a number of fixed points of reference on the skull have been drawn, which indicate the exact length of certain bones, the relationship of the jaws to the skull, of the jaws to the face, of the upper jaw to the lower.

Cephalograms are one of the methods used by oral surgeons to determine in mathematical terms the extent of a patient's jawbone defect. In this case, however, the face-skull relationship is excellent; visible is the delicate proportion of the bones and the perfect alignment of the teeth.

251

plaster model, the surgeon works for hours, as if on a jigsaw puzzle, to determine what section of which jawbone should be moved, and how much, in order to obtain the best results. Until recently, the basic point of reference for the position of the jaws was the proper occlusion of the teeth. But the "right" position may now be determined primarily by aesthetic considerations; a dentist will cap, move or replace some of the teeth, if necessary, to suit the new position of the jaws.

The surgical procedure itself may be relatively quick. However, it sometimes entails five, six or seven separate steps, totaling many hours, that involve reaching the jawbone and cutting at precisely the determined angle at high speed with a knife powered by compressed nitrogen, and then splitting, sliding, repositioning and wiring, sometimes utilizing tiny slivers of bone removed from one side in order to build elsewhere, sometimes using implants of SILICONE rubber.

Surgery is performed either from the outside, through the cheek or the neck, or entirely from inside the mouth, a more complex procedure but one that doesn't leave visible scars. Almost no bandages are used, just secure wiring and rubber bands on the teeth to keep everything in the right position until the bones heal. And of course, the patient can do no chewing while the bones knit into the desired position. The time of recovery varies greatly, depending on the extent of surgery, but usually a patient must stay one week in the hospital and then rest at home for another week. The wires are removed after about eight weeks.

ORGANIC FOOD

"Organic" refers to organically produced crops, i.e., those grown with no synthetic fertilizers, no pesticides and no herbicides. It also refers to livestock free from ANTIBIOTICS and HORMONES, and to food that is prepared without the use of ADDITIVES, PRESERVATIVES or artificial colorants.

Within the past several years, it appears that an increasing number of Americans—mostly young people at first—have joined what could be called the Organic-Food Revolution. Thousands have become alarmed by a relentless stream of reports of environmental pollution and misuse of chemicals in food; by news of contamination by mercury, lead, aluminum, DDT; by BOTULISM scandals among some of the country's most trusted brand names (even incidents involving sodium nitrate, the chemical used to *prevent* botulism). Cyclamates were banned and then rehabilitated—at the expense of saccharine. More and more products are being "demoted" from GRAS, the Generally Recognized As Safe list compiled by the Food and Drug Administration and once considered definitive.

The implications of the organic-food movement are far-reaching. For some, the movement has a strong religious character; for others, it is a necessary fight against complicated allergies; still others are simply attempting to return to a more wholesome way of life and nutrition. With the exception of the fanatics—such as the Zen Macrobiotics and the Vegans (supervegetarians), who are purely and simply malnourished— health-food enthusiasts cannot be dismissed, for it is a sad fact that there is much truth in their convictions about the food we eat. Nevertheless, there are some considerations to be made.

Consider the health-food stores: they have been multiplying throughout the United States at an extraordinary rate. It would be nice to note simply that they are thriving, but the fact is that people who wish to buy organically grown food often are the victims of dishonest storekeepers who call their products organic when they cannot produce any evidence that their products are indeed grown under conditions that would meet an official definition of "organic."

The fraud aspect is important here, because products labeled as "organic" are usually more expensive. And nobody, *nobody* can distinguish at sight an organically grown tomato from a commercial one. Often, not even scientists can distinguish between crops grown with organic fertilizers and those grown with inorganic fertilizers. What is worse, at present, authentic organic foods are not likely to be any less free from contamination by filth, mold, bacterial growth, natural toxins, or such MINERALS as lead and mercury than similar foods sold at regular food stores. In fact, there is a more likely danger of food contamination from some of the organic fertilizers than from chemical fertilizers.

And yet, it is absolutely true that excessive and careless use of chemical fertilizers has aggravated already tragic ecological problems. Organic farming *does* help to prevent water pollution, for instance, by flowing wastes into the soil, though there is no evidence that the compost (manure) yields more nutritious food than chemical fertilizers. Since plants can use only *inorganic* compounds, manure must be broken down by soil bacteria to nitrates, phosphates and potassium before it can be assimilated. Freshly picked vegetables and fruits contain more VITAMINS, but at least one study showed less CAROTENE (the yellow-red pigment in many foods that the body converts into VITAMIN A) in plants from manure-fertilizer soil than those from soil in which synthetic fertilizers supplemented manure.

In addition to organic products, some health-food enthusiasts advocate megadoses of vitamins and mineral supplements in the almost mystical belief that vitamins and minerals, as well as certain other foods such as honey, LECITHIN, rose hips, wheat germ and blackstrap molasses, have special health-giving powers. For example, Zen Macrobiotic dieters ascribe qualities of good and evil to different foods. And raw-food cultists, on the true-enough basis that a large percentage of nutrients in food is lost during cooking, eat only vegetables, fruits, sprouts and seeds—all raw—in order to reduce their "inner pollution."

Returning to the discussion of vitamins, some "health foodists" not only advocate large daily doses of vitamins but often insist on "natural" vitamins, though many vitamins labeled "natural" are often partly synthetic anyway, not to mention the facts that natural vitamins are more expensive and that synthetic vitamins have the same chemical composition, i.e., perform the same biological activity, as the natural. The body, it appears, *cannot* tell the difference between a molecule of VITAMIN C in an orange and a molecule of vitamin C synthetized in a laboratory.

In regard to the sudden popularity of VITAMIN E because of its supposed ability to prevent heart attacks, ease ARTHRITIS pains, cure burns and enhance sexual potency, biochemists can only respond that vitamin E is an excellent antioxidant present in large quantities in leafy vegetables and whole-grain foods, not a miracle drug. But biochemists *do* warn people about the danger of hypervitaminosis, the excessive intake of vitamin A and D, the two vitamins that can be stored in the body and that build up in the liver. Massive doses of most B vitamins, however, do not seem either to harm the body or to provide it with any benefit.

Dermatologists have recently reported that vitamin E capsules intended for ingestion may, when opened and applied to the skin, cause an irritating DERMATITIS instead of erasing wrinkles or reducing scars, as many hopeful people seem to anticipate. But then again, at least one claim made by one of the health foodists' heroes, Professor Linus Pauling, that had been ridiculed and disclaimed by the scientific community is now proving true. When Professor Pauling, who won the Nobel prize for chemistry in 1954, published in 1970 *Vitamin C and the Common Cold*, many scientists and physicians thought that the book marked the "swan song of a great intellect." Professor Pauling's assertion that 1000 mg of vitamin C taken regularly every day will decrease the incidence of colds by about 45 percent and total illness by about 60 percent was dismissed as heresy. Now, "pro-vitamin C" evidence is piling up so rapidly, so unequivocally, that nobody dares mock Professor Pauling any longer, and one article after another is appearing in the medical press to state that, yes, study after study indicates that food *is* an insufficient source of vitamin C and that even a balanced diet does not provide enough vitamin C.

"I suppose all progress is heresy," Professor Pauling is reported to have said in a famous 1973 interview; "any progress involves some rejection of the old ideas and their replacement with new ones."

ORGASMIC DYSFUNCTION (FRIGIDITY)

"Frigidity" was originally a broad expression applied to anything from a *complete* lack of sexual response in a woman to any degree of sexual indifference that was considered disappointing to both a woman and her partner. But today, the term frigidity is more specifically applied to a complete lack of response, while the general condition is referred to as "orgasmic dysfunction."

There are many causes for a woman's—or rather, for a *couple's*—mutual sexual dysfunction: ignorance of a woman's genital anatomy, for instance, and misconceptions concerning the physiology of orgasm; cultural distaste or fear of sexual intercourse; a partner's technique and unhygienic habits; and, in older women, even a CONTRACEPTIVE PILL that contains a high level of progesterone. On the other hand, a dysfunction may be caused by a congenital defect, such as an imperforate hymen (one which completely blocks the vaginal opening), or a physical abnormality such as endometriosis, a condition in which tissue resembling uterine mucous membrane is found in various locations in the pelvic area. And finally, if orgasm (which is a neurovascular response) is inhibited for too long, for either physical or psychological reasons, a chronic pelvic PAIN may result—although women often do not realize that the pain has a sexual origin.

Obviously, congenital defects should be, and presumably are, treated as any other physical condition; however, if the sexual dysfunction is psychogenic—that is, has an emotional origin—it is important that both the woman *and* her partner participate in the treatment, for again, orgasmic dysfunction is a *couple's*, not merely a woman's, problem.

ORTHOMOLECULAR MEDICINE

Orthomolecular medicine is a new, still-controversial type of medical approach formulated by Professor Linus Pauling, the brilliant biochemist and winner of two Nobel prizes (for chemistry in 1954 and for peace in 1962).

Orthomolecular medicine proposes to maintain good health and treat illness on a molecular basis—no longer by employing synthetized chemicals or those derived from plants, but rather by *varying the concentration* (supplementing deficits, subtracting excesses, restoring biochemical balances) of substances that are normally required to preserve good health.

Megavitamin therapy—using the common nutritional vitamins as medicine, but in megaquantities—is one form of orthomolecular medicine. Professor Pauling theorizes that, since many diseases are known to result from defective ENZYMES in the body, and since VITAMINS often act as CO-ENZYMES (the nonprotein part of enzymes), if the body is saturated with large amounts of co-enzymes, enough of them would be available to overcome the hereditary (or acquired) defect caused by abnormal or inadequate enzymes. Thus, biochemical imbalances as diverse as alcoholism, depression and senility could be successfully treated with massive doses of the proper vitamins.

The Huxley Institute for Biosocial Research in New York is the center of orthomolecular medicine. There, three scientists—Dr. Abraham Hoffer, Dr. Humphrey Osmond and, of course, Professor Linus Pauling—are engaged in nutritional and biochemical research that is currently regarded as too nonconformist to be considered "respectable" by many members of the orthodox medical community. Dr. Pauling, for instance, has been working with computer analysis and has been able, using urine samples, to chart biochemical profiles of about three hundred factors, which, if they become standard, could provide physicians with very detailed information about a patient's physiology.

Another field in which this new medical approach is developing is that of psychotherapy. Orthomolecular psychiatry is a theory and treatment of mental illness that is quite different from conventional psychiatric concepts. Professor Pauling points out that the proper functioning of the mind is known to require the presence in the brain of molecules of many different substances. For example, certain mental diseases result from a low concentration in the brain of any one of the following vitamins: thiamine (B_1); nicotinic acid (B_3); pyridoxine (B_6); cyanocobalamin (B_{12}); biotin; ascorbic acid (C); and folic acid. There is also evidence, Professor Pauling points out, that mental function and behavior are affected by changes in the concentration in the brain of a number of other substances, such as glutamic and uric acids.

Schizophrenic patients, for example, generally have no vitamin deficiency by ordinary standards. However, Dr. David Hawkins, director of psychiatric research at the Brunswick Hospital in Long Island, reported that many of his schizophrenic patients who were given large amounts of VITAMIN C (as much as 3 or 4 gm a day) did not excrete the excess vitamin, as normal people do with such massive doses. Schizophrenic patients apparently *retain* doses even as high as seventy-five times the standard recommendation of vitamins C, B_3 and B_6, supporting the orthomolecular-medicine theory that their bodies were suffering from an enormous vitamin deficiency and that the massive doses were indeed meeting their special needs. Dr. Hawkins reported several gratifying results with schizophrenic patients who showed unexpected improvements when megavitamin therapy was added to the traditional psychotherapy.

In theory, orthomolecular medicine is meant not only for the mentally ill but for everybody's normal "maintenance programs" of health and prevention of illness. Consider, for example, the COMMON COLD and its prevention with Professor Pauling's now broadly accepted regimen of vitamin C.

However, simply to ingurgitate massive doses of any vitamin is not advisable. For one thing, the metabolism of vitamins—unlike, let's say, that of PROTEINS—is extraordinarily individual: even normal people seem to have widely disparate needs for vitamins, regardless of age, size, and physical condition. And the rate of a person's vitamin metabolism is not something that can be guessed, not to mention that excessive doses of fat-soluble vitamins could themselves cause abnormalities.

Megavitamin therapy, then, is not for experimenting with at home; it requires the *right* kind and the *right* amount of vitamins under medical supervision.

OVEREATERS ANONYMOUS (OA)

Overeaters Anonymous is a nonprofit, self-help organization patterned after Alcoholics Anonymous (AA). It was founded in the early 1960s in Los Angeles, and as of 1974 it counts more than eight hundred groups throughout the world.

OA's basic concept is that compulsive overeating is a disease affecting a person on the *physical*, *spiritual* and *emotional* levels. Like alcoholics, members of OA believe that will power alone is not enough to control their compulsion.

Most people who join OA have completely lost faith in life and in themselves, as they have repeatedly failed with the traditional methods of weight control. At OA they find friendly people who understand their anguish, have suffered the same compulsion and are now examples that there *is* a solution to the problem.

Although OA's program is strict, members are not pressured but rather made to feel that it is their own desire to hold on to the program that counts. During meetings, members are encouraged to give brief accounts of their experiences. When they recall their former hopelessness and then tell how OA precepts helped them to overcome these feelings, they invariably make a dramatic impression on newcomers.

The first step of the OA program is abstaining from compulsive eating; the second, maintaining recovery *one day at a time* by sponsoring others. (Every newcomer asks someone to be his "food sponsor." A qualified sponsor is someone who has recovered from compulsive eating and has maintained a current state of moderation, having been led through the steps of recovery by another sponsor.)

There are no fees for OA membership; however, each local group is self-supporting through its members' contributions and does not accept outside funds.

OA offers two types of dietary programs, although variations and special diets, such as for diabetics, are accepted.

1) *Low carbohydrate diet*—Three regular meals a day with only sugar-free drinks between meals. All foods are measured and weighed—4 oz. PROTEIN per portion, ½ or 1 cup vegetables and fruits, depending on CARBOHYDRATE content.
2) *Alternate eating plan*—Based on the four primary food types.

The rule is to eat slowly, with small bites and no second helpings; to eat sitting down; not to skip meals, and to weigh oneself only once a month.

On the model of AA—the words "alcohol" and "alcoholics" are replaced with "food" and "compulsive overeaters"—OA offers The Twelve Steps of Recovery:

1) We admitted we were powerless over food—that our lives had become unmanageable.
2) We came to believe that a Power greater than ourselves could restore us to sanity.
3) We made a decision to turn our will and our lives over to the care of God as we understood Him.
4) We made a searching and fearless moral inventory of ourselves.
5) We admitted to God, to ourselves and to another human being the exact nature of our wrongs.
6) We were entirely ready to have God remove all these defects of character.
7) We humbly asked Him to remove our shortcomings.
8) We made a list of all persons we have harmed, and became willing to make amends to them all.
9) We made direct amends to such people wherever possible, except when to do so would injure them or others.
10) We continued to take personal inventory, and when we were wrong, promptly admitted it.
11) We sought through prayer and meditation to improve our conscious contact with God as we understood Him, praying only for knowledge of His will for us and the power to carry that out.
12) Having had a spiritual awakening as the result of these steps, we tried to carry this message to compulsive overeaters and to practice these principles in all our affairs.

Again on the model of AA, OA is guided by The Twelve Traditions:

1) Our common welfare should come first; personal recovery depends upon OA unity.

2) For our group purpose there is but one ultimate authority—a loving God as He may express Himself in our group conscience. Our leaders are but trusted servants; they do not govern.

3) The only requirement for OA membership is a desire to stop eating compulsively.

4) Each group should be autonomous except in matters affecting other groups or OA as a whole.

5) Each group has but one primary purpose—to carry its message to the compulsive overeater who still suffers.

6) An OA group ought never endorse, finance or lend the OA name to any related facility or outside enterprise, lest problems of money, property and prestige divert us from our primary purpose.

7) Every OA group ought to be fully self-supporting, declining outside contributions.

8) Overeaters Anonymous should remain forever nonprofessional, but our service centers may employ special workers.

9) OA, as such, ought never be organized; but we may create service boards or committees directly responsible to those they serve.

10) Overeaters Anonymous has no opinions on outside issues; hence, the OA name ought never be drawn into public controversy.

11) Our public-relations policy is based on attraction rather than promotion; we need always maintain personal anonymity at the level of press, radio, films, television, and other public media of communication.

12) Anonymity is the spiritual foundation of all these traditions, ever reminding us to place principles before personalities.

OVUM (EGG CELL)

The human ovum is the female reproductive cell. It is one of the largest cells in the body—about .135 mm in diameter—and consists of a large nucleus containing a *nucleolus* (germinal spot) and a yolk enclosed by a two-layered cell wall (an inner, thin one, the *vitelline membrane,* and an outer one, the *corona radiata*). Each unripe ovum (there are about thirty thousand unripe ova at the time of puberty) is stored in a small sac in the ovaries called a FOLLICLE.

Every month, throughout a woman's fertile years, one follicle bursts alternately in the *right* or the *left* ovary and one mature egg is released; the corona radiata becomes detached, permitting the sperm to come toward the FALLOPIAN TUBE through fluids surrounding the uterus and the ovaries and finally to enter the uterus. If it has been fertilized, the egg—now called a zygote—attaches itself to the wall of the uterus; if it remains unfertilized, the ovum passes on and out of the uterus two weeks later with the menstrual flow.

P

PAIN

Whether it is defined as a sensation, a perception, or a danger signal of trauma or malfunction, pain is one of nature's greatest mysteries. For one thing, pain can be described only *subjectively* and seldom is proportionate to the extent of the injury—superficial wounds, for example, hurt more than deep ones. Yet, even when a direct injury is involved, pain is not necessarily a simple cause-and-effect phenomenon. Also, when it appears in diseases such as cancer, the disease is usually too far advanced for pain to act as a warning symptom. Moreover, the quality of pain is often determined by previous experience, influenced by its significance in a person's cultural background, and intensified or decreased by psychological factors. And finally, thousands of people suffer from chronic pain with no evident sickness to account for it—pain itself may be a disease.

A conflict has raged among neurologists since the early nineteenth century about whether there are specific nerve endings sensitive to the stimulus of pain or whether *all* nerve endings interpret an extreme stimulus as pain. In 1965 Dr. Ronald Melzack, professor of psychology at McGill University in Montreal, proposed the now-famous (and controversial) Spinal-Gate theory of pain.

The Spinal-Gate theory postulated the existence of a gating mechanism in the spinal cord that can swing shut in a selective manner to block out pain. The gate was thought to be located in the *substantia gelatinosa*, the gelatinous substance present throughout the spinal cord. This theory would explain the analgesic effects of ACUPUNCTURE: the impulses imparted by the acupuncture needles are transmitted by means of large nerve fibers (Class A) to the spinal cord at a much faster rate than the pain impulses, which are transmitted through smaller fibers (Class C). By doing so, the gate closes to information coming over the smaller fibers. Thus, the pain impulses are diminished in intensity or even obliterated when they reach the higher centers.

Even if some aspects of the gate theory are wrong, as many neurologists now believe, it is important because it explores possibilities of blocking pain by means safer than chemicals or the surgical cutting of nerves—such as acupuncture and, as has been recently proposed, electronic analgesia.

In 1968 a neurosurgeon, Dr. Clyde Norman Shealy, director of the Pain Rehabilitation Center at St. Francis Hospital in La Crosse, Wisconsin, modernized a 1918 electrical device—then called the Electreat®—left over from the days when electricity was believed to be not only an analgesic but a miracle cure for a large number of illnesses.

The ability of electricity to relieve pain was known long before the exact nature of electricity was discovered. Scribonius Largus, court physician to the Roman Emperor Claudius, in A.D. 46 used the electric ray of torpedo fish for the treatment of HEADACHE and gout. In the eighteenth century Luigi Galvani demonstrated the effect of direct current on the nervous system, an effect that was well known by the end of the nineteenth century. Crude electrical devices were constructed in great quantities, but too many miracles were predicted in the name of galvanism for the treatment to survive. Despite continual demonstrations of their real abilities in pain relief, the devices became synonymous with quackery and their manufacturers were forced out of business.

With the Spinal-Gate theory of pain, however, the interest in electronic analgesia was revived. As with an acupuncture needle, the larger nerve fibers are activated—electrically, in this case. The electrical impulses apparently set in motion a process that tends to close the gate to information coming over the smaller fibers to the spinal cord, so that the pain message doesn't go through. The device currently used for electronic analgesia consists of a hand-held, battery-operated pulse generator, to which a pair of electrode-tipped wires can be attached. Applied to the skin overlying any painful area of the body, these electrodes provide continuous mild electric stimulations. A ten-minute application apparently can banish a toothache long enough for a dentist to take care of it. Electrodes placed over the nape of the neck for half an hour may prevent MIGRAINE. And the device has apparently proven useful for sciatica and BACKACHE.

Skeptics have argued that a large portion of the reputed relief of pain with this device, especially among patients suffering from chronic pain, can be attributed to a PLACEBO effect, and that some patients don't show any improvement at all. Dr. Shealy agrees that the placebo effect is a factor, but he points out that placebo effects do not last, while many of his patients have shown effects that have lasted many months after the electric treatment.

Even the latest versions of the device, however, are still developmental; the concept of electronic analgesia is still being investigated, and it has a long way to go before it is perfected. But there are reasons to believe that electronic analgesia will be among the most exciting medical news of the next ten years.

PALLIATIVES

A palliative refers to anything that serves to palliate—that is, to give relief. Palliatives don't cure the underlying cause but ease the symptoms. ASPIRIN, for instance, is a classic example of a palliative: it eases occasional PAIN or discomfort.

Essentially, palliatives are used when a disease cannot be cured, either because it is too minor to bother with, such as a temporary HEADACHE, or because it is too serious to offer hope for recovery, as in advanced cancer. In fact, physicians consistently are faced with the basic decision of whether to try to cure a disease or whether it is better to treat only the symptoms and give the patient maximum comfort.

PANTYHOSE

Pantyhose refers to the combination stockings-panties introduced in the mid-1960s to accompany miniskirts, most of which were short enough to reveal garter belts, GIRDLES and even stocking welts.

There is probably no other garment in history that became so popular so fast; many women who never did, or would, wear miniskirts have gladly given up garter belts and stockings for pantyhose. However, from the start, pantyhose were for women a source of what a public-relations director once called "mild desperation." Indeed, to find one's correct size among the dozens of pantyhose brands, with their different concepts of definitions such as "petite," "medium-large," or "duchess," often was a matter of sheer luck. Some manufacturers had six sizes, others had four, and still others had three. A few, depending entirely on the elasticity of the yarn, produced just one size, intended to fit all wearers. Some women solved the problem by wearing panties *over* the pantyhose, though what woman didn't end up, at least once, with pantyhose so long as to fit "like a strapless bodysuit"? Or so short that the crotch wouldn't stretch above the knee?

In 1970 a fourteen-month study called *A Better Fit in Pantyhose* was published by the National Association of Hosiery Manufacturers. The study, headed by Robert Peel, senior research consultant for Hanes Corporation, eventually was translated into unified size definitions to be adopted by the entire industry. The result was a simple chart, placed on each pantyhose package, that finally enabled about 90 percent of all women—whether short or tall, slender or heavy—to find the right size of pantyhose for their height, weight and body structure.

To manufacture exactly proportionate pantyhose is relatively complicated. Stockings need fit only the foot and the leg, but pantyhose must fit the lower part of the torso as well; they must cling like a second skin, and, above all, once manufactured they cannot be altered. To be sure, the stretch yarns that are used to knit pantyhose provide some compensation, but there is a limit to how much they can compensate for an inexact fit.

Among other things, the 1970 study established that "a stocking leg designed to fit a rather short and plump human leg will stretch in length and contract in girth to fit a longer and slimmer human leg, so long as both the plump and the slim legs have the same surface area."

Of course, a woman trying to buy pantyhose in a department store can hardly be expected to calculate the surface area of her legs and hips, or to know the size of her hips or crotch height. But it was also established that the surface area corresponds almost exactly to a person's height and weight; and almost every woman knows approximately her height and weight.

Still, in order to proportion pantyhose correctly, manufacturers had to produce pantyhose that conformed to more subtle relations between measurements. These were eventually worked out in the form of a series of equations. For instance, in an average woman, knee height equals .310 times total height minus 2.61 inches. In turn, the equations were translated into three-dimensional mannequins to be used to test the fit of

This chart, devised by Hanes Corporation of New York City, enables ninety percent of all women—whether short or tall, slender or heavy—to find the right size of pantyhose for their height, weight, and body structure.

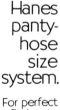

Hanes panty-hose size system.

For perfect fit, locate height at left, then move across to square under weight. The letter in that zone is your Hanes size.

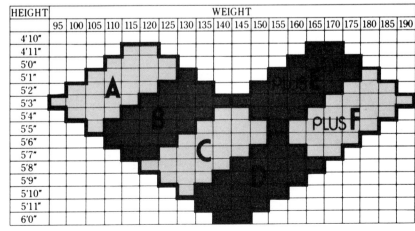

finished pantyhose. The number of mannequins a manufacturer needs depends on the number and range of sizes he markets. (The average is twelve mannequins.)

The first machine-made stockings were knitted flat and sewn up in the back. Shortly before the turn of the century, the circular knitting machine was invented, which made seamless stockings feasible. In practice, contoured seamless stockings had to wait until the 1930s, when nylon was introduced.

For one pair of sheer pantyhose, over a mile of nylon yarn and one million stitches are required. They are knitted on a circular knitting machine that is almost as complicated as a computer and that produces a tube with a knitted-on waistband and an open toe. (The tube is tapered to fit properly throughout the leg and foot surface.) A flat seam is used to close the toe; the stocking is then placed on a flat, leg-shaped form, put in a pressure chamber and exposed to steam at a temperature of 256° F. This gives a permanent shape to the stocking and sets the size that had been originally knit into the stocking. The legs are then matched in pairs and sewn together to form pantyhose. Finally, the pantyhose is dyed, dried, inspected for defects and packaged.

Some manufacturers, such as Hanes and Kayser-Roth, have developed sheer support hosiery, that is, pantyhose whose yarn contains a certain amount of a synthetic elastic fiber called spandex. This fiber has the property of both expanding easily and exerting pressure. For women who suffer from FATIGUE, leg pains, and circulation problems and who have a tendency to VARICOSE VEINS, support pantyhose help to balance the internal pressure of the veins, thus better enabling the leg muscles to pump the blood upward again. To be really useful, of course, compression must be graduated, that is, applied only on certain parts of the leg, such as the foot, the ankle, and the lower part of the leg, while expanding on the hips and the crotch, where compression would hinder circulation.

For pregnant women, special support pantyhose are available, with panty panels that expand on the abdomen as pregnancy advances.

Recent technological developments have also improved the one-size pantyhose. Among the latest superstretch materials is a yarn that, once heated, develops a spiral structure, which allows it to return to its original shape after stretching.

PAP SMEAR TEST

The Pap smear test, devised by the Greek medical scientist Dr. George Papanicolaou, is a method for the early detection of the possible presence of cancerous cells in the cervix or in the vagina. This test is also used to identify the cause of venereal diseases and of VAGINITIS.

The Pap smear test consists of the microscopic study of a smear which the gynecologist first takes from the secretions of the cervix and the vagina with a small aspirator, then places on a glass slide and sends to a pathologist for examination.

All women over twenty—and younger, if they have had children or have contracted a venereal disease—should have regular Pap smear tests. In theory, once a year should be enough; however, in women who have been treated for carcinoma, a smear should be taken every three months for the first years and every six months subsequently.

Menopausal women and those who have a family history of cervical cancer should have the test every six months, because if a Pap test is misread and fails to reveal an early carcinoma, a woman may go for two years without proper attention: long enough for invasive (spreading into the healthy tissue) cancer to develop.

A Pap test is painless, and it takes the gynecologist only a few minutes to obtain the smear.

PAPAIN

Papain is a natural plant ENZYME obtained from the papaya fruit and widely used as a meat tenderizer. Papain is generally recognized as safe for use in food that is subsequently cooked, as the heat required to cook meat readily destroys the papain. In the unlikely event the cooking does not destroy the papain, the gastric juices would do so.

Papain is also used medically as an aid in stomach disorders and is sold in health-food stores as a digestant. Recently, papain extract (known medically as chymopapain) has been used experimentally by a number of orthopedic doctors as an alternative to laminectomy, a delicate surgical procedure in which a ruptured disc, causing severe BACKACHE, is removed from between two vertebrae. In many cases, doctors have found that chymopapain can be injected into the disc, thus breaking down the disc's nucleus, causing it to shrink back into place and consequently easing the pressure on the surrounding nerves.

Chymopapain sometimes causes an allergic reaction, and as of 1974 it has not yet been approved by the FDA. At present, only certain hospitals, such as the Massachusetts General Hospital in Boston, are allowed to use it. However, the doctors report a high percentage of successes, especially in cases of severe sciatica and badly ruptured discs.

PARAFFIN BATH

Paraffin is a waxy, odorless, translucent substance obtained from petroleum. A paraffin bath, available at some of the best BEAUTY SPAS, consists of lying in a shallow tub, having one's body (except the face) coated with a stratum of liquefied warm paraffin to which various oils have been added, and finally being rolled up to the neck in warm covers.

Almost immediately, the body begins to perspire, and the person is left alone to relax in a room that is usually quiet and shaded. About thirty minutes later, when it has hardened and cooled, the paraffin is peeled off and the body gently patted dry and allowed to rest a few minutes.

Sometimes there is a scale in the paraffin-bath room, and a weight-conscious woman may indulge for a moment in the illusion that the paraffin bath has indeed taken off one or two pounds of fat. Naturally, what she has lost in the swift and effortless perspiration in the bath is only WATER, which will be replaced as soon as she drinks a few glasses of liquid.

However, a paraffin bath can be quite soothing: it makes the skin feel smooth and supple, and normally is perfectly harmless.

PATCH TESTING

Patch testing is one of the ways to diagnose whether a person is allergic to certain substances. It consists of taping to the skin, usually on the back or the upper arm, a pad or a patch (often of filter paper) on which is the chemical or substance that is being tested. If a person is allergic to the suspected material, within forty-eight hours the skin at the site of the test shows redness, itching, irritation and tiny blisters—i.e., the reaction is *positive*.

The basic principle of patch testing is simple, and it is the only technique currently available. However, so many mistakes have occurred that many physicians doubt its validity. The reason is that, although the patch test is indeed reliable in principle, it requires great skill and the proper application and interpretation, especially when the physician is testing unknown substances or is searching for an uncommon allergen. On the other hand, testing for standard allergens is now quickly performed and relatively inexpensive.

One of the problems with the test is that it is often difficult to distinguish between a true *allergic* reaction and a simple irritation. And, until recently, many dermatologists used different patches, which led to different results that could not be repeated from clinic to clinic. Also, the patches are often not adhesive enough and fall off before the test is over. More important, the substances used for the test must have a specific concentration, neither too high nor too low, for the wrong concentration is the most common cause of an unsuccessful patch test. When the concentration is *too high*, the patch could produce an inflammation, but this is not necessarily an indication of an allergic reaction; this is called a *false-positive* response. When the concentration is *too low*, there may be no reaction at all—*false negative* response—which is dangerous because the patient will assume that he is not allergic to the material. To prevent these false responses, physicians are now urged to use standard patches, tapes and concentrations, as established by the International Contact Dermatitis Group (ICDG).

In conclusion, the physician cannot accept the patch test at face value: he must evaluate each positive and negative response to make sure there are no false-positives or false-negatives. "With some of the recent standardized information," wrote Dr. Howard I. Maibach of the department of dermatology, University of California School of Medicine in San Francisco, "patch testing is far more objective than a decade ago. With new information becoming available it is likely to become even more objective [1974]."

PERFUMERY

Perfumery is the art of producing scents through combinations of fragrant substances in definite proportions. The perfumer's traditional aspiration was to capture and somehow preserve intact the beautiful natural fragrances of flowers in their living state, which wasn't always easy, since the living odors of flowers cannot be extracted intact. But modern perfumery has solved this problem: it is now possible to synthetize a large number of chemicals whose odors not only resemble portions of those of natural substances but also are stable. This does not mean that perfumery has become computerized; in creating a new perfume, the master perfumer—called a "nose" in the fragrance business—has to be more than a chemist. He is often inspired, the way an artist is by an idea, by a new natural or synthetic product. He then mixes it with three, four or five other carefully chosen substances in an attempt to achieve a blend in which the distinctive character of the main product is not only preserved but enhanced by the combination.

Perfumers use the term *aromatics* (or raw materials) for natural odorous substances, and the term *aromatic chemicals* for their synthetic counterparts. There are two kinds of aromatics:
1) Natural products of vegetable origin.
   a) *Essential oils*, volatile oils found in plants and obtained by distillation;
   b) *Flower oils*;
   c) Natural extracts from *resins, gums* and *mosses*.
2) Animal fixatives.
   a) *Ambergris*, not a gland secretion as was once believed, but an accumulation of material which causes intestinal obstruction in the

sperm whale. After a whale's death, ambergris floats on water even for years. Air and sun make it lighter in color and weight and less pungent in odor. The way ambergris forms is still unknown; one theory is that the process is similar to the formation of pearls by oysters;

b) *Castoreum*, a dried aromatic gland of beaver;

c) *Civet*, a gland secretion of the civet cat;

d) *Musk*, material contained in a gland located under the abdomen of the male musk deer.

Each perfume contains:

1) a *Top Note*—the refreshing scent a perfume gives off when it is first applied (lemon, green bark, muguet, tuberose);

2) an *End Note*—the dominant scent of perfume, which stays with the wearer for a long time; consists of resins mixed with heavy essential oils such as patchouli, sandalwood, artificial musk;

3) a *Middle Note*—also called a modifier, the flowery part of perfume, which forms a bridge between the Top and the End Notes; consists of such scents as carnation, jasmine, lilac, rose, violet.

Perfumes are classified according to their End Notes into the following basic groups:

1) *Floral group*—The most popular flower odors blended in this group are jasmine, rose, lily of the valley, lilac, violet, carnation, hyacinth, gardenia, honeysuckle, narcissus and orange flower. Less frequently it is possible to recognize an odor of jonquil, tuberose, mimosa or acacia. A few of the classic flowery perfumes are:

Quelques Fleurs (Houbigant)	Capriccio (Nina Ricci)
Chanel No. 22 (Chanel)	Diorissimo (Dior)
Fleurs de Rocaille (Caron)	Windsong (Matchabelli)
Paris (Coty)	Joy (Patou)

2) *Spicy blends*—These are easily recognized by an odor of carnation, clove, cinnamon, nutmeg, and small amounts of basil, caraway, estragon. Typical spicy perfumes are:

Early American Spice (Shulton)	Blue Grass (Arden)
Bellodgia (Caron)	Moment Suprême (Patou)

3) *Woody family*—The most important woody odors characteristic for this group are sandalwood, cedarwood and orris root. Their Top Note is usually floral, to balance the basic woodiness. Typical representatives are:

Nuit de Noël (Caron)	Bois des Iles (Chanel)
Antilope (Weil)	Vétiver (Guerlain)

4) *Mossy family*—Oak moss has an odor of forest earth and gives perfumes a warm and lasting End Note. The most famous oak-moss perfumes are:

Chypre (Coty)	Femme (Rochas)
Mitsouko (Guerlain)	Rumeur (Lanvin)
Crêpe de Chine	Ma Griffe (Carven)

5) *Oriental family*—This group consists of perfumes in which woody, mossy and spicy notes are combined with the sweetness of vanilla or of such balsamic resins as benzoin. In order to accentuate the Oriental note, many animal fixatives are used—either musk, civet, or synthetic ambergris compounds. The Middle Note used most frequently for Oriental perfumes is the rose. Typical representatives of this group are:

Tabu (Dana)	To a Wild Rose (Avon)
Youth Dew (Estée Lauder)	Shalimar (Guerlain)

6) *Herbal group*—Members of this group have a very distinctive odor, reminiscent of hay, orchid, clover, and sweet grass. Many colognes for men are in this family. Some classic representatives of the herbal group are:

Jicky (Guerlain)	Aramis (Estée Lauder)
Moustache (Rochas)	

7) *Leather-tobacco group*—Perfumes in this small family can be recognized by their odor of real leather, tobacco, or smoky notes reminiscent of birch tar, a resin from Finnish birch trees. Typical representatives of this group are:

Cuir de Russie (Chanel)	Scandal (Lanvin)
Tabac Blond (Caron)	Bandit (Piguet)

8) *Aldehydic group*—This is a very important family of fragrances. The typical Notes in this group are recognizable not by a natural odor but by the odor of aromatic chemicals called aldehydes. The aldehydes occur in nature in citrus oil and in most floral odors. They can be identified as a sharp or slightly fruity odor. Representatives of this family are:

Chanel No. 5 (Chanel)	L'Aimant (Coty)
Arpège (Lanvin)	Madame Rochas (Rochas)

PERSPIRATION

Perspiration is the moisture (a little less than 1 quart in twenty-four hours) secreted by millions of sweat glands distributed all over the body, close to the skin's surface, to which they are connected by tiny walled passages called ducts.

There are two kinds of sweat glands: eccrine glands and apocrine glands.

1) Beneath the skin's surface are coiled approximately three million eccrine glands, which respond to two kinds of stimulation, *heat* and

emotions—pain, fear, tension, sexual excitement. The eccrine glands on the palms, the soles of the feet, and the underarm constantly secrete *small* amounts of clear, odorless fluid, 99 percent WATER, 1 percent SALT (though emotional stimulation may increase the amount). Those on the rest of the body respond only to physical exertion and heat, except in cases of extreme emotional stimulation, when the whole body may perspire.

2) The apocrine glands are larger and less numerous than the eccrine; they are almost all concentrated in the hairy underarm area (with a few in the pubic hair area), and respond only to emotional stimulation. Apocrine glands are present at birth but begin to function only at puberty, with a decline in their activity in old age. When stimulated, apocrine glands secrete a viscous, milky liquid that is composed of complex organic materials and that also is at first odorless but is subsequently decomposed by bacteria on the skin to form the unpleasant underarm odor.

The most common misconception about perspiration is that it disposes of body wastes. In reality, eccrine glands have one major purpose: to regulate the body temperature. When the salty water of perspiration evaporates, the body's heat is reduced. In cases when an extreme emotional stimulation triggers the eccrine glands on the *entire* body, evaporation causes a chill—the well-known cold sweat—because the body is not heated.

Some people suffer from hyperidrosis—excessive sweating of the palms and soles. The mechanism of hyperidrosis is still little known and is unaffected by available ANTIPERSPIRANTS. One possibility is that the condition may result in part from inherited overactivity of the sympathetic nervous system (a portion of the autonomic nervous system), or to an oversensitivity of the sweat glands to stimulations by the sympathetic nervous system; and that condition can be aggravated by stress and emotion and, in a vicious circle, by the embarrassment caused by the very condition of hyperidrosis.

The human body, physiologists have discovered, is capable of adjusting to prolonged hot weather. After a few days of high temperature, the sweat glands increase their activity so that more heat can be transported to the body's surface for evaporation. The protective mechanism works in this way: when excessive temperature threatens the body's normal 98.6° F. temperature, receptors in the nervous system send a message to the hypothalamus, which in turn signals the blood vessels to dilate in order to deliver a greater volume of heat to the sweat glands, which increase the secretion of moisture to the skin's surface.

The lost fluid, of course, must be replaced by drinking. A minimal amount of body salts, too, is lost with perspiration, and people are sometimes advised to swallow salt tablets to compensate for the reduced supply. However, some doctors feel that an indiscriminate use of salt supplements may be harmful—an extra dash on the next meal, they say, is all that is normally needed to reestablish the balance.

PETROLATUM (PETROLEUM JELLY)

Petrolatum, better known by the trade name Vaseline®, is a neutral, water-insoluble, practically odorless and tasteless substance obtained from petroleum.

Petrolatum is used chiefly as a base for ointments (for minor skin irritations) and for such cosmetics as MOISTURIZERS, hand and hair lotions, and lip pomades. Most moisturizers sold today contain either petrolatum or mineral oil, or a mixture of the two.

Though much more greasy than most cosmetic creams, petrolatum is one of the most inexpensive cosmetic ingredients available and is excellent for its emollient effects.

pH

The symbol pH is used to express the degree of a solution's opposite properties of acidity and alkalinity. The pH scale ranges from 1 to 14, with pH 7 as the *neutral point*. In other words, at normal temperature, a neutral solution such as pure distilled WATER has a pH of about 7; a normal solution of hydrochloric acid, a pH of nearly 1; and a normal solution of a strong alkali such as sodium hydroxide, a pH of nearly 14.

To test the pH of a solution, chemists may use litmus, a blue pigment with a pH range of 4.5 to 8.3 prepared from a lichen called *Roccella tinctoria* and formed with powdered chalk into small cakes. Acids turn blue litmus *red*; alkalis turn red litmus *blue*.

PHEROMONES

Pheromones, or ectohormones, are chemical compounds of volatile acids that function as sex attractants. They have recently been discovered in the vaginal secretions of women and practically all female animals—from insects on up.

Dr. Richard P. Michael, with his team at the Primate Behavior Research Laboratory in Kent, England, in the late 1960s became the first to describe the existence of an odorous cue by which a female in rut signals her sexual condition to the male. Later, Dr. Michael succeeded in isolating the compound and eventually reproduced it in the laboratory.

Unlike HORMONES, which are secreted into the bloodstream, pheromones are excreted to exert specific effects at a distance—such as recognition, danger, alarm, or sexual attraction—on the behavior or physiology of another individual of the same species. The pheromones emitted by the silkworm moth to attract the male, for instance, are so sensitive that one trillionth of a gram can do it.

Dr. Michael reported that when synthetic pheromones are applied to the genitals of a female rhesus monkey (which had been made sexually unreceptive by OVARIECTOMY), it became instantly irresistible to the same male that had previously ignored it.

In 1974 Dr. Michael, now a psychiatrist at the Emory University School of Medicine in Atlanta, Georgia, announced that, as had been long suspected, pheromones are present in humans, too. The vaginal secretions of normal healthy women contain pheromones that are present in the largest amount during a woman's fertile period. What role pheromones play in human sexual behavior is not yet known, but, in Dr. Michael's words, "It is rather interesting that they are there to begin with, have a cyclical production rate and have a function in lower primates."

The Atlanta studies showed that women who take oral contraceptives have fewer pheromones, and that the cyclical changes in their amount are absent. Also, women who douche regularly destroy the bacteria, normally present in the vagina, that produce pheromones. These acid-producing bacteria have an important health function: they help to inhibit the growth of infectious fungi. Thus, whether merely infection deterrents or also sex attractants, human pheromones cannot be ignored. And those women who are so anxious about genital odors that they wash and compulsively deodorize themselves even when preparing for a gynecological examination (thus often making a diagnosis impossible) should protect their pheromones and consider douching only as a prescription, not as a routine hygienic practice.

PHOTOCHROMIC LENSES

Photochromic lenses are special lenses, first developed by the Corning Glass company, which have the property of changing automatically from dark to light and back again, depending on the amount of ultraviolet light to which they are exposed.

There are two kinds of photochromic lenses, trademarked Photogray® and Photosun®.

Photogray®—Photogray® was introduced several years ago and is now manufactured by American Optical Corporation; it is not considered a SUNGLASS lens, since at its darkest it transmits 45 to 34 percent of the light (sunglass lenses should not have more than 30 percent light transmission). When worn indoors, a Photogray® lens will clear halfway in only a few minutes. At its lightest it is almost totally clear: 85 percent light transmission.

Photogray® lenses are often used for tennis or golf because darker glasses tend to obscure a fast-moving object. However, they are mostly worn as "fashion tints" because of their soft and attractive gray tone.

Photosun®—Photosun® is a more recent development that has a range from 20 to 65 percent light transmission. Photosun® lenses do not change quickly but darken gradually; their action depends not only on the degree of ultraviolet radiation but also on the temperature of the atmosphere—the cooler the air, the darker the lenses will get.

Both Photogray® and Photosun® darken to three-fourths of their capacity within the first minute of exposure; about halfway in ten minutes, and about 75 percent in ninety minutes.

Since it is invisible ultraviolet rays, not glare, that cause the change, these lenses darken very little in a car or indoors, no matter how bright the light falling on them.

PHYSICAL CHECK-UP

Many doctors recommend that healthy people *over forty* undergo the following annual physical check-up:

1) Complete physical examination, with special emphasis, in women, on breast examination.
2) Blood pressure.
3) Complete blood count (men and women).
4) Analysis of urine (men and women).
5) CHOLESTEROL and triglyceride determination (men and women).
6) Vaginal examination and, every other year, PAP TEST of the cervix.

For people who have no chronic chest disease, a chest X-ray should be done every three or four years. An electrocardiogram is advisable every year for men, less frequently for women.

For people with a family history of diabetes, a blood-glucose determination is recommended.

For people *under forty*, a general physical examination every two or three years should be sufficient.

PIRARUCÚ

Pirarucú is the world's largest fresh-water fish, found throughout the Amazon Basin, where it is usually harpooned by Brazilian fishermen.

PLACEBO

Native Indian women of the Amazonas reportedly use the scales of the pirarucú to file their nails; and fancy drugstores in the United States sell them for the same purpose. The scales look like giant nails, with a brown, hornlike "half moon" and a finely abrasive, curved white surface, which is the part used as a file.

Pirarucú scales are excellent files. They are less abrasive than emery boards, can be washed and trimmed, last quite a long time and, unlike emery boards, do not get soggy when used in a steamy bathroom.

PLACEBO

A placebo is an inert (that is, no substance in it has any effect on the body) medicament or preparation given for its psychological effect, especially to alleviate momentarily a patient's suffering from a mild form of HYPOCHONDRIASIS or certain types of PSYCHOSOMATIC DISEASES.

Placebos are also used as controls in a variety of experimental series, called double-blind experiments, in which one group of patients participating in a certain study are given the real medication, and a second group, a medication that looks exactly like the real one but is actually a placebo. No member of either group knows whether he is getting the real medication; generally only one person in the research team knows exactly which is which and who is getting what, and the cipher to the experiment is revealed only at the end.

Interestingly, confirming the emotional component of all physical reactions, some patients quite often and with the most disparate substances react to a placebo in a manner similar or identical to those taking the real medication. Further, if the study's "security" breaks down for some reason, allowing the patients to perceive what they are being tested for, they then *cease* to react.

PLACENTA

The placenta is a spongy, disc-shaped organ, covered by a transparent membrane, through which a developing fetus receives nourishment from the mother's body and through which its waste materials are disposed of.

The placenta develops inside the uterus at the point where the fertilized egg attaches itself. Both the blood from the mother and the blood from the fetus circulate in it *separately*. Blood from the fetus flows in and out through two arteries and a vein that are encased in the umbilical cord, which is attached to the surface of the placenta at one end and to the fetus's navel at the other. The waste products of the fetus are carried into the placenta by the arteries, while the vein carries back oxygen and nutrients from the mother.

The placenta is very slender at the beginning; then it becomes thicker and permeable to oxygen and other nutrients from the mother's circulation. It stores IRON, calcium, PROTEIN and GLUCOSE to be used later by the fetus. At the third month of pregnancy the placenta is fully developed; at the last month it begins to deteriorate, and after the baby is born, it comes out of the mother's body, at which stage it is often referred to as the afterbirth.

PLAQUE

Dental plaque is a sticky, colorless layer of bacteria that is constantly forming on teeth. The exact structure of plaque is not clear, though it is known that it contains substances generated by the bacteria mixed with mucin (a component of SALIVA), which the bacteria use as the "glue" that allows them to stick to the teeth.

Certain types of bacteria are especially active in forming plaque. A few seconds after they come in contact with ordinary SUGAR in various foods and drinks, they begin to ferment the sugars, changing them into acids, which attack the tooth enamel.

When it first forms, plaque is 80 percent water and 20 percent solid; but once it has settled on the teeth, more bacteria invade it and proliferate. Before long, plaque turns into a hard, razor-sharp deposit called tartar or calculus that tends to move deeper into the gums and to cause gingivitis (or pyorrhea)—inflammation of the gums. The bacteria in plaque are also considered one of the primary causes of dental caries.

Needless to say, plaque should be removed every day, with a TOOTHBRUSH for the teeth surfaces and with DENTAL FLOSS for the spaces between teeth. As plaque is transparent, it is difficult to know when all of it has been removed. The occasional use of a DISCLOSING SOLUTION helps to locate plaque by briefly dyeing it purple.

PLASTIC SURGERY

Plastic surgery is an extraordinary specialty which is at once at the bottom and at the very top of the scale of surgery.

From the laborer who thinks that plastic surgery is all done with hot plastic to the professor who associates the word "plastic" with implantable materials, believing these to be the primary tools of the specialty, the general public still has numerous misconceptions about plastic surgery—not to speak of the stern, old-fashioned doctor who hesitates to refer a patient to a plastic surgeon because he feels that "nose jobs" and "breast jobs" are unethical, closer to the work of a beautician or a masseur than to that of a real surgeon.

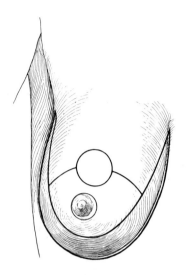

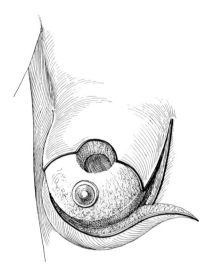

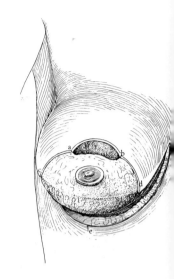

In the upper part of the incision a round portion of the mammary gland is cut out.

A portion of skin and mammary gland from below the nipple is removed.

On the marked breast, the surgeon makes a circular incision around the nipple's areola and cuts the skin along the marked lines.

AUGMENTATION MAMMAPLASTY

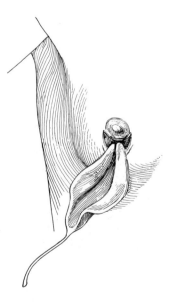

Left: Through a 5 cm. incision along the nipple's lower border, the empty folded balloon implant is inserted behind the mammary gland.

Center: A variable amount of saline solution is injected into the balloon through a small tube, which is then trimmed and sealed.

Right: The incision is sutured.

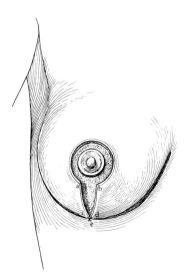

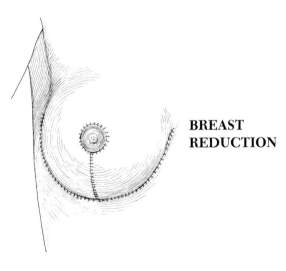

BREAST REDUCTION

The lower corners of the skin flap, C and D, are sutured to E, a previously marked point on the breast fold. Next, the upper corners, A and B, are sutured together.

The areola and the inverted T-shaped incision are sutured in place.

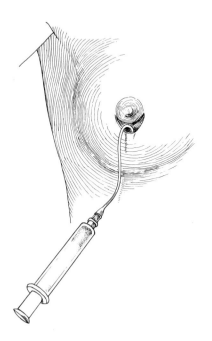

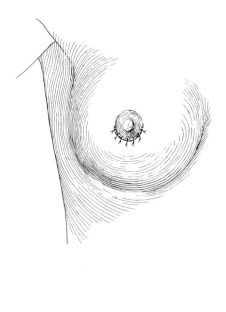

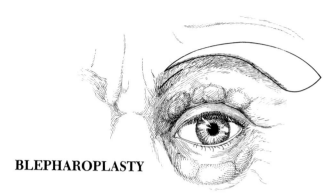

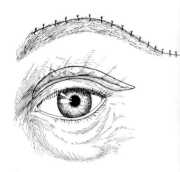

BLEPHAROPLASTY

Drawing illustrating the pockets of fat present underneath the skin in the upper and lower lids. Any combination of these little lumps can protrude as the result of a weakening of a membrane that contains them. An ellipse of skin to be removed in order to elevate a drooping eyebrow is marked in surgical ink.

The ellipse of skin is excised, and the wound is sutured along the eyebrow. The excess skin of the upper eyelid is marked with surgical ink.

COSMETIC SURGERY

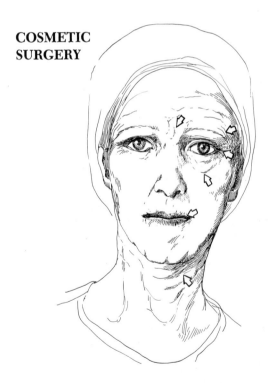

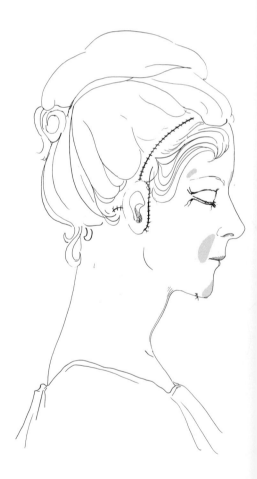

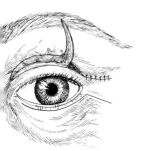
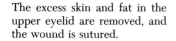

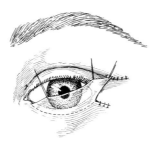

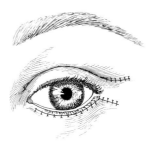

The excess skin and fat in the upper eyelid are removed, and the wound is sutured.

The redundant skin of the lower lid is cut below the lashes line and undermined. The protruding fat is delicately trimmed, and after painstaking measurements, the excess skin is excised.

The final stage of the operation. The suture line in the upper eyelid coincides with the lid's natural fold and with one of the natural creases about the eyes. The one in the lower lid is partially disguised by the lashes and, again, by a natural crease.

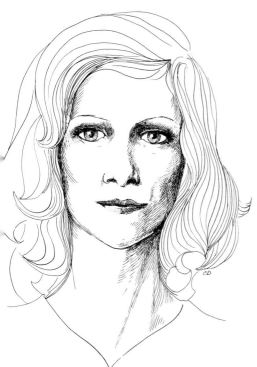

Left: Drawing of a woman approximately fifty years old about to undergo the following cosmetic surgery and adjunct procedures:

Rhytidectomy (face-lift).

Blepharoplasty (eyelid correction).

Submandibular lipectomy (chin correction).

Dermabrasion or chemical peel of the upper lip.

Injections of liquid silicone in the frown lines and other expression lines, such as those above the eyebrows and those encompassing the mouth.

Insertion of a solid silicone implant into the chin.

Center: The same woman shortly after surgery. In practice, of course, each procedure—except for rhytidectomy and blepharoplasty, which sometimes are performed in one session—takes place at a different time.

Right: The same woman after recovery, which is completed approximately six weeks after surgery but can vary considerably, depending on the individual.

279

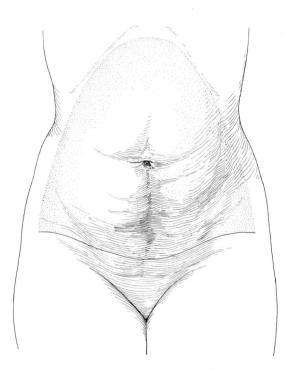

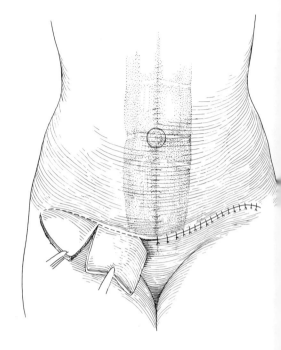

LIPECTOMY

Above: Drawing of a woman's abdomen, which has become flabby following a sudden weight loss, frequent pregnancies or abdominal surgery. The incision line runs along the pubic hair, extending on both sides to the hipbones and then curving slightly downward.

Above right: The skin is undermined up to the ribs and split around the navel, which is then attached to the deeper tissue. The abdomen muscles are reinforced; the skin is pulled downward, and the excess skin and fat are removed.

Right: The navel's new position is marked, and the navel itself is surfaced through a small incision in the skin and sutured in place. Finally, the larger incision is sutured. (The small scar below the navel corresponds to the previous navel's position.)

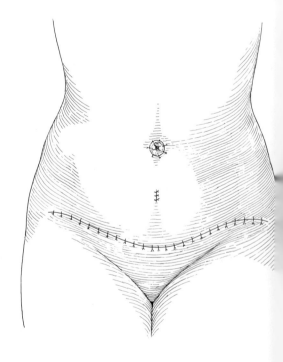

In reality, the word "plastic" derives, in this context, from the Greek *plastikos*, which means "to mold." Plastic surgery is an inventive, unique, diverse surgical discipline that, in an era of superspecialties, draws on several techniques—general surgery, dentistry, otolaryngology, orthopedics, neurosurgery—for the ultimate purpose of restoring normality. And when normality is the starting point, plastic surgery quite naturally strives for beauty.

Surgical reconstruction of the body's structural or functional deficiencies was practiced centuries ago. Ambroise Paré (1510–90), the personal surgeon of Charles IX of France, performed and wrote about surgery with the attitude and sophistication of a modern plastic surgeon; about the same time, Gasparo Tagliacozzi (1546–99), a surgeon from Bologna, wrote a treatise on *The Surgery of Deformities by Transplantation*, much of which extraordinary information is still valid today.

Modern plastic surgery, however, originated in England, and its fathers were two brilliant, eccentric surgeons: Sir Harold Gillies, a Scotsman born in New Zealand, and Sir Archibald McIndoe, an Australian.

A Red Cross surgeon in World War I, Gillies came upon plastic surgery after reading a German book on fractured jaws and watching a French surgeon try to repair mouth injuries. He felt he could help soldiers disfigured by the mutilating but not lethal shrapnel wounds. His original, daring surgical techniques were carried on despite a daily struggle with the British army, whose regulations did not include such procedure as plastic surgery.

With World War II, the usual cycle of medical innovations prompted by war started all over again. This time the victims were burned RAF pilots of the Battle of Britain, and the daring young surgeon at odds with army red tape was Dr. McIndoe. The pilots idolized "Archie" and later founded the Guinea Pigs Club, which met every year to celebrate the man who had invented the impossible in order to rebuild their faces.

Largely for the sake of medical insurance programs, for which a "nose job," for instance, does not yet qualify, plastic surgery today is classified into *reconstructive* and *aesthetic*. Reconstructive surgery is performed in such cases as:

1) *Congenital deformities*, such as cleft lip and palate, malformed jaws, lips, ears, hands, genitals;
2) *Traumas*, such as bone, nerve, tendon and soft-tissue injuries; hypertrophic (very large) scars, burns, unwanted tattoos;
3) *Cancer*, such as malignant tumors of the skin and in the mouth, and MASTECTOMY.

Aesthetic surgery includes:

1) *Rhinoplasty*, operations to correct defects of the nose;

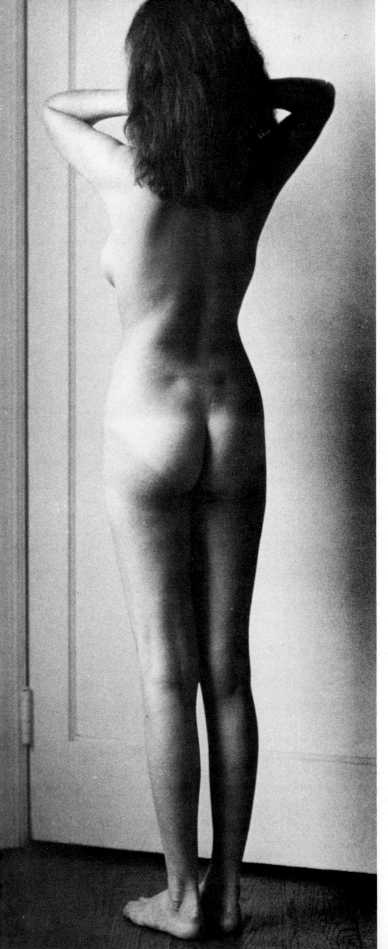

A twenty-six-year-old woman—
who begged her plastic surgeon
never to show her "before" photographs, not even for the most
scientific of lectures—as she looks
six months after undergoing a "riding breeches" operation.

Slender all her life, she used to
have two lumps of fat on her upper
thighs, impervious to diets, massages or exercise. Now, this young
woman's choice whether to wear
bikinis, slinky jersey or the shortest
shorts is entirely up to the whims
of fashion.

2) *Rhytidectomy*, the technical term for a face-lift;

3) *Blepharoplasty*, the correction of redundant eyelid tissue;

4) *Reduction mammaplasty*, reduction of the breast; *augmentation mammaplasty*, enlargement of the breast;

5) *Lipectomy*, excision of excessive fat in the chin, abdomen, arms or thighs.

People seeking reconstructive surgery usually have little trouble finding a surgeon, but when it comes to aesthetic surgery—a highly *elective* procedure—people often "window-shop" for a surgeon, though they rarely know what they are looking for, except, obviously, a good job. They cannot possibly judge the work of a plastic surgeon, and regardless of the surgeon's ability, a prospective patient who is not pressed by emergency has the leisure during the consultation to create in his mind a relationship of trust (or mistrust) with the surgeon. The latter, too, evaluates his visitor; in fact, it is essential that he exercise what amounts to instant psychoanalysis and decide whether the visitor should indeed become his patient. People seek aesthetic surgery for a great variety of motives, of which only some are reasonable.

If the plastic surgeon decides not to operate because of a patient's emotional instability, he has a choice: either politely dismiss the patient, sit and talk with him like an analyst, or refer him to a professional analyst. Either decision has its drawbacks, and it usually depends on the surgeon's temperament, the kind of community he lives in, and, sometimes, on his schedule for that day.

"The continued existence of plastic surgery as a specialty," recently wrote Dr. Jack C. Fisher, associate professor of plastic surgery at the University of Virginia School of Medicine in Charlottesville, "will depend upon not only maintenance of the highest standards of clinical practice but also the inventiveness of its members, who must continue to devise better methods for reconstruction, as they have in the past. This . . . creativity will be possible only so long as reconstructive surgeons apply their skills to the broadest range of problems, rather than focus on the easiest or most lucrative segments of practice."

POISON IVY

Poison ivy and related plants such as poison oak and poison sumac are the most common outdoor sources of so-called allergic contact DERMATITIS in the United States. Each summer about two million Americans suffer from inflammation caused by allergic reaction to the oily resin (sap) found in these plants.

The common belief is that just being near poison ivy causes a skin eruption; in reality, dermatitis occurs only after direct or indirect contact. Sometimes a person suffers an allergic reaction merely by touching the fur of a pet that has brushed against a poison ivy vine, or by touching the clothes of somebody who has come into contact with poison ivy. A reaction may also be caused by contact with the smoke from burning poison ivy plants.

Another misconception is that fluid from the blisters will spread the dermatitis; in fact, this in no way contributes to the ALLERGY.

The dermatitis produced by poison ivy starts between twenty-four to forty-eight hours after a person touches the leaves. The condition consists of reddening and itching of the skin and blisters, which worsen and sometimes become infected from scratching. In severe cases, fever and swollen lymph nodes may occur. The degree of severity depends on the extent and duration of the contact with the leaves and on one's susceptibility to poison ivy. It is therefore important to wash as soon as possible with soap and water all the possible contacted areas of skin, clothes, garden tools, gloves, etc.

Oral antihistamine drugs are often prescribed to relieve the itching, and cortisone preparations for the skin eruption. In severe cases, cortisone pills may be necessary.

POLLENS

Pollen is the male fertilizing element of flowering plants, trees and grasses. It consists of powdery, microscopic grains. As a first step in the formation of the seed, the pollen is brought to the female cell of its species by two basic methods: 1) it may be carried by bees, ants or butterflies as they go from flower to flower; or 2) the pollen may be transported by the wind.

Pollen transported by the first method is sticky and too heavy to be airborne; that transported by the second method is light and—as only one in a million has a chance of reaching female cells—abundant.

ALLERGIC RHINITIS (HAY FEVER) is the common seasonal ALLERGY provoked by sensitivity to pollen. Both kinds of pollen can be allergens, but the first can cause trouble only when a person comes in direct contact with the plant; the second type can cause hay fever through inhalation as well.

Plants furnishing profuse, light pollen are neither fragrant nor colorful—they don't depend on attracting insects to propagate. Spring hay fever is caused by the pollen of trees such as birch, poplar, elm, oak, walnut and maple; midsummer hay fever usually comes from pollinating grasses.

POSTURE

Walking is easier and less fatiguing than standing or sitting, since the process of losing balance and quickly recovering it causes less strain than the effort to keep the body—a very flexible, delicately arranged mechanism—in one position. Indeed, standing or sitting is the result of many small parts cooperating in many small movements.

Postural reflexes are more significant than is usually realized, since they participate and modify other physical processes—everything from walking to the "posture" of internal organs. Breathing and digesting, for instance, are affected by the cumulative effect of stimuli constantly transmitted from joints and muscles to the nervous system. Bad posture may mean a pattern of daily FATIGUE not relieved even by sleep.

Though one may not accept the idea of posture's influencing emotions, certainly the reverse is true: posture does reveal a person's state of mind, habits and, more important, his body image.

Proper posture comes naturally to some people; others have to learn it. A mirror and strong will power may not be enough in planning to change one's postural reflexes—a good teacher can do a better job in less time. The new set of learned movements, performed self-consciously and awkwardly at first, can easily turn into an instinctive, harmonious pattern.

PREGNANCY TESTS

There are several ways of testing whether a woman is pregnant, as so many distinctive changes occur in a pregnant woman's body. In practice, however, proof of pregnancy is usually obtained by one of the following methods:

1) *Direct examination* by a physician (which is not always reliable in the first three months of pregnancy).

2) *Animal tests*, in which a female laboratory animal, such as a mouse, rabbit or toad, is injected with the woman's urine. If the woman is pregnant, her urine contains a hormone called human chorionic gonadotropin (HCG) that produces distinct changes in the ovaries of the injected animal. (These tests, of which several variations exist, were practically the only ones available in the past but have not been used in recent years.)

3) *Immunological tests*, which are quick (ten minutes to two hours), reliable (95 percent accurate as early as ten days after the first missed menstrual period), and the currently preferred pregnancy tests. The test is based on an antigen-ANTIBODY action, i.e., the possible reaction between the HCG in the woman's urine and two reagents in a special preparation; one of the reagents is an *antiserum* (serum containing

antibodies) and the other is composed of preserved red blood cells taken from sheep and coated with HCG. If the woman is pregnant, the HCG uses up all the antiserum and the red cells do not clump (*positive* test); if she is not pregnant, the red cells clump together (*negative* test).

Recently a new pregnancy test was presented by Dr. Brij B. Saxena, professor of endocrinology and biochemistry at the New York Hospital–Cornell Medical Center, which can detect within an hour the existence of pregnancy *before* the first missed menstrual period—as early as six days after ovulation. This test does not entirely supersede the immunological technique but makes it largely supplemental and sometimes unnecessary.

Dr. Saxena's test involves obtaining a few drops of blood from the woman's finger, then analyzing them for the presence of HCG, which apparently may be detected immediately before the fertilized egg's implantation in the uterine wall—that is, before conception, as the medical definition of conception specifically refers to implantation. The only drawback is that in the case of women who have a delayed ovulation, the test may have to be repeated for two or three consecutive days to be accurate.

Because pregnancy can be detected so early, women who fear pregnancy will be able to safely undergo MENSTRUAL EXTRACTION, which is indicated *only* for early ABORTIONS, whereas women who are anxious to become pregnant after experiencing several miscarriages can be helped by immediate administration of the proper HORMONES.

PREMENSTRUAL SYNDROME

Premenstrual syndrome refers to a variety of symptoms that may occur at different phases of a woman's menstrual cycle—a number of hormonal changes that permeate tissues throughout the body and inevitably influence the mind.

Usually the symptoms appear in the four or five days before the onset of the menstrual flow. In about 60 percent of all women, the changes become strong enough to be distinctly perceived. In the remaining 40 percent, the symptoms may be present but so mild that they seem to have little effect on behavior.

Some women experience only *physical* symptoms such as NAUSEA, HEADACHE and blurred vision—all apparently caused by monthly changes in water retention. Others are also affected *psychologically*: they become depressed, emotional, belligerent. Some weep, crave sweets or become lethargic; others experience great bursts of physical and mental energy, and extremes in sexual drive—from total disinterest to nymphomania.

Psychiatrists throughout the United States report that most accidents, recurrence of chronic illness, suicides, crimes and psychotic spells occuring in women take place during their premenstrual period. Some of the findings are contradictory, though, which only reinforces the assumption that many different mechanisms may be responsible for the great variety of premenstrual manifestations.

In addition to the premenstrual syndrome, a small number of women also suffer from the so-called *Mittelschmerz* (German for middle pain), a cramplike, gradual, intermittent PAIN that occurs around the time of ovulation and lasts about two days. A few of these women also display emotional changes similar to those observed in the premenstrual phase.

The premenstrual syndrome is a complex phenomenon not yet clearly understood. However, it is fascinating to note that the entire menstrual syndrome is perhaps the most conspicuous example of the many normal cycles in the human body, in which slight periodic hormonal imbalances are experienced as symptoms; and that it has been used as a prototype for understanding less-obvious cycles.

PREPARED CHILDBIRTH

Prepared childbirth (sometimes misleadingly called natural childbirth) refers to a method of preparing a pregnant woman emotionally, mentally and physically for the delivery of her baby. Though a natural function of women, childbirth is also an extraordinarily intense experience which has the potential of becoming painful and frightening, as women are not equipped with an instinct of how to behave during childbirth, and as most are unaware of the mechanism of labor and delivery.

Specifically, prepared childbirth refers to the Lamaze method, named after the French physician Fernand Lamaze, who learned it in the early 1950s from Russian physicians, followers of Ivan Pavlov's principle of conditioned reflex. The Russians called it psychoprophylaxis and were the first to train women to suppress the brain's instinctive response to uterine contractions and to condition them to controlled breathing and *conscious* relaxation (as opposed to the *passive* loosening of muscles that is normally thought of as relaxation). This technique does not eliminate PAIN but certainly minimizes it—and without ANAESTHESIA.

The Lamaze method is currently practiced throughout Europe, South America and Africa. In the United States it has been modified to a degree: the American version basically maintains that, while a "prepared" woman will need little or no anaesthesia in a normal delivery, she should be assured that the obstetrician is ready to intervene if the delivery presents complications and will administer anaesthetics if necessary.

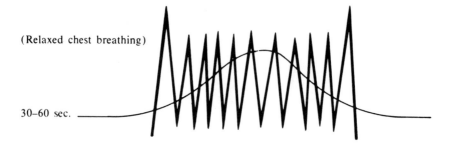

(Relaxed chest breathing)

30–60 sec.

Effacement

The curve represents a contraction during the first stage of labor: effacement. Contractions here have the purpose of softening and thinning out the cervix. They are light and last 30 to 60 seconds, at intervals of 5 to 20 minutes; duration varies greatly with each woman.

The up-and-down lines indicate the kind of breathing with which a woman learns to respond to these contractions: a deep "cleansing" breath at the beginning and at the end of each contraction; in between, slow, deep chest breathing.

This chart illustrates a contraction during the second stage of labor: dilatation. Contractions have the purpose of opening the cervix from 0 to approximately 7 cm. They are strong, last about 60 seconds at intervals of 1 to 3 minutes. They may last several hours.

The response to these contractions should be a shallow, accelerated breathing. Shallow, to keep the diaphragm up, off the uterus; and accelerated, to match the mounting intensity of these contractions and their gradual decrease.

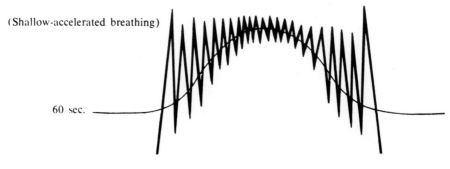

(Shallow-accelerated breathing)

60 sec.

Dilatation

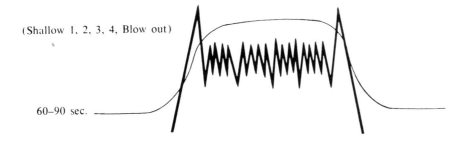

(Shallow 1, 2, 3, 4, Blow out)

60–90 sec.

Transition

This chart illustrates a contraction during the third stage of labor: transition. Contractions have the purpose of continuing to open the cervix from 7 to 10 cm. and of pushing the baby down into the birth canal. They are extremely strong and erratic, last from 60 to 90 seconds at intervals of about 1 minute. Duration is short.

Transition breathing is similar to the dilatation type but with forceful exhalations at intervals.

Illustrations from *Preparation for Childbirth, a Lamaze Guide* by Donna and Rodger Ewy. Courtesy of Pruett Publishing Company, Boulder, Colorado, 1970.

A contraction during the fourth and last stage of labor: expulsion. Contractions have the purpose of expelling the baby. They are weaker, last about 60 seconds at intervals varying from 1 to 3 minutes. Duration varies greatly: from 30 minutes to 2 hours.

Breathing consists of two deep breaths followed by a push, a normal breath, another push and a deep breath.

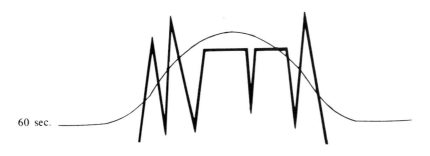

60 sec.

Expulsion

PREPARED CHILDBIRTH

Even if there is pain, however, women who have been properly prepared will not panic and will still regard labor as a time for concentration and for cooperation with the doctor rather than a time for lonely anguish and passive suffering. The atmosphere of cooperation is ensured not only by a hospital team which understands and respects the Lamaze method but also by the presence of the baby's father, who is encouraged to take part in the woman's training and to be a reassuring presence during the entire delivery. One of his tasks is the so-called effleurage, a light massage on the woman's abdominal area that helps her to control the sensation of contraction, which is probably one of the greatest fears a woman has concerning childbirth. Many women seem to think that the process of labor, in which contractions of the uterus must open the tiny cervix wide enough to allow the passage of a baby's head (4 inches in diameter), is almost impossible without excruciating pain. Because of this apparently widespread notion, prenatal training (usually conducted in small classes) begins with a thorough, clear explanation of a woman's reproductive organs. To explain the nature of a contraction, Lamaze therapists use the metaphor of a wave: the contraction starts slowly, increases in intensity, reaches a crest and then subsides—as powerful and uncontrollable as an ocean wave. It is as unwise to try to resist a contraction as it is to stand up to a wave; but by meeting the wave and riding its movement, it is indeed possible to remain on top and safely reemerge. Next, a woman is taught how to relax consciously the muscles of her arms, legs, neck and feet and those surrounding her vagina. She is trained to "feel" each muscle separately by responding to the therapist's directions in contracting, for example, the right arm and the left leg, and vice versa.

During these exercises (which should be practiced daily), the muscles the woman is contracting are simulating the contractions of *involuntary* uterine muscles, and the ones she relaxes represent the body's *voluntary* muscles' withstanding the impulse of tensing the entire body in the presence of uterine contractions.

And finally, the woman is taught to identify the various phases of labor—effacement, dilatation, transition and expulsion—and to practice a special kind of breathing for each phase.

1) *Effacement*—The cervix begins gradually to expand, and the thick, elastic tissue of the birth canal begins to thin down (efface). At first, the contractions are weak; they last thirty to sixty seconds, with intervals of five to twenty minutes. Breathing during this kind of contraction should start with one slow, deep inhalation and a full, emptying exhalation (the so-called cleansing breath), followed by slow, even chest breathing (which keeps oxygen in the system) for

the length of the contraction and ending with a cleansing breath.

2) *Dilatation*—The diameter of the cervix is widening; contractions become increasingly strong and last about one minute, with intervals of one to three minutes. Breathing should begin with one cleansing breath followed by shallow breathing, which is meant to prevent the diaphragm (the thin, disclike muscle that divides the lungs from the abdomen and bears down with each inhalation) from pressing on the uterus. The breathing should accelerate with the mounting of the contraction and slow down when the contraction decreases, ending with one cleansing breath. This phase may last several hours.

3) *Transition*—The baby descends to the bottom of the uterus. Contractions not only become longer and more intense but change in nature: they last one or two minutes, with shorter intervals between them, and the uterus begins to make expulsive efforts. Breathing should start, as usual, with a deep cleansing breath, followed by four shallow breaths and one forceful exhalation—a pattern to be repeated for as long as the contraction lasts. The forceful exhalation is meant to empty the lungs (thus pulling the diaphragm farther away from the uterus), and also as a diversion from a sudden impulse to push, which, since the cervix is not yet completely open, would be premature and painful.

4) *Expulsion*—The cervix is now completely open, and the baby descends into the birth canal, ready to be born. This stage requires greater effort: contractions are strong and varied in duration, with intervals of one to three minutes, but they are usually much faster than the previous phases. By now, the doctor urges the woman to push, which effort is most effective at the apex of contraction. The woman should take two deep, slow breaths, then hold her breath as long as possible while pushing; then another deep breath, more pushing, and a last deep breath, when the contraction subsides. When the baby's head is about to emerge, the woman must stop pushing— the doctor tells her when. Incidentally, to learn to stop pushing in the middle of a contraction, with the baby's head about to emerge, requires a great deal of practice.

After the baby is born, the uterus contracts once more, and the PLACENTA, which had detached itself from the walls of the uterus, is expelled.

PROPHYLAXIS

Prophylaxis refers to any protective treatment or measure necessary to preserve health and prevent the spreading of a disease.

PROSTAGLANDINS

Prostaglandins are naturally occurring, hormonelike substances that are among the most powerful chemical regulators in the body, affecting the reproductive, cardiovascular, nervous and gastric systems. Prostaglandins, which owe their name to the fact that they were originally obtained from the prostate gland, are formed from fatty acids and are found in nearly all tissues of the body, with the highest concentration in the semen.

Sixteen prostaglandins have been discovered so far and classified into subgroups: A, B, C, E and F. As of 1975, only a few have been thoroughly investigated clinically. However, several studies are being conducted dealing with the use of prostaglandins as vasodilators and vasoconstrictors to enhance fertilization, to induce ABORTION or labor in late pregnancy, to inhibit ulcers, and to prevent ASTHMA, nasal congestion, MIGRAINE, HYPERTENSION and male sterility.

Prostaglandins, which are believed to stimulate or inhibit the action of many HORMONES, are not a new discovery; as early as the 1930s, two physicians reported the effects of these strange compounds on the muscle of the uterus. But, as often happens, prostaglandins remained laboratory curiosities for many years. In fact, because of the complexities of their chemistry, it really was not technically possible to isolate and identify them until 1956 (in Sweden). They gained sudden attention because of their use in fertility control.

The first prostaglandin released in the United States for commercial medical use was PG F_2, manufactured by the Upjohn Company and given the name Prostin F_2 Alfa. PG F_2 has been approved by the FDA for use in second-trimester abortions. The great advantage of the prostaglandin over the saline injection—the commonly used procedure for late abortion—is that it is safer for the patient and easier for the physician: the former consists merely of an injection into the amniotic cavity, whereas the latter entails replacement of the amniotic fluid with the saline solution.

In the future, it is very possible that prostaglandins, among other things, will become the ideal CONTRACEPTIVE, replacing the indignities of the mechanical contraceptives and the hazards of the hormonal ones. A small dose of prostaglandins, applied at home on the twenty-seventh day of the menstrual cycle, would automatically bring about a menstrual flow after a few hours, whether a woman is pregnant or not.

PROTEINS

Proteins are a very large class of naturally occurring and extremely complex combinations of the elements carbon, hydrogen, nitrogen, oxygen, sulfur and occasionally phosphorus, IRON, and other elements. Proteins are essential constituents of all living cells, both animal and vegetable, and also essential to the diet of the human organism.

Protein is not merely a basic nutrient, such as CARBOHYDRATES and FATS, but the *only* basic nutrient capable of building, repairing and maintaining all of the body tissues. This is because proteins contain nitrogen, which is indispensable for life and growth on earth and possibly throughout the universe.

Although protein is the most complex substance known to man, it begins simply, with only twenty-two components—the amino acids. Plants and bacteria manufacture their own special amino acids from carbon, hydrogen and oxygen in the air and water, but humans cannot make their own proteins (or their own VITAMINS) and must get them from eating plants or the flesh, milk and eggs of animals. These complex food proteins are then broken down by digestion into the twenty-two original amino acids, which in turn are reassembled into the many different proteins needed by different tissues for life and growth.

This process of rearrangement, Dr. Jean Mayer, professor of nutrition at Harvard University Medical School, wrote in the August 1974 issue of *Family Health,* "can be likened to a typewriter's reproducing as many of each letter as necessary to form all the words of a language . . . for whatever is being written. The twenty-two amino acids are the equivalent of the twenty-six letters of the English alphabet. . . . Just as English uses more e's and o's than x's and z's, so we need certain of the amino acids in greater quantity than others. . . . And the different proteins are like the final products of a typewriter: some of them are as short . . . as an advertising slogan—two or a few amino acids; others contain thousands.

"The body's 'typist' who puts together the final products . . . is also a protein, a complicated molecule that . . . exists in the center of every cell, is shaped like a double helix, and is called . . . deoxyribonucleic acid. Its popular name is DNA, and it contains the genetic code, which is not only different in each species but slightly different for each individual within a species."

When specific amino acids are required, the DNA sends out the appropriate message; the amino acids are gathered and assembled in the proper sequence, and the new protein is sent to wherever in the body it is needed.

The human body needs all twenty-two amino acids, but only the so-called *essential* amino acids—leucine, isoleucine, lysine, methionine, phenylalanine, tryptophane, threonine and valine—have to be taken from food. Nonessential amino acids can be manufactured from other substances in the body. Foods with the right amount of all eight essential amino acids are called complete proteins and have a very high biological value. Human breast milk has probably the highest biological value of all foods. Eggs and cheese, too, are very high. Cow's milk, beef and fish follow. Vegetable proteins have lower biological value than animal proteins, but when mixed together they can reach quite high values. For instance, wheat has several amino acids but very little lysine; thus, it can be mixed with beans, which are low in methionine but contain lysine. Also useful for a balanced diet are a mixture of animal and vegetable proteins, as long as they are consumed at about the same time.

The need for proteins is determined by body size and weight; proportionately, children need more because they are still growing.

One popular misconception is that protein helps "burn off" fat. This is due to a misinterpretation of a famous laboratory experiment in which volunteers who ate pure protein spent 30 percent of the calories as heat immediately after the meal. However, in practice, except for egg white, no food is ever *pure* protein; and as soon as other foods are added to pure protein, calories are burned at the normal rate; i.e., only 10 percent is spent as heat after a meal.

PRURITUS (ITCHING)

Pruritus, the medical term for itching, is a phenomenon resulting from irritation of nerve endings in the skin, either in a single spot or on more or less large areas of the body. Itching represents a defense mechanism and often is a warning signal of the presence of some irritant in the system—a virus, a fungus, an allergen or a parasite. Sometimes, however, itching seems to occur for no reason at all—idiopathically, as a neurosis.

Persistent itching may also be the first sign of many other systemic diseases, such as liver and kidney disturbances, diabetes, leukemia or Hodgkin's disease.

Another, less dramatic form of pruritis is the so-called xerosis (winter itch), which refers to the reaction of susceptible skin made excessively dry by overheated rooms in winter.

The irresistible reaction to itching is scratching, and indeed, scratching seems to relieve the itching—at least temporarily. In reality, we simply substitute the itching with another sensation: PAIN. People at times go so far as to scald the itching skin, or to scrape it until it bleeds, and sometimes infection sets in.

Removing the underlying causes eventually removes the pruritus, too. However, there is still no prompt scientific remedy for the symptom itself. Only PALLIATIVES are available, such as cortisone compounds, certain lotions such as calamine, or low temperature, which decrease the itching by affecting the nerve endings in the skin but do not really cure the itch.

PSORIASIS

Psoriasis is a chronic, recurrent disorder of the skin that affects approximately one out of fifty persons in the United States. It is characterized by well-demarcated, red, scaling patches on the skin that generally appear on the scalp, elbows, nails and knees. The skin eruption results from an increased rate of production of cells in the outer layer of the skin and is almost always hereditary.

Psoriasis is neither infectious nor contagious; it may amount to a few small lesions or cover large areas of the body; it affects every race at any age, except very young babies and elderly people. Sometimes a scratch may result in the formation of a psoriatic spot at the site. A few patients develop ARTHRITIS in those areas.

Psoriasis does not leave scars and is *not* precancerous. It tends to clear up spontaneously—it may disappear and never reappear, or it may disappear and reappear months or years later. In some cases, seasonal changes, sunshine, emotions and other factors seem to play some role in both the clearing of the skin lesions and their reappearance. Incidentally, there are other skin conditions that resemble psoriasis; anyone who thinks he has psoriasis should consult a dermatologist.

There is no specific cure for psoriasis; all treatments are PALLIATIVES. Nevertheless, the proper treatment can be so effective as to result in a complete clearing of this skin disorder. The method of therapy depends on the severity and duration of the psoriasis, as well as the age of the patient and his past experience with the condition. Often, therapy must be used intermittently or even continuously to keep the disease under control.

Treatment of psoriasis includes:

1) Locally applied creams, ointments, lotions or tinctures such as mercury compounds, tar derivatives, salicylic acid, and steroids (cortisone derivatives). The last named may be injected directly into the lesions.

2) Exposure, twice a day, to superficial X-rays called Grenz rays, or ultraviolet light in a specially constructed "light box," an advanced, potent form of ultraviolet rays. After the light treatment, the patient takes a medicated bath to remove excess scales.

3) For severe cases, certain powerful drugs known as antimitotic agents (inhibiting mitosis, the typical way cells divide and multiply) are used. This treatment is used only under the strictest supervision of the physician who prescribes it.

PSYCHOACTIVE DRUGS

Any drug that acts on the mind is called psychoactive. Most modern psychoactive drugs are synthetic, i.e., chemically manufactured, but a few are still extracted from plants, herbs, and other natural sources as they have been for centuries. The science that studies psychoactive drugs is called psychopharmacology. A discipline as old as the first man who first chewed on a leaf that made him feel as if he could fly with the eagles or else made him unmindful of enemies and beasts, modern psychopharmacology was born, technically speaking, in the early 1950s when a team of French chemists isolated chlorpromazine, with the specific intent of producing a nonaddictive compound that would relax anxious patients awaiting surgery. What was meant to make surgery a less traumatic experience also changed the course of psychiatry: the first tranquilizer had been discovered.

Psychoactive drugs have been variously named and often confusedly classified, but basically they can be divided into two categories: 1) those with a predominantly *calming* action, such as sedatives, also called tranquilizers, and hypnotic drugs (or sleeping pills); and 2) those which are mainly *uplifting*, such as stimulants and antidepressants.

There are two kinds of tranquilizers: major tranquilizers, such as Thorazine®, and minor tranquilizers, such as Miltown®, Librium®, and Valium®. Tranquilizers act on the central nervous system, but just how they relieve anxiety is still a scientific mystery. One theory is that they lessen the level of norepinephrine and serotonin—two HORMONES formed in the hypothalamus and involved in the regulation of mood—when these overflow because of anxiety. Conversely, antidepressants may lift mental depression by stepping up these hormones' abnormally reduced levels. However, neither tranquilizers nor stimulants actually destroy or produce hormones; these drugs seem to have the power to discourage or encourage the hormones' availability at critical sites of the brain. This means that psychoactive drugs, while not *curing* mood disturbances, cut through syndromes to control the basic symptoms, regardless of their combination. In the case of "agitated depression," for instance, in which anxiety and depression are concomitant, a mixture of tranquilizer and antidepressant must be used, since a single drug that would treat both symptoms has not yet been found. In a category of its own, unclassifiable as yet, stands the most extraordinary of psychoactive drugs, LITHIUM CARBONATE, a salt of lithium, a highly reactive alkaline metal used in the treatment of manic depression.

Psychoactive drugs cannot help psychopaths—probably nothing can be done for a mind that has lost, or has never had, any reference point to reality. However, they can be helpful to neurotics *who are extremely ill*—something like penicillin, which is successful with pneumonia but almost useless in treating the COMMON COLD. They don't work instantly, ASPIRIN-like; it may be days, even weeks, before any effects become evident. This is good enough: release mental depression from INSOMNIA, apathy, FATIGUE, stupor, loss of weight or OBESITY; calm the agitation, tremor, irrational fears and the fury of anxiety, and life will be bearable again. Psychoactive drugs can spell the difference between life and death for the deeply depressed person with suicide on his mind. And because they come in the form of pills and tablets and are prescribed as ordinary medications, psychoactive drugs give the patient the feeling of being in control—he can take or ignore the pills as he pleases—and also release him from the shame of considering himself insane, an outcast. Sicknesses that are treated with prescriptions always seem respectable.

Few drugs are as overused as tranquilizers, and few are as controversial as antidepressants. Unlike lithium, whose therapeutic benefits are well established, the status of these drugs is less certain. Both anxiety and depression are strongly rooted in life experience, which means that psychoactive drugs should always be considered no more than an adjunct treatment. Psychotherapy and changes in the environment sometimes may be more to the point than drugs. Also, since anxiety and depression are often episodic, drugs should not be used indefinitely but only when the symptoms are disabling. And the knowledge that relief is available may in itself sustain a patient. And finally, by limiting the treatment to short courses, one can avoid such problems as tolerance, dependency, side effects, loss of efficacy, and the need to increase doses.

No drug will always do exactly and only what it is supposed to do for everyone; and tranquilizers, stimulants and antidepressants are all powerful and complex chemicals that can induce many side effects in different people or in the same person at different times.

PSYCHOSOMATIC DISEASES

Any illness resulting from the interaction between mind (or emotions) and body is called psychosomatic. But since the onset and the course of practically any sickness can be influenced by personality—and even in the case of an infectious disease, emotional disturbances can undermine the body's defense mechanism—in a sense, most illnesses are psychosomatic to a certain degree.

This vagueness of meaning is probably one of the reasons why the term psychosomatic seems slightly disreputable to certain physicians. Also, the word had an instant success when it was coined about forty years ago; it entered the layman's language so enthusiastically that it was bound to be misused. By now, however, though they don't always accept the concepts of psychosomatic medicine (opinions differ even within the specialty), physicians agree that health and disease cannot be considered simple phenomena. In either case, complicated cellular and biochemical functions are involved, which occur in individuals who live in social environments and are subject to psychological experiences. "Cultural factors may also be influential," recently wrote Dr. Adam J. Krakowski, chief of the division of psychiatric liaison and research at the Champlain Valley–Physician's Hospital Medical Center in Plattsburgh, New York. "For instance, in some people illness provokes an immediate motivation to seek medical help, while others seek help only as a last resort; finally there are those who may believe that cure comes from religious, not medical, healings."

A good internist, then, has to deal with each patient as a unique body/mind unit; he has to know when to prescribe specific drugs, or just a PLACEBO; when it is dangerous to dismiss a woman obsessed with the fear of BREAST CANCER, for instance, by insisting that there is nothing clinically wrong with her. Often the localized and realistic physical PAIN a patient complains about is the symptom of a so-called "masked" depression.

A good psychiatrist has to play many roles, too, and play them by ear. He has to know when and to whom to suggest depth analysis, short-term psychotherapy, PSYCHOACTIVE DRUGS or a referral to a specialist such as a gynecologist or an allergist.

PTOSIS

Ptosis refers to the falling down of an organ or its parts. It also indicates the drooping of the upper eyelids due to paralysis or merely the effect of gravity and old age, and the sagging of breasts from their normal, youthful position.

PUERPERIUM

Puerperium is the condition of a woman immediately after childbirth. It also refers to the approximately six-week period from the time of delivery to the time when the uterus regains its normal size.

PUMICE STONE

Pumice stone is a white, gray, or yellowish volcanic glass; it is light in weight because it is full of cavities produced by the expulsion of water vapor at a high temperature as lava comes to the surface.

Pumice can be powdered and pressed into a textured solid form to be used for polishing and smoothing the rough skin of elbows, knees, and soles of the feet.

QR

QUACKERY

The "health practitioner" who has a "miracle cure" but no medical training is a quack, and quackery is his business. But old-fashioned quacks—flamboyant confidence men pitching their products at a carnival—are rare these days; modern quackery is often subtle, elegant, expensive, difficult to recognize, a mixture of real chemical and medical terms and misleading claims. Quackery sometimes is embedded in otherwise legitimate labels. Often it is simply an *omission* of information. In the field of beauty care, quackery may be harmless but also useless—except for the illusion of beauty it sells. And, of course, a few "miracle cures" may turn out to be extraordinary discoveries of maligned geniuses. After all, the history of medicine is full of such stories.

The most common types of quackery are:

1) false claims for drugs and COSMETICS, such as cures for baldness; drugs that "melt" fat without dieting or lift faces without surgery; unproven treatments for cancer;

2) food fads and unnecessary food supplements;

3) fake medical devices, such as bust developers, machines said to reduce excess weight by vibration or radiation, and special suits or bandages that purport to reduce fat only in certain parts of the body, as well as usually legitimate devices such as EYEGLASSES or dentures that may become quackery if fitted by mail order.

As a rule, any product or service that is offered as a "secret remedy," advertised in sensational magazines, or sold from door to door by a self-styled "health adviser"; or any drug whose sponsor claims that he is battling the medical profession (which will not accept his wonderful discovery) and who readily produces testimonials from other people who benefited from its miraculous effects, may be considered quackery.

The FDA suggests that any person who suspects he is the victim of quackery inform his physician or the county medical society of his

299

district; ask the Better Business Bureau about the reputation of the promoters; inform the local post office in case the drug or device is promoted through the mail, and, finally, get in touch with the FDA's headquarters: 5600 Fisher Lane, Rockville, Maryland 20852.

RADIATION

Radiation is energy moving through space as invisible waves. The frequency of these waves helps to determine radiation characteristics and how the radiation will affect people.

Frequency also is a basis for classifying radiation as X-rays, light, ultraviolet and infrared rays, or microwaves. The frequency scale from least energetic to most energetic is called the electromagnetic spectrum.

The two major categories of radiation are *ionizing* and *nonionizing*.

Ionizing radiation—X-rays are an example of this type. Ionizing radiation has the ability to strip electrons from atoms, creating electrically charged ions capable of disrupting life processes. Adverse effects on people exposed to ionized radiation seems directly proportioned to the amount of radiation received.

Nonionizing radiation—Light and microwaves are examples. Nonionizing radiation lacks the ability to create ions but may disrupt body processes through other mechanisms. The relationship between amount and effect of nonionizing radiation is unknown.

A variety of radiation-producing machines and radioactive materials are currently used in medical and scientific techniques for the purpose of detecting and treating diseases. However, scientists do not completely understand how radiation interacts with living tissues. They have learned that radiation can disturb the balance in a cell so that it can no longer perform its function. If enough cells are affected, processes in the entire body may be disrupted. And if radiation harms the reproduction cells, the damage may be passed on to future generations.

The human body is able to repair minor radiation damage to normal cells; but if the dose is large, repair will not be complete.

Most of what is known today about the effects of radiation on humans is the result of observation of people exposed to large amounts of radiation. Some of these effects are harmful, such as a burn from a sunlamp, or SKIN CANCER from chronic exposure to ultraviolet rays, and some are useful, such as the destruction of cancer cells during RADIOTHERAPY.

Not much is known about the effects of small amounts of radiation, such as emissions from radio transmitters for instance. Specifically, it is not definitely known whether there is an amount of radiation below which deleterious effects *do not* occur. Also difficult to establish is the relationship between exposure and long-term effects, partly because the effects are similar to those of diseases which may not be related to radiation, and partly because the effects may not appear until years after exposure.

The kind of radiation to which a person is exposed, the amount of radiation, and the area of the body irradiated are very important in determining the effects of the radiation on the body, especially in the case of radiotherapy for cancer, where the basic purpose is to destroy cancer cells while limiting as much as possible the damage to the surrounding healthy cells. In general, rapidly dividing cells appear to be more sensitive to radiation than nondividing cells, and highly specialized cells are less sensitive than nondifferentiated ones.

Among the best-known types of radiation are X-rays. However, some X-ray examinations are unnecessary and can be avoided. To make sure people receive an X-ray examination only when necessary, the FDA advises:

1) Don't decide on your own to have an X-ray examination, such as at a mobile unit for detecting tuberculosis.

2) Don't insist on an X-ray when you visit your doctor or dentist; let him judge whether you need one.

3) Tell your doctor and dentist about previous X-rays.

4) Women who are pregnant or who think they might be pregnant should tell their physicians. Radiation may affect the fetus, and knowledge of possible pregnancy may affect the doctor's decision as to whether to use X-rays or not.

5) In the case of X-ray examination of the lower abdomen, lower back, or hip areas of men of reproductive age or younger, including children, the X-ray technician should be asked to protect the reproductive organs with a special lead shield. To protect the reproductive organs of a woman is often impossible, because the lead shield can obscure needed diagnostic information on X-ray film.

RADIOTHERAPY

Radiotherapy is the use of RADIATION for the treatment mostly of cancer, as radiant energy destroys cancer cells.

In BREAST CANCER, the treatment usually chosen for those with early tumors is MASTECTOMY; it is debatable whether radiotherapy should be given. In those women with advanced disease, radiotherapy is usually the main treatment for the breast and, when the cancer has spread, for other tissues such as bone.

Radiotherapy is also extensively used for other forms of cancer, such as SKIN CANCER and many cancers of the head and neck.

RAGWEED POLLEN INDEX
FOR THE UNITED STATES

Any city or community having an index above 10 is poor for allergy sufferers;
between 5 and 10 is fairly good; below 5 is good; below 1 is excellent.
Figures in parentheses are best possible estimates.

ALABAMA

Birmingham	(49)
Foley	4
Mobile	8

ALASKA

Fairbanks	0
Juneau	0
Nome	0

ARIZONA

Grand Canyon	
National Park:	
North Rim	
(Fall only)	0.15
South Rim	
(Fall only)	0.12
Phoenix	
(Fall only)	0.21
Tucson	
(Spring)	2
(Fall)	3

ARKANSAS

Gassville	45
Little Rock	62
West Memphis	(81)

CALIFORNIA

Alpine	3
Arcata	3
El Centro	1
Escondido	1
Lassen Volcanic	
National Park	0.03
Los Angeles	
(Spring)	0.22
(Fall)	0.8
Monterey	0.24
Oakland	0.2
Pasadena	0.68
Sacramento	0.2
San Diego	1
San Francisco	0.2
Santa Barbara	3
Sequoia National Park	0.03
Tujunga	1.4
Yosemite National	
Park	0.3

COLORADO

Burlington	(23)
Colorado Springs	4
Denver	19
Glenwood Springs	0.8
Mesa Verde	
National Park	0.5
Pikes Peak	0.9
Rocky Mountain	
National Park:	
Estes Park	1
Grand Lake	0.2

CONNECTICUT

Bridgeport	26
Fairfield	26
Hartford	54
New Haven	25
Sherman	13
Stamford	28
Stratford	26
Waterbury	27

DELAWARE

Wilmington	(54)

DISTRICT OF COLUMBIA

Washington	42

FLORIDA

Bradenton	4
Clearwater	7
Coral Gables	2
Daytona Beach	3
Everglades National	
Park	4
Fort Lauderdale	
(Beach)	6
Fort Myers	0.19
Fort Pierce	5
Gainesville	20
Jacksonville	6
Key West	0.12
Live Oak	5
Melbourne	21
Miami	2
Miami Beach	0.26
Ocala	13
Orlando	3
Panama City	32
(Sunnyside Beach)	2
Pensacola	10
(Santa Rosa Island)	0.054
St. Petersburg	4
Sebring	3
Tallahassee	6
Tampa	6
West Palm Beach	5
(Morrison Field)	31

GEORGIA

Atlanta	24
St. Simon Island	77
Valdosta	8

IDAHO

Boise	5
Moscow	(0.5)
Pocatello	5
Sun Valley	0.3

ILLINOIS

Bloomington	89

Chicago	62
Chicago Water Crib	66
Decatur	114
East St. Louis	(100)
Elgin	73
Evanston	73
Grayslake	63
North Chicago	74
Peoria	122
Quincy	98
Rockford	98
Rock Island	113
Springfield	73
Streator	78
Urbana	80

INDIANA

Cicero	76
East Chicago	(64)
Evansville	136
Fort Wayne	107
Indianapolis	92
Jeffersonville	(102)

IOWA

Ames	87
Cedar Rapids	122
Council Bluffs	(148)
Des Moines	69
Iowa City	93
Waterloo	125

KANSAS

Goodland	23
Kansas City	(101)
Wichita	58

KENTUCKY

Covington	(122)
Lexington	151
Louisville	99
Trappist	86

LOUISIANA

New Orleans	43
Tallulah	(33)

MAINE

Alfred	15
Allagash	1.4
Auburn	13
Augusta	9
Bar Harbor	5
Bethel	1.6
Belfast	1.3
Boothbay Harbor	5
Camden	9
Deblois	1
Eagle Lake	2
Eastport	6
Enfield	1
Grand Lake Stream	1.4

Greenville Junction	0.35	Escanaba	57	**NEVADA**	
Houlton	3	Flint	76	Lake Mead	
Jackman	4	Frankfort	65	(Hoover Dam)	
Kineo	27	Gaylord	54	(March, April)	4
Lincoln	2	Gladwin	99	(Fall)	0.3
Machias	4	Grand Haven	90	Reno	0.1
Macwahoc	0.46	Grand Rapids	126		
Millinocket	0.38	Grand Traverse	37	**NEW HAMPSHIRE**	
Newagen	1	Grayling	52	Bath	3
Newport	3.5	Harbor Bay	61	Berlin	8
New Portland	1	Hillsdale	78	Bethlehem	5
North Augusta	10	Houghton	9	Blue Job Mt.	2
Oquossoc	2	Ironwood	17	Carrol	0.9
Orono	10	Isle Royale		Charlestown	14
Poland Spring	12	National Park	0.29	Claremont	7
Portland	24	Lake City	33	Colebrook	1.4
Presque Isle	0.44	Lansing	94	Concord	7
Quoddy Head	0.6	Ludington	60	Conway	3
Rangeley	9	Mackinac Island	19	Crotched Mt.	5
Rockland	8	Mackinaw City	13	Derby	2
St. Francis	0.09	Mancelona	39	Dixville	3
Southport	8	Manistee	54	Dover	5
Speckle Mt.	2	Manistique	12	Errol	0.5
Stonington	12	Marquette	12	Exeter	26
Upper Dam	2	Menominee	37	Federal Hill	7
York	8	Mt. Pleasant	74	Franklin	5
		Munising	16	Groveton	2
MARYLAND		Newberry	20	Hampton	4
Annapolis	32	Northport	25	Hillsboro	5
Baltimore	51	Ontonagon	13	Hinsdale	11
Bethesda	65	Owasippe	8	Holderness	5
Frederick	82	Petoskey	30	Jeremy	18
Perry Point	65	Port Austin	107	Keene	7
Takoma Park	(41)	Powers	21	Laconia	1
		Rogers City	19	Lancaster	0.75
MASSACHUSETTS		Roscommon	21	Lebanon	17
Amherst	25	St. Ignace	8	Lincoln	2
Annisquam	3	St. Joseph	103	Littleton	3
Boston	16	Sault Ste. Marie	4	Manchester	9
Boston		Stambaugh	24	Moosilaukee	0.45
General Hospital	24	Traverse City	39	Nashua	29
Gloucester		West Branch	31	New Ipswich	8
(A & G Hospital)	7			New London	5
E. Gloucester	5	**MINNESOTA**		North Conway	3
W. Gloucester	5	Duluth	44	Ossipee	3
Magnolia	5	Minneapolis	99	Pawtuckaway	0.5
Nantucket Island	5	Moorhead	125	Peterborough	27
Newton Center	44	Rochester	89	Pittsburgh	2
Northampton	20	Tower	6	Plymouth	4
Rockport	5	Virginia	8	Rochester	17
Winchester	19	Winona	124	Rye	15
Worcester	9			Warren	2
		MISSISSIPPI		Weirs	9
MICHIGAN		Biloxi	7	Whitefield	2
Alpena	20	Vicksburg	33		
Ann Arbor	119			**NEW JERSEY**	
Bad Axe	40	**MISSOURI**			
Baldwin	41	Kansas City	109	Asbury Park	18
Bay City	72	St. Louis	78	Atlantic City	30
Benton Harbor	110			Caldwell	88
Big Rapids	57	**MONTANA**		Dover	36
Blaney	16	Glacier National Park:		East Brunswick	38
Boyne City	35	Belton	0.1	East Orange	34
Cadillac	31	Many Glacier	0.1	Flemington	101
Charlevoix	21	Miles City	4	Fort Dix	53
Cheboygan	23	West Yellowstone	0.2	Freehold	72
Coldwater	190			Haddonfield	74
Copper Harbor	5	**NEBRASKA**		Hightstown	87
Crystal Falls	14	Lincoln	63	Jersey City	5
Detroit	66	North Platte	13	Linden	58
East Tawas	75	Omaha	148	Madison	62
		Scottsbluff	38		

Maplewood	21	Raquette Lake	6	Springville	49
Marlboro	40	Redford	7	Syracuse	25
New Brunswick	60	Sabattis	8	Utica	32
Newark	18	Santa Clara	15	Watertown	43
Paterson	44	Saranac Lake		White Lake	67
Pitman	51	(Rogers Hospital)	23	Woodridge	21
Red Bank	69	Saranac	19	Eldred (Yulan)	35
Sandy Hook	39	Schroon Lake			
Sparta	16	(Severance)	8	**NORTH CAROLINA**	
Summit	42	Speculator	12	Asheville	57
Teaneck	31	Ticonderoga	29	Charlotte	42
Trenton	26	Tupper Lake	8	Great Smoky	
Verona	33	Turin	12	Mountains	
Westwood	18	Wanakena	7	National Park:	
Wildwood	34	Wells	13	Newfound Gap	(4)
		Wilmington	16	Hatteras	71
NEW MEXICO				Raleigh	28
Albuquerque	7	Catskill area:			
Roswell	4	Big Indian	4	**NORTH DAKOTA**	
		Fleischmanns	10	Fargo	(125)
NEW YORK CITY		Haines Falls	5		
Metropolitan area:		Hunter	29	**OHIO**	
Battery	27	Phoenicia	13	Akron	115
Bronx	24	Pine Hill	5	Cincinnati	122
Brooklyn	22	(Funcrest)	3	Cleveland	56
Croton	29	Tannersville	11	Columbus	75
Farmingdale	44	Windham	28	Dayton	104
Fire Island		Zena	12	Toledo	122
(Ocean Beach)	11			Youngstown	77
Flushing	30	Statewide:			
Garden City	28	Albany	48	**OKLAHOMA**	
Huntington	44	Binghamton	31	Fort Sill	(73)
Jamaica	35	Buffalo	54	Henryetta	(75)
Manhattan	25	Celoron	41	Muskogee	85
Northport	31	Cortland	37	Oklahoma City	73
Pomona	26	Dannemora	19	Okmulgee	57
Rockaway	40	East Berne	32	Pawhuska	31
Staten Island	30	Elmira	43	Tulsa	65
White Plains	32	Elsmere	49		
Yonkers	38	Fairport	32	**OREGON**	
		Forestburg	15	Coquille	0
Adirondack area:		Fremont	38	Corvallis	0
Ausable Forks	20	Geneva	57	Crater Lake	
Big Moose	6	Gloversville	29	National Park	0.1
Blue Mt. Lake	3	Hornell	34	Milton-Freewater	6
Chateaugay Lake	8	Jamestown	65	Portland	0.55
Chilson	6	Jeffersonville	26	Turner	2
Elk Lake	4	Kauneonga Lake	48		
Ft. Ticonderoga	21	Lake Huntington	23	**PENNSYLVANIA**	
Hague	16	Liberty	16	Altoona	52
Hudson Falls	37	Lockport	71	Broomall	40
Indian Lake	6	Lowville	20	Erie	65
Inlet	8	Mamakating	22	Hatboro	48
Keene	5	Margaretville	15	McKeesport	95
Keene Valley	1	Minnewaska	20	Meadville	75
Keeseville	26	Montauk	10	Philadelphia	55
Lake George	23	Monticello	24	Pittsburgh	90
Lake Kushaqua	15	Newburgh	40	Pittsburgh (Brentwood)	74
Lake Placid	10	Ogdensburg	46		
Long Lake	6	Olean	42	**RHODE ISLAND**	
Loon Lake	5	Oneonta	33	Block Island	31
McColloms	6	Oswego	35	Providence	26
McKeever	10	Perry	114		
Mt. McGregor	18	Port Washington	27	**SOUTH CAROLINA**	
Newcomb	9	Remsen	40	Charleston	11
North Creek	20	Riverhead	70	Columbia	40
Northville	27	Rochester	60		
Old Forge	22	Roscoe	14	**SOUTH DAKOTA**	
Owl's Head	9	St. Regis Falls	33	Aberdeen	17
Paul Smiths	7	Schenectady	27	Mobridge	10
Port Henry	14	South Fallsburg	47	Pierre	14

Rapid City	12	Yakima	0.18	Fredericton	0.43
Sioux Falls	52			Fundy National Park:	
		WEST VIRGINIA		Haslam Farm	3
TENNESSEE		Charleston	32	Waterside	5
Great Smoky Moun-		White Sulphur Springs	19	Lakeview	3
tains				Gagetown	11
National Park:		**WISCONSIN**		Grand Manan	1.6
Headquarters	13	Eagle River	13	Jemseg	4.39
Newfound Gap	4	Kenosha	51	McAdam	1.5
Johnson City	51	Madison	98	Moncton	1.43
Knoxville	49	Milwaukee	81	Newcastle	0.21
Memphis	73	Plum Island	40	Perth-Andover	0.93
Nashville	69	Sheboygan	90	Pointe du Chene	9
		Superior	(44)	Sackville	1.7
TEXAS				St. Andrews	1.2
Amarillo	41	**WYOMING**		St. George	1.09
Big Spring	5	Grand Teton		St. John	0.9
Brownsville	24	National Park	0.1	St. Stephen	1.4
Corpus Christi	30	Lander	23	Shediac Cape	0.8
Dallas	115	Yellowstone		Sussex	2.93
El Paso	15	National Park:		Tracadie	1.9
Fort Worth	71	Mammoth	0.2	Waterside	5
Galveston	36	W. Yellowstone		Welsford	1.13
Houston	68	(Montana)	0.2	Woodstock	0.68
San Antonio	16				
		VIRGIN ISLANDS		**NEWFOUNDLAND**	
UTAH		St. Thomas	0.025	Corner Brook	0.1
Bryce Canyon				St. John's	0.3
National Park	0.9	**CANADA**		
Hurricane	4			**NOVA SCOTIA**	
Salt Lake City	8	**ALBERTA**		Antigonish	0.43
Salt Lake City:		Banff	0	Baddeck	0.44
Airport	2	Beaver Lodge	0	Cape Breton	
Canyon Rim	18	Calgary	0.028	Highlands	
Downtown	7	Coleman	0.028	National Park	0.36
Midvale	37	Cypress Hills	0.012	Chester	0.41
South Salt Lake	2	Drumheller	1	Digby	4
Vernal	3	Edmonton	0	Highlands	
Zion National Park	0.7	Jasper	0	National Park	0.48
		Lake Louise	0.009	Ingonish Island	2
VERMONT		Lethbridge	1	Kentville	5
Burlington	47	Manyberries	0.2	Meteghan	3
		Medicine Hat	7	Middle West Pubnico	0.29
VIRGINIA		Vermilion	0	Truro	0.21
Alexandria	(41)	Waterton Lakes Park	0.012	Yarmouth	5
Charlottesville	35				
Norfolk	50	**BRITISH COLUMBIA**		**ONTARIO**	
Richmond	42	Saanichton	0.06	Algonquin Park	16
Roanoke	85	Summerland	0	Bancroft	8
Shenandoah		Vancouver Island	1	Barry's Bay	2.2
National Park:		Victoria	1.19	Bellville	30
Big Meadows	10			Black Sturgeon Lake	2
Headquarters	35	**MANITOBA**		Blind River	3
		Brandon	2	Cedar Lake	6
WASHINGTON		Dauphin	5	Chalk River	2
Mt. Rainer		Morden	12	Cochrane	2
National Park:		Pierson	6	Cornwall	23
Longmire	0	Riding Mountain		Dorset	6
Paradise Valley	0.1	National Park	0.155	Espanola	3
White River	0.04	Russell	1	Fort Francis	1.6
Olympic National		The Pas	0.1	Fort William	0.11
Park	0.1	Winnipeg	7	Georgian Bay	
Seattle	0.02			Islands National	
Seattle-Tacoma		**NEW BRUNSWICK**		Park	16
Airport	0	Bathurst	0.24	Gravenhurst	17
Spokane	0.1	Campbellton	0.06	Haleburton	3.20
Walla Walla	3	Chipman	1.44	Hamilton	89
Wenatchee	46	Dalhousie	0.4	Honey Harbor	7
Wenatchee Valley		Doaktown	0.71	Huntsville	11
Experiment Station	84	Edmundston	0.90	Kapuskasing	0.34

Kenora		Central Etobicoke	77	New Carlisle	3
(Cedar Lake)	9	N.E. Etobicoke	114	Nominingue	7
Lake Joseph	4	Westport	5	Normandin	3
London	40	Windsor	(59)	Outremont	29
Madoc	13			Perce	2
Magnetawan	5	**PRINCE EDWARD**		Point au Trembles	36
Mallorytown	41	**ISLAND**		Pointe-Claire	32
Mindemoya		Cavendish	0.5	Quebec	18
(Manitoulin Island)	8	Charlottetown	2	Rimouski	8
Muskata Falls	5	Mantague	1	Riviere-du-Loup	8
New Liskeard	0.26	O'Leary	2	Ste-Agathe	10
North Bay	8	Prince Edward		Ste-Anne-de-Bellevue	42
Ottawa (district)	17	Island National		Ste-Anne-de-la	
Parry Sound	19	Park	4	Pocatiere	9
Peterborough	35	Souris	1	St-Jovite	6
Picton	38	Summerside	1	St-Lambert	5
Point Pelee		Tignish	1	St-Martin	55
National Park	29			Sherbrooke	26
Port Arthur	7			Tadoussac	2
Port Carlings	9	**QUEBEC**		Victoriaville	30
Rosseau	3.3	Baie Saint-Paul	4		
Sault Ste. Marie	6	Berthierville	33	**SASKATCHEWAN**	
Smith Falls	19	Cap-de-la Madeleine	45	Nelford	0.1
St. Lawrence		Carleton	2	Prince Albert	0.1
Islands National		Caughnawaga	58	Prince Albert	
Park	38	Chandler	0.1	National Park	0
South River	1.74	Charlesbourg	2	Regina	0.3
Sudbury	4	Dorval	59	Saskatoon	0.51
Temagami	3	Farnham	64	Scott	0.1
Tobermory	4	Father Point	1	Swift Current	1
Toronto	45	Gaspe	0.2		
Metropolitan		Grand Riviere	0.2	**BERMUDA**	
Toronto areas:		Iles-de-la-Madeleine	0.1	Hamilton	0
Toronto Island	29	Jonquieres			
City Hall	42	(Chicoutimi)	4		
Mimico	43	Lac-des-Plages	7	**CUBA**	
West Toronto	47	Lac-des-Seize-Iles	11	Havana	0.2
S.E. Etobicoke	54	Lennoxville	4		
West Scarborough	59	Matane	3		
North Scarborough	62	Matapedia	0.1	**MEXICO**	
S.W. Etobicoke	62	Mont-Albert Caspesie	0.1	Juarez	16
East Scarborough	65	Mont Joli	0.2	Matamoros	(24)
Weston	65	Mont-Laurier	7	Mexico City	4
Willowdale	70	Mont Tremblant	8	Tampico	4
Dufferin-Lawrence	72	Montreal	62	Torreon	4

Compiled by Oren C. Durham of the American Academy of Allergy.
Courtesy of The Allergy Foundation of America.

RAGWEED

The members of the ragweed family are the second most common plants, after POISON IVY, responsible for contact DERMATITIS. In the ragweed, both *leaf* and *pollen* may produce the allergic reaction: the pollen causes a hay-fever type of ALLERGY, which means that a person is allergic to a substance in the pollen—probably a PROTEIN—which dissolves in the watery secretions of the nose. But a contact dermatitis from ragweed means that a resin or a fatlike ingredient present in the leaves has dissolved in the natural oil of the skin.

Treatment of mild cases of ragweed dermatitis is relatively simple: cold compresses applied to the affected areas of the skin. But no one can decide better than the physician what remedies to use in a specific case. In general, treatment consists of cooling lotions, anti-itching drugs, cortisone creams and immunizing injections.

RECOMMENDED DAILY DIETARY ALLOWANCES (RDA)

The RDA were established by the Food and Nutrition Board, a division of the National Research Council, National Academy of Sciences, in May 1941. The allowances are designed to maintain good nutrition in healthy people in the United States under current living conditions. Their original standards have been reevaluated several times as new scientific evidence has become available.

RDA are not to be confused with the Minimum Daily Requirements established by the Food and Drug Administration, which merely reflect the quantities necessary for the prevention of *deficiency diseases*. The recommended allowances imply neither minimum nor optimum requirements, but rather a recommendation that substantially covers all individual variations in the needs of normal healthy people.

RELATIVE HUMIDITY

Relative humidity is the amount of moisture in the air compared to the maximum amount that the air could contain at the same temperature.

Rh FACTOR

The Rh factor is a substance present in the blood cells of a large proportion of people. It is found in the blood of about 85 percent of white women and about 95 percent of black women.

This factor is a matter of concern only if it is *absent* in the pregnant woman while being *present* in the husband's blood. In this "incompatible" couple, the infant—which may inherit the factor from its father—

307

RECOMMENDED DAILY DIETARY ALLOWANCES

Persons	Age in years From up to	Weight in pounds	Height in inches	Food energy (cal)	Protein (gm)	Calcium (gm)	Iron (mg)	Vitamin A (I.U.)	Thiamin (mg)	Riboflavin (mg)	Niacin equivalent (mg)	Ascorbic acid (mg)
Infants	0–⅙	9	22	lb. x 54.5	lb. x 1.0	0.4	6	1,500	0.2	0.4	5	35
	⅙–½	15	25	lb. x 50.0	lb. x .9	0.5	10	1,500	0.4	0.5	7	35
	½–1	20	28	lb. x 45.5	lb. x .8	0.6	15	1,500	0.5	0.6	8	35
Children	1–2	26	32	1,100	25	0.7	15	2,000	0.6	0.6	8	40
	2–3	31	36	1,250	25	0.8	15	2,000	0.6	0.7	8	40
	3–4	35	39	1,400	30	0.8	10	2,500	0.7	0.8	9	40
	4–6	42	43	1,600	30	0.8	10	2,500	0.8	0.9	11	40
	6–8	51	48	2,000	35	0.9	10	3,500	1.0	1.1	13	40
	8–10	62	52	2,200	40	1.0	10	3,500	1.1	1.2	15	40
Boys	10–12	77	55	2,500	45	1.2	10	4,500	1.3	1.3	17	40
	12–14	95	59	2,700	50	1.4	18	5,000	1.4	1.4	18	45
	14–18	130	67	3,000	60	1.4	18	5,000	1.5	1.5	20	55
	18–22	147	69	2,800	60	0.8	10	5,000	1.4	1.6	18	60
Men	22–35	154	69	2,800	65	0.8	10	5,000	1.4	1.7	18	60
	35–55	154	68	2,600	65	0.8	10	5,000	1.3	1.7	17	60
	55–75+	154	67	2,400	65	0.8	10	5,000	1.2	1.7	14	60
Girls	10–12	77	56	2,250	50	1.2	18	4,500	1.1	1.3	15	40
	12–14	97	61	2,300	50	1.3	18	5,000	1.2	1.4	15	45
	14–16	114	62	2,400	55	1.3	18	5,000	1.2	1.4	16	50
	16–18	119	63	2,300	55	1.3	18	5,000	1.2	1.5	15	50
Women	18–22	128	64	2,000	55	0.8	18	5,000	1.0	1.5	13	55
	22–35	128	64	2,000	55	0.8	18	5,000	1.0	1.5	13	55
	35–55	128	63	1,850	55	0.8	18	5,000	1.0	1.5	13	55
	55–75+	128	62	1,700	55	0.8	10	5,000	1.0	1.5	13	55
Pregnant				+200	65	+0.4	18	6,000	+0.1	1.8	15	60
Lactating				+1,000	75	+0.5	18	8,000	+0.5	2.0	20	60

SOURCE: Courtesy of UNITED STATES DEPARTMENT OF AGRICULTURE, House and Garden Bulletin No. 72, 1971. NAS-NRC Publ. No. 2216, Food and Nutrition Board, 1974.

may cause the mother to develop ANTIBODIES against the Rh factor. Antibodies are manufactured by the mother's body as a protection against foreign substances introduced into her blood—in this case, the baby's red blood cells, which contain the Rh factor.

Ordinarily, the first baby that causes this reaction in the mother is not affected by the mother's antibodies; but if she has already developed these antibodies *before* her first pregnancy—because of a transfusion of Rh-positive blood, for instance—even the first baby may be affected. However, this happens very rarely, since the Rh factor is always checked carefully before any transfusion; even still, a problem may arise with women who have had a transfusion many years previous, before anything was known about Rh.

When antibodies are present in a woman's blood, usually after one or more pregnancies, they are inherited by the baby and may destroy its red cells, that is, cause ANEMIA or other changes.

Even among Rh-negative women married to Rh-positive men, the antibodies appear in the blood of only one in every twenty. In severe cases, labor is sometimes accelerated in order to reduce the baby's exposure to the mother's antibodies, and the baby receives a blood transfusion right after birth.

If the condition is not recognized, the baby may die at birth or be born with severe jaundice.

RHINOPLASTY (NOSE SURGERY)

Rhinoplasty—plastic surgery of the nose—can reduce the size of, straighten, build up, lengthen, shorten, scoop out, tilt up or tilt down a "wrong" nose. It can do everything from reconstructing tissue and bone to correcting the slightest malfunction in breathing, smelling, or uttering a vocal sound.

The most popular operation, so common that many people immediately associate it with fleshy-nosed teenagers, is *reduction* rhinoplasty. The actual steps of this operation are relatively easy for an expert plastic surgeon. The difficulty lies in deciding just how much to remove and how much to retain. It is this decision, measured within sixteenths of an inch, that makes rhinoplasty one of the most delicate and at times unpredictable operations ever undertaken.

Surgery is performed from inside the nose and under a local anaesthetic painlessly administered after the injection of a BARBITURATE whose effects last only a short while. This prevents the patient from bleeding as much as he would under general ANAESTHESIA and keeps the face looking natural during the operation, thus providing a guide for the surgeon, who constantly has to consider the future relationship of the nose to the face.

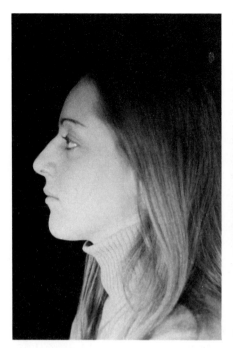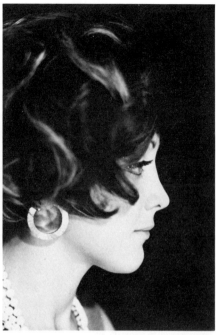

Left: A twenty-five-year-old woman photographed shortly before undergoing rhinoplasty.

Right: The same woman, two months after surgery. The new, delicate shape of her nose inspired her to change hairdo and to experiment with makeup. The result—though some people may find the "before" profile stronger, more personable—is truly stunning.

Left: Drawing of a long and hooked nose, with slightly too fleshy nostrils and a large tip. Visible is the bone segment of the nose bridge and the upper and lateral cartilages. Indicated is the amount of cartilage to be shaved off in order to correct the profile. The dotted line near the nose tip indicates where the cartilage is cut in order to slim the tip.

Center: The dotted lines indicate, respectively, where the cartilage is cut in order to shorten the nose and where the nostrils are narrowed.

Right: The operation is completed. With the exception of the nostrils, surgery is performed from inside the nose.

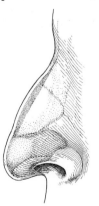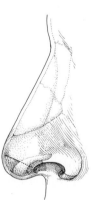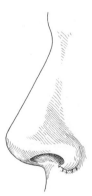

Usually, the nose tip is reshaped first; second, the hump of the bridge is removed; third, the septum (the sheet of cartilage dividing the nose lengthwise) is cut shorter or straightened and, particularly in thick-skinned, hooked noses, also scooped out to compensate for the inevitable telescoping of the skin over a suddenly shortened framework.

Excision of a triangle from the septum tilts the nose; excision of a rectangle shortens it; excision of a trapezoid shortens *and* tilts it; excision of an ellipse repairs a hanging columella (the midline tissue between the tip and the floor of the nose).

To narrow the nose, the surgeon performs a carefully designed fracture of the bone plates and presses them, often with his thumbs, into a new, slender position. The last step is the suturing of the mucosa (the nose lining), which requires extremely light stitches. The very last step, necessary only in case the lowering of the bridge has made the nose wings collapse, requires a triangular or diamond-shaped excision at the base of each nostril, which will draw the wings together, leaving only two barely visible scars.

Reduction rhinoplasty is a forty-five-minute operation followed by one week of bandages. The dreaded black-and-blue aftereffect and the swelling vary greatly according to the patient's skin and healing capacity. It varies also with the skill of the surgeon; particularly if he narrows the nose, a knowledgeable handling of the bones is important to avoid bruises and to prevent the bones from resuming their previous position.

Augmentation rhinoplasty, a less common but more dramatic procedure, is required for a nose twisted or flattened by an accident, for an abbreviated nose with an exaggerated upward-tilted tip and large soft-edged nostrils, or for a nose overly trimmed by previous surgery.

Through an incision within one of the nasal passages, the surgeon dissects straight along the depressed bridge a pocket in which he later

Excision of a triangle (A) from the septum tilts a nose; excision of a rectangle (B) shortens it; of a trapezoid (C) shortens and tilts it; of an ellipse (D) repairs a hanging columella, the tissue between the tip and the floor of the nose.

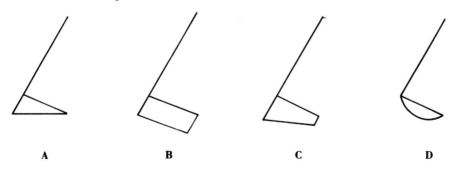

A   B   C   D

inserts an implant to build up the bridge. A sliver from the patient's hipbone or rib cartilage, or else a piece of SILICONE rubber provides the implant. The implant is carved with great precision so as to fit exactly where the nose is depressed without later shifting. On the upper surface, which will become the new contour of the nose, it is adjusted to fit the patient's face. If the tip also needs support, the implant is L-shaped and is inserted through an incision in the columella or the lower part of the septum.

The operation is followed by a few days of ANTIBIOTIC therapy, five days in the hospital, and biweekly checking of the bandages until the incision has healed—three or four weeks in all.

RHYTIDECTOMY (FACE-LIFT)

Unlike most of the other PLASTIC SURGERY procedures, which were developed at one time or another in Europe, the face-lift was invented in the early 1900s probably by Dr. Charles Conrad Miller of Chicago. He was a quack and a genius, an embarrassment to the American medical profession of his time, yet a man who today is considered one of the fathers of modern cosmetic surgery. Dr. Miller performed not only face-lifts but also such unheard-of surgical extravaganzas as reducing large mouths, narrowing wide nostrils and creating dimples, whose location on the face he selected "after having the patient smile."

In 1912, Madame le Docteur Suzanne Noël, a Parisian physician with a penchant for dermatology, read in the newspapers that an aging French actress had just returned from a tour in the United States, where she had undergone an extraordinary operation on the scalp that had restored her youth. The news, as Madame Noël wrote later in a delightful little book about aesthetic surgery, excited her so much that she begged the actress to allow her to examine the scars. It turned out that the actress had undergone something similar to today's mini-lift. Madame Noël immediately put aside dermatology and dedicated herself completely to surgery—the face-lift had thus crossed the Atlantic.

Since Madame Noël's day, though surgery has become bolder and the results more striking, not much has been added to the technique of face-lift. To reassure her patients of their progress, she even thought of preoperative and postoperative photographs, a practice all modern plastic surgeons follow. It is an unwritten law that photographs should always be taken: they are the surgeon's—or the patient's—best evidence, in case of a malpractice suit, of what the operation was all about. In general, however, the surgeon needs preoperative photographs to discuss the possible improvements with the patient, and later takes them to the operating room as a guideline during surgery.

Ear surgery, nose surgery and ORAL SURGERY are far more intricate matters than a face-lift, working as they do on the very framework of the face. The face-lift's purpose is just the opposite: to "tidy up" the face without altering its configuration, and in this lies the challenge. There should never be a *new* face, just a face imbued with new life—in other words, an illusion of youth, which in the face-lift becomes substantial and, within its limitations, permanent.

In the face-lift, the surgeon is concerned primarily with the skin; the nose, the chin, the ears, the jaws and the scalp are landmarks around which he works, using them as points of reference *and* as anchorage for the sutures. The first thing the surgeon must decide when planning an operation for an aging face is whether to perform a rhytidectomy (standard face-lift), a BLEPHAROPLASTY (correction of wrinkles around the eyes), or both. In the latter case, he further has to decide whether to perform them in a single session and which to do first. Also to be taken into consideration is whether the excess skin in the lower lid is indeed a defect of the lid and not part of the sagging of the cheek, in which case the face-lift alone might take care of it. Finally, in case of a pronounced double chin or extremely loose skin on the neck, a standard face-lift may not be enough, and a SUBMANDIBULAR LIPECTOMY (correction of the chin) might be required in addition to the face-lift or instead of it.

The choice of whether to perform the operations in one session depends, in part, on the endurance of both the patient and the surgeon. Also, the temporary swelling caused by an eyelid correction could mislead the surgeon about the actual condition of the rest of the face. There is, however, no *best* solution.

A standard face-lift starts with an incision in the hair-bearing scalp, about 3 cm above the "widow's peak" along a small strip of scalp, previously parted, with the hair on either side placed out of the way. The incision proceeds downward in front of the ear, parallel to a little crease, which is usually present, and curves around the earlobe. It continues upward and then sharply back, reaching into the neck hairline, along a second previously prepared strip of scalp.

The second step is to separate the skin from the superficial subcutaneous tissue, starting from the back of the ear and proceeding toward the jaws, taking care not to injure the facial nerves, the muscles or the blood vessels. On the temples the surgeon must undermine a little deeper in order not to damage the hair FOLLICLES.

Often the surgeon gathers the subcutaneous tissue upward and backward toward the ear and sutures it firmly to the fascia (the tissue protecting the facial muscles), which has become as inelastic as the aging skin. Over this smoother ground, the surgeon gently rotates and redrapes the skin. Two key sutures are placed near the ear, one slightly above it, the other somewhere behind it, and the excess skin is cut off. The incision in front of the ear is the last one to be closed. The surgeon rotates the skin upward without pulling it, cuts off the excess skin and sutures it delicately in place. The same is done on the other side of the face, once the surgeon has assured himself of the symmetry.

Some surgeons favor general ANAESTHESIA, but many prefer a local anaesthetic combined with an intravenous ANALGESIC. For one thing, the general anaesthesia tube might conceal a portion of the face and mislead the surgeon in his judgment of the face's overall condition.

A firm dressing that exerts a slight pressure is placed over the face, with cotton pads around the ears, and removed after forty-eight hours. The sutures in front of the ears are usually removed after three to five days; those behind the ears should not be touched for at least ten to twelve days.

"RIDING BREECHES" OPERATION

"Riding breeches" is a popular English expression (the French call it CELLULITE) for lumps of solid fat that women sometimes have on their thighs and buttocks and which are impervious to DIETS, MASSAGE or EXERCISE. The riding-breeches operation is a relatively new—at least in the United States—PLASTIC SURGERY procedure that corrects this defect by trimming the excess fat and skin.

American plastic surgeons have always known about riding breeches. Some call it trochanteric lipodystrophy; others call it simply fat, pointing out that lipodystrophy is something completely different. But most of them do not concern themselves with treating the condition, though many, at least once in their careers, have surgically removed excess fat from an obese patient. As recently as the mid-1960s, most plastic surgeons in this country were reluctant to correct riding breeches because the known techniques involved lateral, vertical scars that were visible on women wearing bathing suits and did not correct the appearance of either the front or the inner portion of the thighs. The few who had an idea of how to slice off the fat in a more aesthetic way were almost never asked by patients to perform the operation.

In 1964 *Plastic and Reconstructive Surgery*, the journal of the American Society of Plastic and Reconstructive Surgeons, published an article by Dr. Ivo Pitanguy, a Brazilian surgeon who described his own method of removing riding breeches.

As often happens—for good or for bad—with certain innovations, laymen showed the way to the experts. In this case, hordes of women from all over the world, including the United States, began to fly to the Pitanguy clinic in Rio de Janeiro to be operated on for riding breeches.

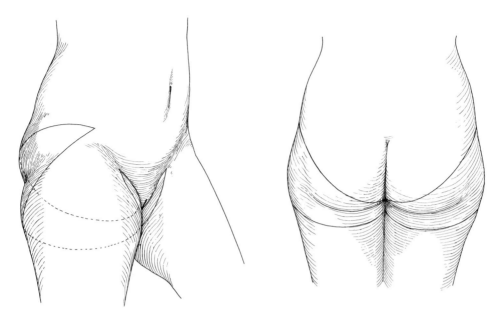

Above: Three-quarter and back views of a case of "riding breeches." Two lines have been drawn on the buttocks, one above and one below the gluteal fold, to show where the incision will be made and where the skin will later be sewn together. The lines are sometimes extended to the inner side of the thighs in order to correct the flabbiness often present there.

Below left: One step in the operation showing how a crescent-shaped section of fat tissue is being lifted and rated, to be subsequently removed.

Below right: The patient after the operation. The sutures coincide, in the inner side of the thighs, with the inguinal fold, and in the back with the gluteal fold, and extend on the outer side of the buttocks in a curve that almost reaches the height of the hipbone.

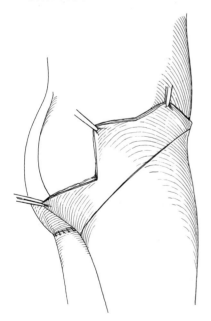

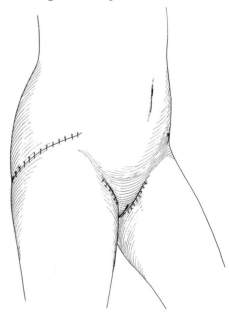

315

"RIDING BREECHES" OPERATION

Only recently have American plastic surgeons stopped ridiculing Dr. Pitanguy, and some of them have begun successfully to perform more and more riding-breeches operations themselves.

The first step in this procedure is the calculation of the quantity of tissue to be cut off. For this purpose, two curved lines, indicating the site of the incisions, are marked in surgical ink on each buttock of the patient. The upper line is traced above the buttock's fold to establish the height of the future fold; the lower, just beneath the fold. These lines describe an ellipse (comprising the characteristic depression on each buttock that sets off the bulge of the riding breeches) bent upward on the outer side of the thigh, more or less near the hipbone, depending on the amount of tissue to be cut.

With the patient anaesthetized and lying on her stomach, the surgeon cuts the skin along the tracings and removes an ellipse of skin and fat tissue. He then bevels the superfluous fat and slightly undermines the skin along the margins of the two incisions. Next, the surgeon pulls the lower flap upward to fill the concavity and, after rotating them (to avoid tension on the inner side of the thigh), he approximates the two skin edges with subcutaneous sutures, and finally sews them neatly together on the surface.

To correct the flabbiness often present on the inner side of the thighs, a strip of skin can be removed in addition to the ellipse. Its lower margin is gently pulled upward, rotated (to avoid tension on the outer side of the thigh), and sutured with stitches coinciding with the inguinal fold.

Several pounds of lumpy fat can be removed from each thigh with this operation. It lasts about three hours and requires general ANAESTHESIA but almost never a blood transfusion. This surgery does not interfere with the lymphatic circulation and in no way endangers the muscles of the legs.

Recovery, compared to other plastic-surgery procedures, is relatively slow and a bit irksome: for three or four days the patient has to stay wrapped in elastic bandages from her waist down to her knees. She may leave the hospital after eight days, but for at least a few days more she won't be able to bend her legs or sleep on her back. Climbing stairs will seem an impossible task for a week, and sitting on a hard chair will be comfortable only after three weeks. In six weeks, however, the patient will have forgotten her discomfort and begin to enjoy her new silhouette.

The two symmetrical scars that, in the back, coincide with the buttocks' folds can be well covered by even a small bikini bottom, and if the patient is a good healer, they will pale with time.

RUBBER GLOVES

Cotton-lined rubber gloves (or disposable thin plastic gloves) offer adequate protection against what dermatologists informally call house-wives' DERMATITIS—rough, reddened hands and cracked skin around the fingers and nails caused by daily exposure to WATER, SOAPS, DETERGENTS, dust, fruit and vegetable juices, bleaches and polishes.

There are, however, some definite rules regarding the wearing of rubber gloves, warns Dr. Bedford Shelmire, Jr., in his book *The Art of Looking Younger.* "If you don't know the rules and observe them, the gloves will make your problem worse instead of better."

First, rubber gloves should be worn consistently and should be replaced immediately when punctured or torn, which seems to happen quite often, regardless of their quality. Second, rubber gloves should be worn without rings and should be one size too large to allow space for a pair of washable cotton gloves to be worn under them, since the lining becomes dirty quickly and tends to remain moist, as it absorbs very little sweat. Hands perspire considerably when they are covered with rubber, "and a layer of warm sweat next to the skin can be almost as irritating as a detergent," notes Dr. Shelmire.

Rubber gloves should not be immersed in hot water or worn for more than half an hour at a time. After removing the gloves, a woman should always rinse her hands in cool water, dry them thoroughly and apply a hand cream.

S

SALABRASION

The removal of unwanted tattoos by using table salt is called salabrasion. It is a relatively new, simple technique that consists of rubbing the tattoo briskly and firmly with a moist salt-impregnated sponge. Abrasion is continued for about thirty to forty minutes, or until the skin becomes red. Sometimes a so-called "tattoo gun" is used to puncture the skin, which is then covered with salt.

After the salt is rinsed away, an ANTIBIOTIC ointment is applied and the area is covered with a sterile dressing. In about forty-eight hours, the area becomes dry and forms a crust that thickens and becomes brown in a few days. After one or two weeks, the crust, which has absorbed most of the tattoo's pigment, separates from the underlying skin.

The tattoo will by then have faded considerably or, in some cases, be completely removed, without showing scars. In four to six weeks the procedure can be repeated if necessary.

Salabrasion differs from other conventional methods of tattoo removal in that very little pigment is actually removed during the procedure; rather, the skin appears to be stimulated to do a sort of "biological removal" during the healing process.

SALIVA

Saliva is a clear, alkaline secretion produced by three glands in the mouth: one under the tongue, behind the lower front teeth, and one in each cheek, opposite the last two upper teeth.

Saliva keeps the mouth moist so that food may be lubricated, and also helps speech and swallowing. It contains ENZYMES that initiate predigestion of starchy foods before they reach the stomach, and it neutralizes any food that may be either acidic or alkaline, as both can irritate the mouth mucosa.

Saliva helps to prevent tooth decay by neutralizing the acids produced by germs. However, it also contains certain PROTEIN-like substances, as yet not entirely identified, that are absorbed by tooth surfaces, thus promoting the formation of PLAQUE.

Saliva disinfects and heals wounds and cuts, but *only* within the mouth.

SAUNA

The traditional Finnish sauna bath is a little cabin made of natural timber, built ideally on a lake shore. Inside are a platform and tiered benches made of pourous, slow-heating wood, usually aspen. In a corner, a pile of hard, nonexpanding stones—*kiuas*, in Finnish—are heated over a cast-iron or brick stove. The oldest saunas were called "smoke saunas" because the smoke from the stove's wood fire actually had to make its way out through the cabin itself. Later, however, a chimney was added.

A dim light (bright lights are not conducive to the atmosphere of a sauna), a wooden pail *(kiulu)* filled with WATER, a wooden-handled copper ladle, and a whisk made from birch or eucalyptus twigs *(vihta)* are all the furnishings needed in a classic sauna.

The cabin is heated to approximately 90° or 100°C. The sauna bather lies naked on one of the benches (the higher the bench, the hotter the air), where he perspires copiously for as long as he can stand it, occasionally whipping himself with the fragrant whisk (which is first dipped into hot water) to promote blood circulation and to increase PERSPIRATION.

At intervals, to further increase perspiration, conscientious sauna bathers throw a ladleful of water on the stones to produce a *loyly*, which feels like a wave of unbearably hot air, but which in reality briefly lowers the cabin's temperature and raises its HUMIDITY. In five or ten minutes the humidity is absorbed by the wooden roof and walls, and the temperature climbs back to its previous level.

Modern saunas usually have an electric stove and a washroom adjacent to the cabin, where bathers may come out a few times to catch their breath and eventually to get a thorough scrubbing. The last stage of the sauna ritual is an ice-cold shower, a roll in the snow, or a plunge into a wintry lake followed by a brisk swim. The very last stage, though it is rarely mentioned in sauna manuals, should be lots of moisturizer over the entire body.

The walls and the benches of the sauna should be unpainted: heated paint has an unpleasant smell and prevents the wood from drying.

The best sauna towels, the Finns recommend, are rough-textured tow cloths or pure linen—thick, soft towels will not absorb the moisture and will make one perspire more in the effort of getting dry.

The best way to preserve birch twigs after collecting them in midsummer is to put them in plastic bags and keep them in a deep freezer. Shortly before use, they should be thawed at room temperature.

After a sauna, to correct the body's dehydration and loss of salt, Finns eat a *saunapala:* smoked salmon, salted herring with boiled potatoes, and lots of cold beer. No Finn fools himself into thinking that the few pounds he loses in the sauna are the equivalent of an instant diet; what is lost is only water, and the balance is quickly reestablished as soon as the inevitable post-sauna thirst is quenched. However, most sauna *aficionados* tend to believe that perspiration will somehow wash out their bodies' "impurities." The truth is that the three million eccrine glands coiled beneath the skin surface have one purpose only: to regulate body temperature.

SCLEROSING SOLUTION

Sclerosis basically means hardening of tissue. Sclerosing solution is a chemical solution—usually a sodium salt known by the trade name Sotradecol ®—that is injected into stretched veins (varices) for the purpose of erasing them. The solution acts as an irritant, causing the blood to clot and the walls of the vein to turn into scar tissue.

Vascular surgeons and dermatologists favor this technique for obliterating small peripheral VARICOSE VEINS, those unsightly winding blue lines many women have on their legs and thighs. This procedure, however, is not advisable when major veins and their branches show extensive damage to their valves.

With the patient standing erect (the varices are most prominent in this position), the vein is punctured and the leg raised to a horizontal position in order to empty the vein. Then a small amount of sclerosing solution is injected, and the leg is kept in the horizontal position a few more minutes. In order for the solution to be dissipated more quickly, the patient is asked to stand, move his toes rapidly, and immediately resume his usual activities. A mild form of phlebitis (inflammation of the vein) accompanied by some swelling in the leg may occur, but it usually subsides after about a week. The complete clearing of the injected vein takes about six weeks.

Some physicians recommend a variation of this procedure for slightly larger varicose veins. The patient lies down, and the affected leg is raised to a 45° angle. Before injecting the solution, the physician inserts a needle into the varicose vein and withdraws blood until no more blood backs up. Leaving the needle in place, he attaches a second syringe and, while exerting a slight pressure with the thumb and forefinger above and below the injection site, he injects a small amount of Sotradecol ®. The whole procedure lasts about fifteen minutes, and the patient is allowed to get up after a five-minute rest.

SHAMPOOS

Shampoos are preparations made of surface-active ingredients that remove superficial grease, dirt, skin debris and residues of hair-grooming products from the hair shaft, without affecting the hair, the scalp or the body's health in general.

A man with a crewcut can wash his hair with a SOAP bar and rinse it in the shower, but everyone else—women *and* men—requires a hair-washing product that not only cleanses the hair but also makes it glossy, soft and manageable. A good shampoo also minimizes eye sting, does not irritate the scalp, and does not remove too much of the scalp's natural oil. Naturally, the more delicate the condition of hair—bleached, tinted, suffering from DANDRUFF—the more complex the shampoo's formula.

The original shampoos were soluble soaps, i.e., the products of chemical reactions between lye or potash and the fatty acids of animal or vegetable oils. The disadvantage of soap shampoos is that they deposit on the hair shaft a dull film of insoluble calcium or magnesium salts, especially when used with hard WATER.

Modern shampoos are usually made with various synthetic DETERGENTS, though they too utilize fatty acids. The difference between these and the pure soap shampoos is that the portion of the fatty acids that react to form insoluble soap residues are replaced in the detergents with a unit that does not form insoluble mineral salts.

Shampoos are manufactured in various forms: liquids, lotions, gels, creams and pastes. Liquid shampoos are the most popular because they are easy to apply and to rinse. A typical formula for shampoo may include coconut oil, olive oil, ethyl alcohol, potassium hydroxide, water and a soft detergent. Among the additives are foam builders to increase lather stability; CONDITIONERS, such as LANOLIN or SILICONES, to coat and lubricate hair; preservatives to prevent the growth of MOLDS; ANTIOXIDANTS; anti-DANDRUFF agents; PERFUMES; color additives. Incidentally, foam is not a sign of effectiveness in a shampoo; however, it has a psychological factor, as most people find an abundant lather much more satisfying than a scanty one, the shampoo's ultimate efficiency notwithstanding.

Frequent shampooing does not in any way affect hair growth, and it does not cause people to lose hair; the slightly increased number of loose hairs usually found during washing results from the dislodging of previously lost hairs that are still entrapped among the others, or from the shedding of hairs that are about to be lost owing to natural processes. In fact, hair may be washed daily without harm and the frequency depends only on an individual's habits. Naturally, the oilier the scalp, the more frequently a person would want to wash his hair. Incidentally, because water neutralizes one of the strengthening bonds in hair—the hydrogen bond—wet hair is weaker than dry hair and breaks more easily when combed or brushed.

Regular shampooing may be supplemented with the use of a waterless or dry shampoo. These products usually consist of absorbent powder and a mild alkali; they have been greatly improved in recent years and give better results than previously available dry shampoos. The method of applying dry shampoos varies depending on the brand, but the principle is the same: the product is applied to the hair, left for a few minutes and then brushed away.

SHAVING

Among women in the United States, shaving is one of the most popular methods for temporarily removing superfluous hair from legs and underarms. All women who use a safety razor presumably know that a sharp blade is best for satisfactory shaving, but some seem to overlook the fact that warm water and shaving soap (or chemically heated lather) are necessary, too. Any man will confirm how painful it is to shave a dry beard.

Regardless of the type of product, a good shaving soap should produce an easy and copious lather, as its primary function is to retain moisture on the area in order to thoroughly wet and soften the hair. Shaving soap also provides a film that protects the skin from the irritation of the razor, sufficient viscosity to hold hairs erect (thus facilitating the cutting), and enough lubrication to make the razor glide easily and painlessly over the skin.

Some women, however, find it difficult to shave around the shinbones and prefer an ELECTRIC SHAVER to puttering with lather and dull razor blades. Although they may be of daintier design, efficient electric shavers for women should be constructed essentially like men's shavers. The ideal electric shaver for women should be light, simple to operate and to clean (all shavers work better when clean), quiet and nonirritating, especially on the skin of the underarms. They should also be equipped with adapters for power-outlet sockets in foreign countries. But, according to the *Consumers' Research Magazine* for 1974, this ideal shaver "has still to be designed."

The most common misconception about shaving is that it makes new hairs grow faster, thicker and darker. In truth, the hair only *appears* to be thickened by shaving, because a short hair is less flexible than a long one and thus feels coarser. Shaving has no effect on the structure of the hair shaft, which is determined solely by the root, the papilla, the only living part of hair.

SILICONES

Silicones (dimethylpolysiloxane) are a large family of chemically related synthetic materials whose basic formula is derived from sand and a carbon compound. Their most common source is quartz rock. Silicones were accidentally discovered in the 1920s by Frederick Stanley Kipping, a British chemist who dismissed them as "unattractive gels," not realizing that they would one day revolutionize both industry and surgery.

Silicones, which can be liquid, oily, gelatinous, spongy or rubberlike, have been commercially available since the early 1940s and are currently used for thousands of different products, from the astronauts' boots to molds of TV-set frames. And since the early 1950s, the medical community has recognized their potential as a biomaterial, i.e., a strong, stable and chemically inert substance that can be implanted in the body as a substitute for human tissue, as it is able to withstand the body's hostile reactions and will not adhere to or damage adjacent tissues, promote bacterial growth or induce blood-cell and ENZYME destruction.

A magnified cross-section of an acne pit, showing the injections of droplets of liquid silicone between the deepest stratum of the skin and the fat tissue.

The silicone is injected with a very slender needle and with swift, contiguous, perpendicular or diagonal injections into the skin indentation.

Each droplet eventually will be capsulated in fibrous tissue by the body and will resemble the delicate but substantial globules of fat tissue, thus leveling off the acne pit.

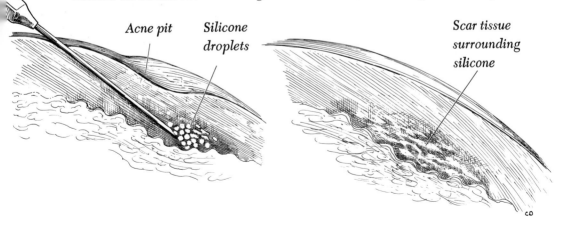

Acne pit   Silicone droplets

Scar tissue surrounding silicone

SILICONES

Though the perfect biomaterial has still to be discovered, materials such as dacron, teflon and other fibers are currently being used to repair arteries, tendons, bladders, heart valves and bile ducts. As for the silicones, they can double for adipose tissue, cartilage and even bone, which makes them very important to PLASTIC SURGERY for permanent implants and injections.

While the various forms of *solid* silicone have been part of every plastic surgeon's equipment for a number of years, *liquid* silicone has only recently become legal in this country. In the mid-1960s, Dow Corning, the American company that first manufactured medically purified silicones with the name of Silastic®, became alarmed by international reports of mishaps as a result of injections of liquid silicone and decided to investigate. It turned out that several unscrupulous doctors were injecting it in large quantities *directly* into the breast tissue

Left: A breast prosthesis made of a translucent silicone gel wrapped in a thin-walled envelope approximating the softness, mobility, weight and shape of a real breast. The prosthesis is inserted behind the mammary gland through an incision in the breast fold and is secured to the chest wall by the ingrowth of fibrous tissue through a backing of Dacron net.

For women who have undergone mastectomy and need breast reconstruction, custom-made prostheses can be designed to fill the armpit defects caused by the removal of lymph glands. *Courtesy of Heyer-Schulte Corporation of Santa Barbara, California.*

Right: Silastic® breast prosthesis—the first silicone breast implant, developed in 1963 by Dr. Thomas D. Cronin of Baylor University in Houston, Texas. *Courtesy of Dow Corning Corporation of Midland, Michigan.*

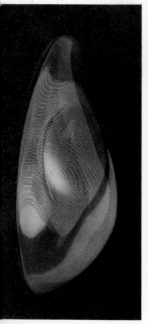
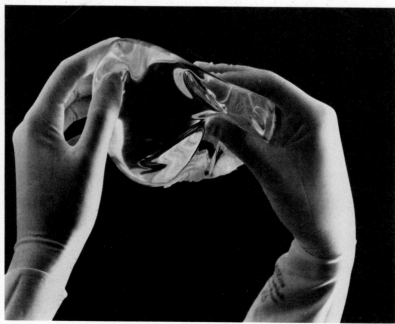

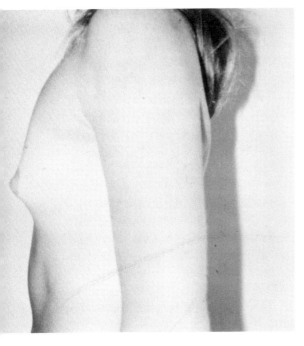

A twenty-four-year-old patient of Dr. Franklin L. Ashley of Los Angeles, California, with underdeveloped breasts.

The same patient, eighteen months after insertion of a silicone breast implant.

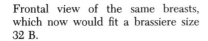

Frontal view of the same breasts, which now would fit a brassiere size 32 B.

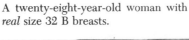

A twenty-eight-year-old woman with *real* size 32 B breasts.

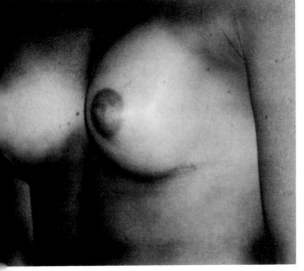

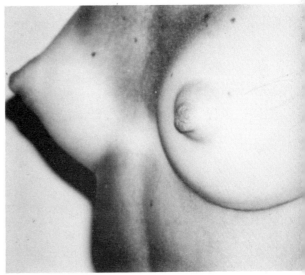

of flat-chested women. This often caused the slick, free-moving fluid to wander, drawn by gravity, along the smooth planes of muscles, either disappearing into the tissue or collecting in the abdominal cavity or in clumps under the skin, which not only could not be removed but caused complications such as CYSTS, infections and tumors. And when they tried to prevent silicone from slinking off by mixing it with various ingredients, those doctors obtained even worse results.

Dow Corning then voluntarily listed liquid silicone with the FDA, which meant that this compound ceased to be an "implant material" (as the solid silicone is) and was classified as a "drug," subject to much stricter regulations. Seven well-known plastic surgeons and one dermatologist were asked to investigate and experiment with liquid silicone, and after a few years they filed essentially favorable reports. As of 1975, liquid silicone, too, has become available to most physicians, provided they inject it in microscopic quantities and under no circumstance into breast tissue.

Liquid silicone—Liquid silicone is used to obliterate deep wrinkles, furrows, ACNE and chickenpox scars, and to build up cheekbones. It is injected into the deepest stratum of the skin with a fine needle, one droplet at a time—no more than twenty drops in one session, no more than one or two sessions a week. After it lodges in the skin, each droplet is automatically surrounded by a tiny fibrous capsule, which is the body's way of healing around anything that intrudes into the pattern of its tissues. If the droplets are evenly distributed, rather than rushed close to each other in a small area, the body will create a lacing of fibrous tissue and silicone which will resemble the delicate but substantial lobules of human fat tissue.

Liquid silicone is of great help, too, in the treatment of facial hemiatrophy and facial lipodystrophy, two mysterious, though fortunately infrequent, disturbances of fat metabolism that cause the wasting away of the soft tissue of the face. The hemiatrophy strikes on only one side; the lipodystrophy extends to the entire face and neck and often to the upper part of the arms and to the torso.

Vulcanized silicone—Vulcanized silicone is produced by a technique, still being tested, in which liquid silicone is injected along with the proper catalyst, thus producing a gelatinous deposit beneath the skin. It is hoped that vulcanized silicone will be applied successfully in the near future to the treatment of pectus excavatum, a defect of the chest that bizarrely bends a man's or a woman's ribs, or gives to the chestbone an unattractive funnel-like appearance.

Silicone gels—These are used for certain types of breast implants, such as the Cronin prosthesis, named after Dr. Thomas Cronin of Baylor University in Houston, Texas, who developed the first breast implant.

The Cronin prosthesis consists of a thin mold of silicone rubber shaped approximately like a "falsie" and filled with silicone gel; it resembles the weight and consistency of real breasts. The implants are easily inserted through an incision in the fold beneath the breast and are placed in a pocket *behind* the mammary gland. On the side that adheres to the chest muscle, the implant often has a backing of dacron-mesh discs, into which the body, in its healing process, will intertwine strands of fibrous tissue, thus securing it in place without the need for sutures.

Breast implants are used to enlarge very small breasts (augmentation MAMMAPLASTY) or in the reconstruction following radical, simple or subcutaneous MASTECTOMY, i.e., removal of all or part of the breast tissue because of cancer or chronic cystic mastitis, a recurrent inflammation of the mammary gland. The implants are also used to build up the smaller of severely asymmetric breasts (the larger breast often requires reduction mammaplasty).

Silicone rubber—As it can approximate the consistencies of both cartilage and bone, silicone rubber can be used as a framework for the reconstruction of malformed or damaged ears, for artificial joints replacing those deformed by ARTHRITIS, and to build up the depressed bridge of a nose or the bone of an uneven or too small chin.

SKIN CANCER

Cancer of the skin is the most common of all cancers but also the least dangerous, because, unlike most other types of cancer, its causes are well established, its development is relatively slow, and, more important, it is visible and can be treated while still premalignant.

Skin cancer may develop from repeated exposure to X-rays, from burns or disease scars, but mostly from exposure over a long period of time to intense sunlight.

The so-called "high risk" skin-cancer patient is a person over fifty with fair or freckled skin, a genetic predisposition to skin cancer, and a year-round suntan. On his face, ears, hands, neck, and forearms, he is prone to develop heavily wrinkled and atrophied skin, blotches of various shades, and certain skin growths called actinic keratoses—i.e., growths produced by ultraviolet rays—from which malignant tumors may later develop.

Actinic keratoses are an irregular reddish thickening of the epidermis. The lesions have flat surfaces that are often covered by small, thin gray or brown scales. The earliest keratoses are no larger than a few millimeters; several may appear at once and later run together as they gradually increase in size, and they bleed when the scale is peeled off. (Incidentally, if they *don't* bleed, they may be seborrheic keratoses, which have nothing to do with sunlight.)

Not all actinic keratoses turn into skin cancer, yet most dermatologists feel that it is best to destroy all of them as early in their development as possible, because they are premalignant and could develop cancer within ten years. The choice of therapy—cryotherapy, electrodesiccation or chemotherapy—depends essentially on the size and nature of the lesions. For a few isolated keratoses, cryotherapy or electrodesiccation is the preferred technique; chemotherapy is recommended for keratoses that are numerous and spreading.

Cryotherapy—This refers to the therapeutic use of extremely cold temperature. It consists of applying liquid nitrogen with a cotton swab applicator held sixty seconds on the lesion—enough time to freeze the tissue. The treated lesion will sting for a few minutes, then start to swell and to crust. The crust comes off after a few days, and the lesion heals after about ten days. Some dermatologists prefer to use carbon dioxide, either in capsules or as loose dry ice pressed into a stick and applied on the lesion for fifteen seconds. The lesion will blanch and then solidify. Later, the dermatologist lightly scrapes it off with a small curette. The lesion heals in about two weeks, leaving no scar, although people with dark complexions may be left with a tiny depigmented area.

Electrodesiccation—This consists of brushing and slightly charring the previously anaesthetized keratosis with a high-frequency electric needle. The charred tissue is then scraped off with a curette. A small crust will develop and peel after two weeks.

Chemotherapy—In chemotherapy, a chemical called 5-Fluorouracil® (5-FU) is rubbed liberally not only on the lesions but on the entire affected area twice a day for ten days to two weeks. During this time the patient should avoid direct sunlight, as this chemical is a photosensitizer. (In the southern regions of the United States, dermatologists prefer to prescribe 5-FU only during the winter months.)

The chemical acts *only* against abnormal tissue and is harmless to healthy skin, though care should be taken not to rub it on the eyelids and the lips. After three or four days, the lesions treated with 5-FU react as they would to a severe sunburn. Sometimes the patient feels a burning sensation even where there are no visible keratoses, which means that the chemical is affecting cells that have just begun to be transformed into future keratoses. The burning sensation is often so strong that the dermatologist should reassure the patient that it is a sign of healing. After about ten days, the lesions become bright red and develop crusts, which peel off after several days. The new skin underneath is pink, smooth and resistant to the development of further keratoses.

Any growth of the lesion, a thickening or a change in its color, the development of itching, or a tendency for it to bleed without quick healing may be a sign that the keratosis is turning malignant. The most common types of malignant tumors are basal cell carcinoma and squamous cell carcinoma. The former starts as a small, translucent, hemispheric growth of about 1 or 2 cm in diameter that eventually breaks down in the center, forming a tiny ulcer. The latter is more serious because it can metastasize, i.e., spread to distant organs. It usually starts with a keratosis which ulcerates, develops a ragged edge, and finally becomes very hard and firm. (The most dangerous of all types of skin cancer is the melanoma, because it often metastasizes with enormous rapidity.)

The choice of therapy for either basal-cell or squamous-cell carcinomas is surgical excision, the simplest, surest (though a scar-forming) treatment for skin cancer, provided *all* cancerous tissue is removed. For an older patient who cannot tolerate surgery, or whose tumor is particularly deep, X-ray therapy is sometimes used.

When cryotherapy is used, the liquid nitrogen is applied with a small spray gun, because the tumor is larger and deeper than a keratosis, and a cotton swab would not be sufficient. (And since it is difficult to calculate exactly the depth of the tumor or the amount and freezing time of nitrogen needed to destroy it, the dermatologist may first insert into the tumor a thermocouple, a needle tipped with a device that measures small temperature variations.) The frozen area blisters and becomes red; a scab forms a few days later and peels after about four weeks, leaving the area free from cancerous tissue.

SLEEP CLINICS

The following eight clinics are currently offering diagnosis and treatment of common sleep disorders:

CALIFORNIA: Sleep Disorders Clinic and Laboratory, Stanford Medical School, 780 Welch Road, Suite 203, Palo Alto, California 94301, (415)497-6601

MARYLAND: Laboratory of Clinical Psycho-Biology, National Institute of Mental Health, National Institutes of Health, Bethesda, Maryland 20014, (301)496-6886

MASSACHUSETTS: Sleep Disorder Clinic, Department of Psychiatry, Peter Bent Brigham Hospital, Boston, Massachusetts 02115, (617)734-8000, Ext. 420

NEW HAMPSHIRE: Dartmouth Medical School, Hanover, New Hampshire 03755, (603)643-4000, Ext. 3642

OKLAHOMA: Veterans Administration Hospital (183), 921 North East Thirteenth Street, Oklahoma City, Oklahoma 73104, (405)272-9876, Ext. 263

PENNSYLVANIA: Sleep Research and Treatment Center, Department of Psychiatry, Milton S. Hershey Medical Center, Pennsylvania State University, Hershey, Pennsylvania 17033, (717)534-8529

TEXAS: Baylor Sleep Laboratory and Clinic, Department of Psychiatry, Baylor College of Medicine, Texas Medical Center, Houston, Texas 77025, (713)747-3000, Ext. 145

VIRGINIA: Sleep and Dream Laboratory, Box 347, University of Virginia Hospital, Charlottesville, Virginia 22901 (804)924-2365

SMEGMA

Smegma is a thick, bad-smelling secretion consisting mainly of shed epithelial cells. Smegma may be found under the prepuce (the foreskin of the penis) and around the labia minora (the folds of skin surrounding a woman's genital area).

One of the reasons for men's circumcision is to prevent the accumulation of smegma in the folds of the prepuce. In women, smegma can be completely avoided by a thorough daily cleansing of the external genital area with water and soap.

SOAPS

The chemical reaction that occurs between selected fatty acids (such as stearic acid or oleic acid) and alkalis (such as sodium hydroxide or potassium hydroxide) results in the formation of a substance called soap.

The quality and the texture of soap depend on the careful blending of high-quality vegetable- and animal-fat mixtures, while the type of soap depends on the different methods of manufacture the soap curd is subjected to.

Milled soaps—These are the most common and most inexpensive types of soap. Perfume and color are added to the curd; the compound is milled once, compressed, cut into bars and packaged.

French soaps—The initial chemical reaction is controlled to yield a milder curd, i.e., one with a low alkali residue. Perfume is of high quality, and the soap undergoes several millings.

Floating soaps—These contain a great deal of moisture and many air bubbles (which make them float) and undergo no milling procedure. The quality is good, but the soap bars melt rapidly, and some tend to deteriorate during storage.

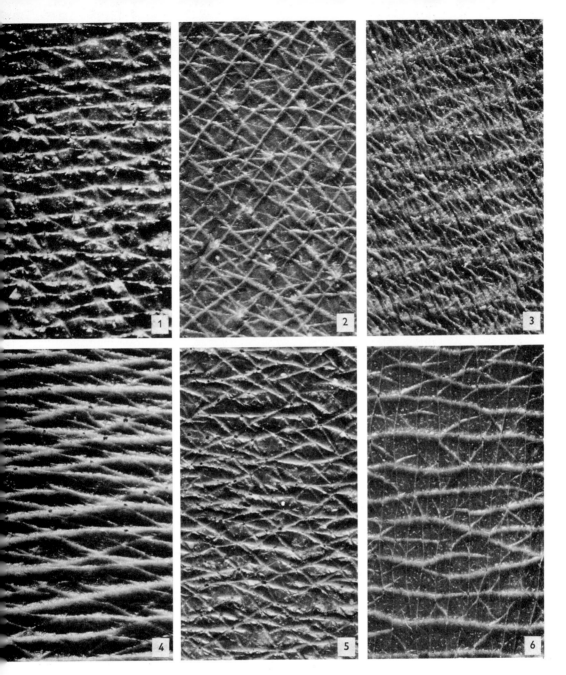

Replicas of human skin from different parts of the body. The ridges and furrows of the skin surface patterns—dermoglyphics—vary according to the anatomical structure and the function of the skin.

The replicas are obtained by pressing a fast-drying silicone rubber material against the skin and photographing the impressions at different magnifications. To be able to examine the magnified dermoglyphics is of great significance both in criminal investigation and in scientific research. Chromosomal disturbances, for instance, are revealed by dermoglyphics. Also, certain skin diseases, such as ichthyosis, cause irregular arrangements of the ridges.

1) The skin of the cheek (magnification: 10 times)
2) The skin of the forearm (magnification: 7 times)
3) The skin of the inside of the elbow (magnification: 7 times)
4) The skin of the wrist (magnification: 7 times)
5) The skin of the thigh (magnification: 7 times)
6) The skin of the ankle (magnification: 7 times)

SOAPS

Transparent soaps—These contain little color additive and a larger proportion of vegetable fats than the opaque milled soap. During their manufacture other ingredients such as sugar, resin, alcohol, and glycerin are added. Transparent (or glycerin) soaps are often advertised as "neutral" and therefore less drying or irritating to the skin than the more alkaline milled soap.

Superfatted soaps—These are milled and contain an additional proportion of fatty materials (such as LANOLIN), which account for a thin film deposited on the skin. One of the best superfatted soaps, Neutragena®, also contains a buffer that lowers its alkalinity. Superfatted soaps do not cleanse as well as ordinary soaps, but they are much milder.

Special soaps—These may contain various additives such as deodorants, cold cream, antibacterial agents, antiseptic medicaments, abrasive granules, alcohol and a variety of fragrances or "natural" ingredients. However, deodorants, synthetic colors and fragrances are a frequent source of ALLERGY and may cause irritation as soon as the skin is exposed to sunlight (photosensitivity). Hexachlorophene, for instance, which for years was the most common antibacterial additive in soap and talcum powder, has been found to have toxic effects (apparently it can be absorbed into the blood through normal, unbroken skin). As of October 1972, hexachlorophene has been limited to products available only on prescription.

For nonallergic people and people who don't sunbathe, there are many special soaps, both domestic and imported, available at fancy drugstores. Some of these are listed below. Their lovely scents add no cleansing power to the soap—they just make it smell nicer.

Almond Cold Cream Soap	Milk-and-Sulphur Complexion Soap
Beeswax Soap	Mink-Oil Soap
Birchleaf Sauna Soap	Mountain-Pine Soap
Camellia-Plum-and-Honey Soap	Oatmeal Soap
Carrot-Juice Soap	Olive-Oil Castile Soap
Cinnamon Soap	Rose Soap
Cucumber Soap	Royal Jelly Soap
Coal-Tar Soap	Sandalwood Soap
Cyclamen Soap	Seaweed Soap
Honey-and-Glycerin Soap	Sesame-Oil Soap
Lemon Soap	Strawberry-Juice Soap
Lettuce Soap	Swiss Buttermilk Soap
Lilac Soap	Tomato Soap
Maize Soap	Violet Soap

A soap should always be used with lukewarm (never hot) water on an already wetted skin. It should be applied evenly, including in the folds of the skin; it should never be massaged into the skin (unless one is advised to do so by the dermatologist for a specific reason) and should be rinsed off quickly and thoroughly.

SOFT CONTACT LENSES

Soft contact lenses, which were developed in Czechoslovakia in the late 1950s but first appeared on the American market in 1971, are thin, curved shells of water-absorbing plastic called hydroxyathyl methacrylate (or hydrogel).

When soft contact lenses are dry, they have the brittleness of a cornflake, but they become soft and pliable when saturated with water. When placed on the eye, they mold themselves to the shape of the cornea, the transparent tissue that covers the colored iris and pupil, adapting quickly to the eye without applying pressure to the cornea's surface. Because of this quality, soft contact lenses recently have become available for therapeutic use as a comfortable, transparent, moist bandage for a damaged cornea, while also providing the eye with some vision. Also, since they are slightly larger than the cornea (unlike hard contact lenses), they can protect it better and have less tendency to shift position when a person blinks.

The soft contact lens is made from a molded blank, or "button," of hard plastic material; the button is cut with a precision lathe and polished to prescription in the hard form, then soaked in a saline solution (water mixed with salt in the same proportion as in tears). During this hydration process, the dimensions of the lens increase about 20 percent.

There are, however, some drawbacks: soft contact lenses are damaged more readily than the hard ones, and if chipped or scratched, they may be penetrated by bacteria and therefore become more difficult to sterilize. They are useless when dehydrated and are easily disturbed by atmospheric conditions such as wind or heat and by changes in the tear flow. They cannot be made to precise optical specifications, and in clinging to an irregular cornea—as in the case of astigmatism—they partially mirror the irregularity. And finally, the care of soft lenses is more complicated than that of hard lenses; because of their tendency to retain harmful chemicals, soft lenses have to be either steamed in distilled water, sterilized in hydrogen peroxide or stored in a sodium chloride solution.

Nevertheless, hydrogels are safe, nontoxic, well tolerated by most people, relatively easy for experienced ophthalmologists to fit, and much more comfortable than hard lenses, especially when first compared to the recommended half-hour for hard lenses. They tend to minimize small

SOFT CONTACT LENSES

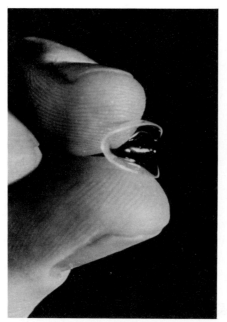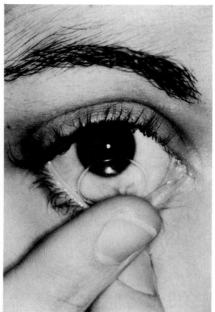

Left: A soft contact lens manufactured by Warner-Lambert Company of New Jersey, with the trademark Softcon®. Because of its water-absorbing qualities, this type of lens has been found to be an excellent transparent bandage for certain eye injuries. As an alternative to prescription hard contact lenses, however, soft lenses are still being perfected.

Right: How to place a soft contact lens. *Courtesy of Warner-Lambert Company, Morris Plains, New Jersey.*

irritations such as swelling of the cornea and the abrasions sometimes caused by hard lenses. A major problem with hard lenses—dirt particles lodging under the lens—seldom happens with soft lenses. Also, since soft lenses cling to the eye, they are less likely to fall out accidentally, which makes them very suitable for sports and strenuous activities. Finally, soft lenses allow people to switch back to eyeglasses with little or no blurring of vision, something hard-lens users often experience for as long as a week.

Before inserting or removing hydrogels, a wearer must wash his hands thoroughly, rinse them of soap residues and dry them with a lint-free towel. After removing it from the case, without touching the surface that is applied to the eye, the wearer should flex the lens between the thumb and forefinger to make sure it is not inside out. Then, with the lens on the tip of the forefinger, he pulls down the lower eyelid, looks upward and places the lens on the lower part of the eye. Then he closes the eye and lightly massages the lid to help center the lens. To remove it, he again looks upward, slides the lens down, and pinches it lightly between thumb and forefinger while pulling it away from the eye.

At present, ophthalmologists do not agree as to whether soft lenses are sufficiently permeable to oxygen. Some believe that the oxygen passing through a soft lens is insufficient and that, as is the case with hard lenses—which are completely impermeable to oxygen—the cornea of a soft-lens-wearer receives oxygen dissolved in the tears, which are pumped under the lens with each blink. Others feel that because the soft lens adheres closely to the cornea, very little oxygen actually gets through. Still others hold that enough gaseous oxygen permeates the soft lenses to nourish the cornea adequately.

The future of soft contact lenses looks good. Not only are the hydrogels being improved but SILICONE rubber lenses are currently undergoing clinical investigation. The silicone lens—called Silcon®—is harder than the hydrogel and softer than the hard lens, is nontoxic, is highly permeable to oxygen, doesn't need to be steamed or stored in saline solution and never loses its original curvature.

As Dr. Jules L. Baum, associate professor of ophthalmology at Tufts University School of Medicine, wrote in 1973, "Today, we are at the Wright-brothers'-airplane stage of development in soft contact lenses . . . it is too soon to know or to predict their full potential. But even at this early stage one thing is clear: soft contact lenses will have a definite place in ophthalmological theory."

SOMATOTYPE

During the last thirty-five years, Dr. W. H. Sheldon, a renowned physical anthropologist, has developed a system of classifying the various human body types with respect to their physical components, called their somatotype, which is considered the most practical method of establishing the relationship between the physique and disease in general.

According to the shape of their bodies, human beings are classified as endomorphs, mesomorphs and ectomorphs. Most people fit into one of these three major body types, though few are pure endomorphs, mesomorphs or ectomorphs; rather, most people have characteristics belonging to more than one type.

When endomorphy predominates, a person has a more or less plump body, with short arms and legs, small hands and feet, and delicate joints. Endomorphs may be slender in youth, with relatively inactive fat cells. But as they reach thirty, endomorphs tend to become overweight. Women have round hips, large bosoms, and not a sharp feature in their entire body. Endomorphic men have large abdomens and narrow chests.

Mesomorphs are more aesthetically proportioned: broad shoulders, straight bodies of medium height, strong chests in the men; firm, small breasts and boyish hips in the women. In general, mesomorphs have

335

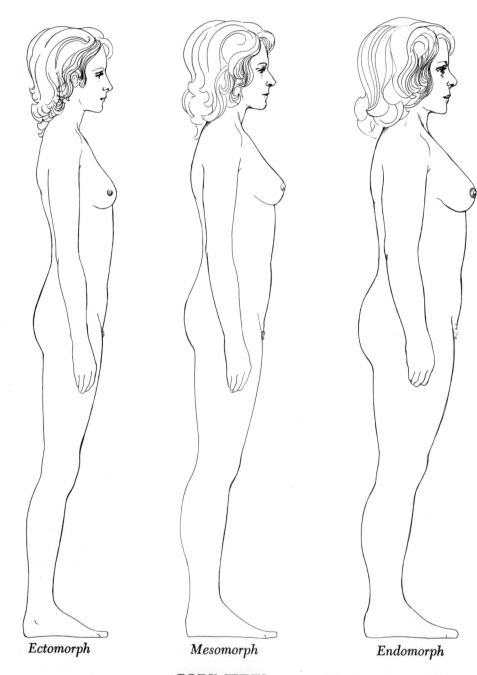

Ectomorph   *Mesomorph*   *Endomorph*

BODY TYPES

According to the shape of their bodies, human beings can be classified as:

Left: Ectomorphs—small bodies, long legs, narrow hands and feet.

Middle: Mesomorphs—broad shoulders, strong arms and legs, strong chests (men), small breasts and boyish hips (women).

Right: Endomorphs—plump bodies, short arms and legs, delicate joints.

Most people fit into one of these three major body types or a combination of them, though few are pure ectomorphs, mesomorphs, or endomorphs.

square faces and strong arms and legs—in a word, people in this category, both men and women, are the athletes.

Ectomorphs have relatively small bodies, with long legs and arms, narrow hands and feet, and tapering fingers. They have a delicate bone structure and long muscles. Faces are often small and triangular.

Somatotype ratings were used in a study of obese young girls conducted by Dr. Jean Mayer, one of the world's foremost authorities on nutrition. The girls were rated for endormorphy, mesomorphy and ectomorphy according to Sheldon's 7-point scale. For instance, a girl with very high endomorphy, fairly high mesomorphy, and very low ectomorphy, was rated 7:5:1. (A pure endomorph would be 7:1:1; a pure mesomorph, 1:7:1; and a pure ectomorph, 1:1:7.)

One of the conclusions that Dr. Mayer reached at the end of the study was that overweight adolescent girls are more endomorphic than, considerably less ectomorphic than, and somewhat as mesomorphic as normal girls of comparable age chosen at random from the general population. Despite the fact that, in adults, OBESITY is a much more complex syndrome, Dr. Mayer's findings may well apply to obesity in general: endomorphs are genetically prone to accumulating fat; meso-morphs can go either way; and ectomorphs practically never become fat, no matter how much they eat.

SOYBEANS

Soybeans are an annual legume with a high content of PROTEIN (nutritionally somewhat less complete than meat) and FAT (extracted as soybean oil). Even though the fat content—18 to 20 percent—is less than that of other oil-seed crops, the yield per acre is often higher than that of other oil seeds because soybeans have a richer harvest. When the oil is removed, what is left of the soybeans is turned into livestock feed.

The soybean plant originated in China, but, unlike other crops, it did not spread around the earth during the era of geographical discoveries. Until the early part of this century, nearly all soybeans were grown in eastern Asia, and they remained of small importance in the United States until World War II brought a shortage of butter and an increased interest in soybean oil. In 1943 there were in this country more than ten million acres planted with soybeans, a number which jumped to forty million by the late 1960s, thus making the United States one of the largest producers of soybeans.

In the last few years a trend has developed toward a more intensive consumption of soybean protein in human food, either as artificial meat or in other forms. For artificial meat, soybean protein is spun into fibers, partitioned to resemble whatever kind of meat intended, and flavored accordingly. The name of the fiber-textured vegetable protein is TVP. As defined by the U.S. Department of Agriculture, the material must have "a structural integrity and identifiable texture such that each unit will withhold hydration and cooking and other procedures used in preparing the food for consumption." In other words, once boiled or fried, it must not cease to look and taste like meat.

As of 1974, imitation meat is available to the public as imitation bacon bits, flavored and colored to resemble crisp bacon; and as unflavored textured vegetable protein, used as a meat "extender" in hamburgers. However, except for vegetarians, most consumers at present do not seem to be very much interested in soybeans.

SPIDER VEINS

Very tiny dilated veins are called spider veins. They are not, and never will turn into, VARICOSE VEINS. They never hurt, though sometimes at the end of the day they may cause a slight sensation of heat or a mild discomfort. However, spider veins are unattractive, and some physicians are skillful in injecting a SCLEROSING SOLUTION that coagulates the blood and turns the walls of the small veins into scar tissue. Sometimes new spider veins develop in the same area after a while, but the procedure is safe and, in general, aesthetically very satisfactory.

SPONTANEOUS ABORTION (MISCARRIAGE)

Spontaneous abortion, or miscarriage, as laymen prefer to call it to distinguish it from *induced* abortion, refers to the spontaneous loss of an embryo (or a fetus) before it has matured enough to live in the outside world, usually before the fifth month of pregnancy. At least one pregnancy in ten comes to an end this way; about two-thirds of these occur in the first three months. Usually the embryo dies about six weeks before the miscarriage is completed.

Miscarriages may result from abnormalities of the OVUM (or, more rarely, of the fetus); anatomical defects of the uterus or the cervix; hormonal defects; nutritional problems; extrauterine pregnancy, or SYPHYLIS.

Although miscarriages occurring early in pregnancy can rarely be prevented, many of the causes can be recognized and treated before the next pregnancy, and there is a good chance that they will not recur. However, a woman should not consider this an absolute rule and should be thoroughly examined by a gynecologist before planning another pregnancy. But sometimes the precise cause of a miscarriage cannot be established.

Miscarriages used to be blamed on falls or blows to the mother's abdomen, but in fact these rarely cause a miscarriage, as the fetus is well protected within the uterus and normally is not hurt even when the mother is injured. Nor is the fetus hurt by a pelvic examination, as some women sometimes fear.

Miscarriages that are attended to promptly by the doctor (especially the so-called incomplete abortions, in which a part of a fetus remains in the uterus after the miscarriage) are rarely dangerous to the mother, and recovery is usually rapid.

STIM-U-DENT®

Stim-u-dent® is the popular trademark for balsalike medicated tooth-picks. They are soft, nonabrasive, pleasantly flavored, with one flat side, and are compressible enough to adapt to all shapes of teeth, including ones that are closely spaced. Stim-u-dent® is used for removing food particles from surfaces not reachable with a TOOTHBRUSH and for gently stimulating gums without injuring them.

STRIAE (STRETCH MARKS)

The skin has a number of elastic fibers that give it firmness and prevent it from sliding, but which can also extend, shrink and follow the movements of the body. However, when rapid weight gain and loss follow each other, as in pregnancy or a crash DIET, these fibers become distended for too long and may break. A stretch mark is the tiny scar that appears when the elastic fiber has broken in the skin.

Stretch marks appear most frequently on the breasts, the thighs and the abdomen; they are pink at first and later turn white, and are usually lighter when the surrounding skin is suntanned.

Since some people tend to develop stretch marks more readily than others, the predisposition to them is probably genetic. HORMONES, too, may play a role in causing stretch marks. For instance, when hormones are administered as medication, or when their production is increased because of some glandular disturbance, stretch marks similar to those resulting from pregnancy may appear.

Whatever their cause, stretch marks seem to be indelible.

SUBMANDIBULAR LIPECTOMY (CHIN CORRECTION)

Chin correction is a PLASTIC SURGERY procedure often performed in conjunction with a FACE-LIFT. A 3-cm horizontal incision is made in one of the creases under the chin, and the skin is separated from the fat down to the level of the thyroid cartilage. A thin stratum of fat—at least 2 to 5 mm thick—should be preserved; otherwise the skin will attach itself directly to the muscle, creating a sharp and uneven chin contour.

The plastic surgeon trims the rest of the fat all the way to the neck, off the cordlike bands of the platysma (a broad, thin layer of muscle in the front of the neck), carefully avoiding the lower ramifications of the facial nerve, whose course is very close to the muscle. If fat is the major defect being corrected, and if the skin is not overstretched, this is the only surgery required, and the incision is simply closed—subcutaneously with catgut, which is absorbed by the body, and on the surface with silk stitches. A pressure bandage is applied, and the sutures are removed after five to seven days.

Quite often, however, a "double chin" is accompanied by loose skin; for years surgeons have offered different solutions for this problem. Some have suggested the excision of a vertical ellipse of skin and fat, or a long horizontal ellipse of skin alone; others recommend a simple vertical skin incision; still others call for two horizontal incisions—one under the chin and one on the lower part of the neck—joined at their midpoints by a vertical cut.

All of these methods, however, often leave noticeable scars on the neck, especially if a certain tension is being exerted on them. Besides, in some cases, there really is no excess skin once the fat has been removed: all the available skin is needed to adhere to the remodeled chin-neck angle that had been obliterated by the presence of fat. Sometimes the chin fat extends on both sides as far as the jaws, in which case the fat has to be removed from there, too, in order to keep the face contour as smooth as possible. If the "double chin" is also receding, the surgeon adds a solid SILICONE implant.

SUN PROTECTION

Of all the sun's rays that manage to penetrate the earth's atmosphere, 1 percent are in the ultraviolet range. Human skin tans and burns when ultraviolet rays strike and disperse the melanin (natural pigment) in the outer layer of the skin. About two days later, the rays penetrate the deeper layer to the melanocytes (pigment-producing cells), causing them to produce more melanin, which migrates to the surface of the skin and becomes visible as a tan.

Ultraviolet rays are invisible and penetrate only a fraction of an inch, but because they are shorter than the visible light waves of the sun, their effect on the skin is relatively slow, though powerful and potentially dangerous. How much a person tans or burns depends in large part on how much ultraviolet radiation the skin is exposed to, which in turn depends on the latitude, the season, the altitude, the time of day, the presence of reflecting surfaces such as snow, sand, or water, and, naturally, on the amount of pigment in the skin.

Ultraviolet rays affect the skin's inner layer irreversibly and cumulatively, even after a tan has faded. Though not so harmful as air pollution, sunlight can be one of the most negative environmental influences on the human skin: its radiant energy can precipitate or aggravate a number of diseases, such as certain inheritable skin conditions. It can also be one of the major factors in the development of SKIN CANCER in susceptible people. Certain prescription drugs—ANTIBIOTICS, sulfonamides, diuretics, tranquilizers—may cause some people to overreact to sunlight, i.e., become photosensitive. And finally, years of overexposure to sunlight inevitably renders the skin more leathery, dry and blotchy than warranted by a person's age. Sun protection, therefore, is necessary not only in case of illness but also for the healthy person who identifies good looks more with the condition of his skin than with a deep tan. As of yet, there are no preparations available that prevent sunburn while at the same time encouraging rapid tanning.

Sun protection can be obtained at three levels: with suntan lotion, sunscreen and sun block.

1) *Suntan lotions*, such as Coppertone®, Tanya® and Sea and Ski®, permit tanning while providing a minimum of burn protection.
2) *Sunscreens*, such as Presun®, Pabanol®, Sungard® and Uval®, provide adequate burn protection but keep tanning to a minimum.
3) *Sun blocks*, such as Noskote® and zinc oxide ointment, allow no tanning but offer an almost total protection against sunburn.

As suntan lotions have only a limited effect, and as sun blocks are so thick and opaque that most women hesitate to cover large parts of their bodies with them, the most realistic sun protection at present comes from the sunscreens. There are many brands of sunscreens available; however, these differ little, as all essentially contain a *chemical screen* (which absorbs some of the ultraviolet rays) and a *base* (which can be an oil, a cream, a lotion, a spray, or WATER mixed with ALCOHOL). Sunscreens are all more or less effective for sun protection; the only difference is that a greasy base is not so easily washed away by PERSPIRATION or sea water as an alcohol-and-water base. The most effective chemical screen reportedly is para-aminobenzoic acid, called PABA for short, which has only one drawback: it is not very soluble, and the alcohol needed to keep it in solution may have too much of a drying effect for delicate skin. Slightly less effective are iso-amyl and glycerol (two para-aminobenzoic derivatives) and benzophenone derivatives. The only drawback to these screens is that they are likely to cause a photoallergic reaction in sensitive skin.

In recent years, lotions called artificial tanners have been devised. The major ingredient in these preparations is a chemical called dihydroxyacetone (DHA), and the color achieved results from a reaction between DHA and amino acids in the skin. These lotions only color the skin and provide no protection against sunlight, unless they also contain a chemical screen. Moreover, the color is difficult to control, and even if applied carefully, the "tan" is streaked and uneven and often has an unnatural yellow hue.

More recently, artificial tanners called bronzers have become available. These contain a water-soluble stain that simply colors the skin and which can be readily washed off with soap and water. Bronzers, too, fail to protect the skin from the sun, and their prolonged use sometimes dries out the skin.

However, a comprehensive sun protection is on its way—at least for women—as many medicated COSMETICS are now being produced with a sunscreening agent to protect the skin at all times, even when it is exposed to the sun.

SUNGLASSES

"True" sunglasses (as opposed to "cosmetic" glasses) have lenses that are tinted or vacuum-coated for the purpose of filtering out *visible* rays (brightness and glare) as well as *invisible* rays (ultraviolet and infrared) of sunlight, to which the eye is sensitive.

To be effective, sunglass lenses should not let pass more than 30 percent of light—19 to 20 percent is the ideal quantity. Both lenses in the sunglasses should be carefully matched to provide the same density, shade of color, and optical quality for both eyes.

True sunglass lenses are made of prescription-quality materials with a precise curvature, accurately ground and polished to eliminate defects that may produce eye strain. At present, there are no sunglass (or eyeglass) lens materials available that are completely unbreakable or shatterproof; however, since January 1972, people have been able to demand lenses that are impact-resistant, i.e., made of laminated, heat-treated or chemically hardened glass that at least prevents them from shattering spontaneously (because of steam or sudden changes in temperature) or breaking after a slight impact. Plastic lenses are impact-resistant, too, though they do not filter out infrared rays.

Neutral gray or sage green are the colors recommended for best color perception, best protection from sun glare, and least color distortion. Truly neutral gray lenses, such as True-Color® of American Optical, provide nearly natural color perception, absorb ultraviolet and infrared rays, and transmit all colors in their true relationship.

Other colors are of lesser or no value in sunglasses: *blue* absorbs too much yellow and red, therefore reducing sharpness of vision and quality of perspective; *red* absorbs too much blue and green, as does *yellow*, though yellow (and brown) lenses are quite effective in sharpening contrast and detail for a person who skis, boats, or drives under hazy conditions. (By absorbing practically all the blue light, yellow can penetrate the haze.)

Sunglass lenses can be substituted for regular lenses in the making of prescription glasses, including bifocals. Another choice for people who wear prescription glasses is clip-on sunglasses worn over regular glasses. But even if of excellent quality, clip-ons have a number of disadvantages: they add extra weight to frames; their surface, combined with that of the eyeglasses, can produce confusing reflections; and they generally fail to give adequate protection because they are only as large as normal-size eyeglasses. (This disadvantage applies also to sunglass lenses inserted into a prescription frame.) Sunglasses should always be large enough so that the wearer does not have to look over or around them.

Inexpensive sunglasses (and some of the expensive ones, too) are usually inadequate; even if they are very dark, they do not absorb ultraviolet and infrared rays, and are more damaging to the retina (the perceptive structure of the eye) than the other extreme: clear lenses that do not reduce *visible* light at all but filter out only the *invisible* rays.

Cosmetic glasses, which for a while were called "fun" glasses, usually have thin pastel-colored lenses of several possible shades—pink, violet, bright green. The latest are gradient, with color fading from top to bottom, or one color running into another. These lenses are quite attractive; however, despite their primarily cosmetic function, they too must be impact-resistant. As long as they are free of distortion and have sturdy, well-balanced frames, these sunglasses are excellent for protecting the eyes against the grime, dirt and dust of city air (although they provide minimal protection against light rays), for wearing over CONTACT LENSES to prevent additional irritation to the eyes, for shielding the eyes from wind and for keeping eye makeup in place.

SYNDROME

A syndrome is a group of symptoms that occur together and are typical of a disease.

SYNERGISM

Synergism refers to the combined action of agents such as drugs so that their combined effect—which is not necessarily beneficial—is greater than the sum of their individual effects.

SYPHILIS

Together with GONORRHEA, syphilis is the most common of the venereal diseases (diseases spread by sexual contact). However, syphilis is very different from gonorrhea: the latter is basically a localized condition that affects the sexual organs themselves, whereas syphilis quickly enters the bloodstream and is carried throughout the body.

Syphilis may be transmitted by direct contact with an infected lesion or with transfused blood, or passed from a mother to her unborn child (congenital syphilis). The organism responsible for human syphilis is a spirochete called *Treponema pallidum*—a combination of bacterium and protozoon—with the characteristic corkscrew shape so familiar to medical students but so diaphanous as to be barely visible under the microscope except in the dark.

Syphilis seems benign at first, causing merely a sore at the point of infection. Yet it takes only a few hours for syphilis to become systemic, i.e., to invade the entire body, though no test could find evidence of the disease at that point (latent syphilis).

At three to four weeks after exposure, an ulcer—the chancre—appears at the site of infection. This persists one to five weeks and then heals spontaneously. About six weeks later, a localized or generalized skin rash may appear and also quickly heal. (At this stage, syphilis can be diagnosed from blood tests.)

If untreated, the disease will eventually—as many as five to fifteen years later—reappear as a violent and catastrophic attack that may affect the central nervous system (causing paralysis) or the heart.

By the late 1960s, syphilis seemed to be disappearing from the United States, but by the early 1970s it had again risen to epidemic proportions. Still, the available methods for diagnosing and treating syphilis are excellent: the disease responds promptly to penicillin and, for people allergic to this drug, to such ANTIBIOTICS as tetracycline and erythromycin.

Public health officials currently are trying to contain the damage of syphilis by tracing, tactfully and efficiently, each infection. But some people who contract syphilis are never treated or even diagnosed. One typical situation is that of an infected person who presents himself for treatment but does not name *all* his contacts, for fear of having to admit, for instance, a secret homosexual relationship. Also, in cases of anonymous relationships, it may be impossible for a long time to trace a "carrier," i.e., an individual harboring syphilis organisms in his body without apparent symptoms.

Ever since the spirochete was discovered in 1905, microbiology texts have classified *Treponema pallidum* as anaerobic, i.e., growing only in the absence of OXYGEN. Recently, however, Dr. Charles D. Cox of the

University of Massachusetts discovered that the syphilis organism, while it does indeed die more quickly when exposed to air, requires oxygen to thrive. This means that scientists may soon be able to grow this organism in the laboratory and ultimately develop a VACCINE against syphilis. Until a vaccine becomes available, however, the control of syphilis will depend on prevention (hygienic measures, the use of condoms) and early treatment of infection. The key to both is, of course, *education*—not only of the public but of such people as schoolteachers, pharmacists and nurses, who can often be more successful than physicians in gaining the necessary confidence from people—especially young people—to impress on them the gravity of the disease *and* how easily it can be cured.

Photomicrograph, magnified 34,000 times, of a *Treponema pallidum,* the organism responsible for human syphilis, with its characteristic corkscrew shape so familiar to medical students.

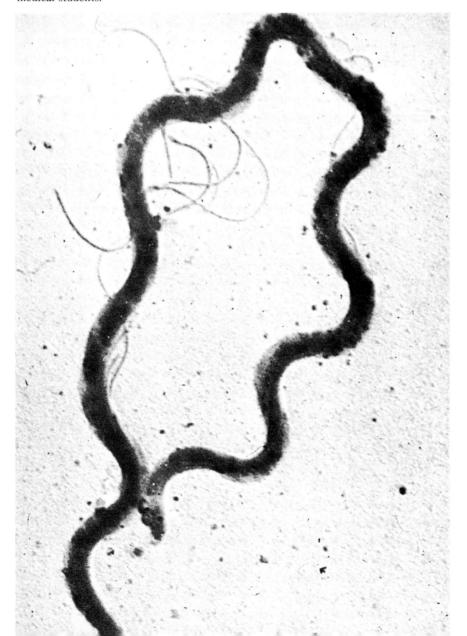

345

T

TENNIS TOE

Tennis toe is a disorder that occurs when a tennis player stops short, after dashing to the net, for instance, and jams his big toe hard against the front of his sneakers. The result is the rupture of small blood vessels beneath the toenail, producing discoloration, swelling and pain.

The risk of tennis toe is greater during play on cement or other hard-surface courts that, unlike clay or grass surfaces, do not permit the foot to slide during sudden stops.

Pain usually subsides after a few days. Tennis toe can be prevented by wearing comfortable sneakers and, if possible, by playing on surfaces other than cement.

THERMOGRAPHY

It was first noted in 1956 that BREAST CANCER is associated with an elevation of temperature of the skin over the lesion, owing to the increased metabolism and blood requirements of the cancer. Thermography is a measurement of this skin heat translated into a pictorial representation of the infrared radiations of the skin. In other words, the breast is scanned with an infrared camera, and the heat energy is transformed into a light pattern that can be recorded by a Polaroid camera.

The accuracy of thermography in detecting breast cancer is not perfect (as in MAMMOGRAPHY, about 85 percent); very large lesions, for instance, may show little temperature change because of calcification and the density of the tissue. On the other hand, very small tumors have been found with thermography alone, often after negative mammography.

In the last few years, color thermograms have been devised, which are easier to interpret than the shades of gray on the standard thermograms and which may prove to be more accurate.

THINNERS

Thinner is a generic name for any agent that removes from the skin the superficial stratum of dead cells and the pigment contained in them. Thinners have the purpose of opening pores blocked by dirt that has not been entirely removed by CLEANSERS and by the natural buildup of cells, which with age tend to stick together and are not so easily shed as young cells. Because of this, the outer layer of the skin of mature women tends to become thick and rough, filled with irregularly distributed pigment. Thinners, then, prevent the formation of blackheads and whiteheads and generally improve the skin's texture, giving it a lighter and more uniform color.

Thinners can be either *abrasive* or *chemical.*

1) *Abrasive thinners*—These include rough washcloths, or wet washcloths sprinkled with ordinary salt; PUMICE; LOOFAH or camel-hair mittens, and cleanser to which abrasive particles of almond meal, pumice or plastic have been added to the cleansing base. In a way, SHAVING is a thinning process, too: shaving of men's cheeks and women's legs prevents cellular buildup. And, technically, DERMABRASION—performed with rotating stainless-steel brushes—is an abrasive thinner as well, though, of course, it is quite a drastic procedure, with the purpose of removing from the face wrinkles, tattoos, freckles, and ACNE and smallpox scars.

2) *Chemical thinners*—These work by dissolving the cells of the outer layer with a chemical caustic, usually phenol. The process is called CHEMICAL PEEL, and its purpose is similar to that of dermabrasion, though it is a less traumatic process.

Dermabrasion and chemical peel, then, are exceptional thinning processes that should be performed only for specific reasons and by skillful dermatologists; the only type of thinner which can safely be used at home is the ordinary abrasive thinner. Indeed, together with cleansing and moisturizing, thinning should be part of the basic routine of every woman interested in maintaining a young-looking skin for as long as possible.

TOOTH REPLANTATION

Few people are aware that a tooth that has been knocked out often can be replanted. The most important consideration in a successful tooth replantation is *time:* the tooth must be replanted in its socket within thirty minutes after it has left the mouth. The longer the tooth remains out of the socket, the greater the chance for root absorption, a process in which root substance is lost because of pathological changes.

If a person loses a tooth in an accident, he should find it, wrap it in a wet cloth, and take it immediately to a dentist. He should not attempt to clean it, because the tissues clinging to the tooth are necessary for a successful replantation. The dentist will prepare it under sterile conditions before replacing it.

Some replantations are temporary—the tooth survives from one to ten years. Others survive as long as forty years.

TOOTHBRUSHES

Toothbrushing removes PLAQUE and other debris from the outer, inner and biting surfaces of the teeth. The most practical manual brushes have a straight handle, a flat brushing surface, and soft, end-rounded bristles. Brushes should be replaced frequently, because a worn-out brush cleans poorly and its bent bristles may hurt the gums. The head of the brush should be small enough to reach every tooth.

Electric toothbrushes, which some people consider just another gadget, are in reality quite pleasant and more thorough than manual toothbrushes in removing plaque from all tooth surfaces. They are also particularly useful for handicapped people. For delicate or hypersensitive teeth, however, the best brushes are still the manual ones, preferably with natural bristles. Electric brushing for people with these kinds of teeth should be reserved for the biannual professional tooth-cleaning by the dentist.

TUBAL LIGATION

Tubal ligation is a sterilization procedure in which a woman's FALLOPIAN TUBES are closed, in order permanently to prevent an egg cell from passing through the tube to the uterus each month, and to prevent any sperm from moving up the tube past the point of closure. After the operation a woman will continue to ovulate, and her hormones will function as usual; the only difference will be that the mature egg can no longer be fertilized.

Traditional tubal ligation is a major operation performed through an incision in the abdomen. Recently, however, two new methods have been developed, and tubal ligation can now be performed by an expert gynecologist with either of these simpler, safer and less traumatic techniques: laparoscopy or hysteroscopy.

Laparoscopic sterilization—The laparoscope is a narrow tube equipped with a viewing lens and a light. It is inserted into the pelvic cavity through a tiny incision near the navel, thus enabling the gynecologist to have a direct view of the ovaries and the uterus *without* the need for a major incision. Incidentally, laparoscopy not only is a new method of sterilization but has been used for many years for diagnosis—to evaluate infertility or unusual bleedings, for instance—and, more recently, for such surgical procedures as BIOPSIES (when cancer is suspected) and removal of CYSTS and misplaced IUDs.

In either case—diagnosis or tubal ligation—the surgeon makes a small transversal (vertical) incision just below the navel and inserts a tube into the cavity, through which carbon dioxide is passed in order to expand the cavity. The tube is then pulled out and the laparoscope inserted. In the case of tubal ligation, a slender forceps carrying electric current is inserted through the same incision or another tiny one. Looking through the laparoscope, the surgeon clasps one of the Fallopian tubes with the forceps, approximately in the middle. Electric current is passed through the forceps, severing the tube; a small portion of the tube is removed, and the two ends are cauterized. The procedure is then repeated with the other tube. The carbon dioxide is allowed to escape, and the incisions are sutured and bandaged. The patient is usually able to go home a few hours after awakening from the general ANAESTHESIA.

To make laparoscopic sterilization even more gentle, the Obstetric-Gynecological Department of the University of North Carolina uses, instead of electrocautery, tiny plastic clips to cut the Fallopian tubes. The clips are placed around the tubes and are held together with a gold-plated, stainless-steel spring designed to let the clip gently cut the tube over a few days.

Hysteroscopic sterilization—In this technique, a fiberoptic endoscope—a narrow metal tube equipped, like the laparoscope, with lens and cold lights—is inserted into the uterus through the cervix. The uterus is then filled with a GLUCOSE solution (or carbon dioxide) to distend the cavity. This permits the surgeon to locate the two tiny openings of the Fallopian tubes. With an electrode on the end of the endoscope, the surgeon cauterizes the two openings. Scar tissue later blocks the tubes and prevents the passage of sperm.

Only local ANAESTHESIA is needed for this procedure, which takes about ten minutes, and the patient recovers within hours. Six weeks later the patient returns for a pelvic examination, and three months later for X-rays, to make sure that the tubes are indeed closed. During this three-month period, a woman should use other means of CONTRACEPTION until the success of the operation is confirmed.

UV

UNDERWEIGHT

Chronically underweight people, unless they suffer from ANOREXIA
NERVOSA, are generally ignored by physicians, despite varying degrees of
HYPERTENSION, nervousness, sleeplessness, lack of appetite and, ulti-
mately, a distorted self-image that may be associated with disorder.

There are tens of thousands of people who are trying to gain weight
but who, even on supplementary diets, are unable to do so. The problems
of the very thin are not unlike those of the very fat, and in a way they are
even worse: not only is there little doctors and nutritionists can do about
them, but they seem less urgent (and less visible) than those of obese
people.

The very fat often can lose weight if placed on a strict low-calorie
diet. However, it is almost impossible for the very thin to fatten up. For
one thing, they are usually quite active and are easily satiated by very
small meals. Constitutionally, thin people stop feeling hunger quite
abruptly, as if one more mouthful of food would make them gag. Also,
underweight is often determined genetically, by a lack of adipose cells in
which to store surplus fat. Ordinarily, for every 3500 unburned CALORIES,
one pound of fat is accumulated—except in chronically underweight
people, who don't have enough adipose cells.

EXERCISE, although it burns fat, often promotes a weight increase.
However, once underweight people have been reassured that their
thinness is not due to a chronic disease such as diabetes, ANEMIA or
tuberculosis, all they can do is make the best of it—not unlike fashion
models who learn to do so.

URTICARIA (HIVES)

Urticaria, commonly called hives, is a very common condition. It consists
of swollen lesions of different shapes that are pinkish or almost white.

Hives can be small, medium or large; they itch maddeningly, but they are always transitory—they never last more than a few hours. However, new hives may form for several days in a row or even keep forming chronically. Hives may cause swelling of the eyelids, of the mouth and of the hands and feet. They may be accompanied by HEADACHES and difficulty in breathing or swallowing.

Hives are usually caused by drugs, such as ASPIRIN, TRANQUILIZERS and ANTIBIOTICS, or by food, although any substance—animal, vegetable, or chemical—may cause them in people sensitive to the substance.

In a very large number of instances of hives, particularly of the chronic type, no allergic cause can be found. Sometimes the swelling has to do with release of histamine in the tissue, triggered by local irritation; sometimes it is caused by sensitivity to temperature changes. Often, however, the reason for urticaria cannot be traced at all. Some allergists speculate that once these enigmatic hives are explained, some of the other baffling ALLERGIES will be understood.

VACCINE

A vaccine consists of a suspension (particles mixed with, but not dissolved in, a fluid) of weakened or dead microorganisms such as bacteria or viruses that is injected under the skin for the prevention or treatment of infectious diseases.

VAGINITIS

Vaginitis, or leukorrhea, as it is called medically, refers to an *abnormal* discharge from the vagina, which should not be confused with *normal* discharge: a clear, odor-free secretion from the glands of the cervix or the vagina that may increase at the time of ovulation or just before MENSTRUATION, and which requires no treatment other than normal hygiene. Unlike normal vaginal discharge, vaginitis is excessive and irritating, may cause swelling and has an odor. It may originate in the tissues of the vagina, in the cervix, or in the lining of the uterus as a result of several different conditions. Among the most common are trichomoniasis, moniliasis, hemophilus bacteria, GONORRHEA, atrophic vaginitis, viral infection, tumors, venereal warts and childbirth.

Trichomoniasis—Infection of the vagina by an organism known as *Trichomonas vaginalis*, which may occur at any age. It may be found by the gynecologist on a routine examination in patients who have no apparent symptoms other than the discharge. It is transmitted by sexual contact; the *Trichomonas* organism can survive in the male urethra without causing symptoms and therefore can be spread back and forth by intercourse. Treatment is simple, including oral and local medication.

Moniliasis—Yeastlike fungus which produces a thick discharge and causes itching, burning, painful intercourse, and bladder symptoms. Treatment is simple, consisting of an antifungal preparation and a cortisone ointment.

Hemophilus—Bacteria whose presence are determined by special laboratory techniques. It is treated with sulfonamides for several weeks.

Gonorrhea—Vaginal discharge due to gonorrhea may be mild, although at times it causes frequent and uncomfortable urination. Often, there is no pain, no swelling, no irritation; therefore, gonorrhea may go unnoticed, especially in young girls.

Symptoms usually appear two to five days after intercourse. Gonorrhea may exist along with other vaginal infections and may be accurately diagnosed only when special cultures are taken. Treatment requires ANTIBIOTICS.

Atrophic vaginitis—Usually occurs after MENOPAUSE, but sometimes also after HYSTERECTOMY or removal of the ovaries.

Viral infection—Caused by a virus called *Herpes genitalis,* which is acquired by sexual contact. It manifests itself as small blisters that rupture and may result in ulceration in the cervical and vaginal region. They are very painful and are made worse by moisture. It may last six weeks and frequently recur. No definite prevention or treatment is yet available.

Tumors—Vaginal discharge mixed with blood may be the only symptom in cases of benign and malignant tumors of the cervix or of the uterus. Smears and biopsies are indicated for this type of discharge.

Venereal warts—Also called genital warts, caused by a virus. They are acquired by sexual contact and are different from other WARTS. They first appear outside of the vagina and spread inside the vagina around the clitoris and the urethra. A very small wart may grow and rapidly proliferate. At times they may not appear for several weeks after sexual contact, and a man may not be aware he is infected. If treated early and effectively, these warts are readily cured.

Childbirth—Following delivery, there is a vaginal discharge that may persist for about four to six weeks. Usually it is due to the healing of the cervix and the lining of the uterus.

Mild vaginitis may become more serious in the presence of diabetes, menstruation (with the blood functioning as a culture for bacteria), pregnancy, and CONTRACEPTIVE PILLS (because they cause similar congestions in the cervix and the vagina); INTRAUTERINE DEVICES (through which infection may spread to the uterus); vaginal sprays (if a woman is allergic to the perfume in the spray, this may cause infection and worsen vaginitis); antibiotics taken for other infections (because antibiotics destroy the normal bacteria in the vagina, thus allowing the fungal infection to grow); GIRDLES, tight pants, or wet bathing suits (because constricting garments increase PERSPIRATION, and most of the microorganisms that cause vaginitis grow in a moist environment). Vaginitis is the most frequent condition for which a woman consults her gynecologist. More than 50 percent of all women have a mild or severe form of vaginitis at some time during their lives. Once considered one of the inevitable misfortunes of womanhood, vaginitis is still neglected by some women, although most of the time it can be treated with speed and efficiency.

VALIUM®

Valium® (diazepam), together with Librium®, is a PSYCHOACTIVE DRUG, belonging to the category of the minor tranquilizers.

Valium® was introduced in 1963 by Hoffmann-La Roche, one of the largest pharmaceutical companies in the United States, and is currently widely prescribed for the prompt, temporary relief of symptoms of anxiety, tension and preoperative medication, and as a muscle relaxant. Valium® is manufactured both as a pill and as a liquid for intravenous injection.

The major reason for the popularity of Valium® is its relative safety: unlike BARBITURATES, it is not addictive and it would be almost impossible to commit suicide with Valium®. However, like most tranquilizers, Valium® is meant to handle only acute, temporary conditions; large doses or a prolonged use of this drug may cause tolerance in some patients, i.e., more and more of it may be required to produce the initial effect. Also, in excessive doses it may cause such side effects as sleepiness and loss of coordination, which are enhanced when mixed with ALCOHOL. Withdrawal symptoms may follow abrupt discontinuance.

Because of the relative safety and quick action of Valium®, it is very useful as a premedication, for it reduces apprehension and tension in patients about to undergo general ANAESTHESIA or in a woman during labor. Valium® has also been found to be useful in relieving the pain of muscle spasms resulting from BACKACHE and slipped discs, and in reducing muscle spasms resulting from emotional factors. And finally, Valium® is often prescribed as an adjunct for the therapy of heart disease and epilepsy.

Valium® should not be given to very young children, pregnant women, psychotic patients, people who are known to be hypersensitive to this kind of drug, or people who are engaged in occupations requiring complete mental alertness.

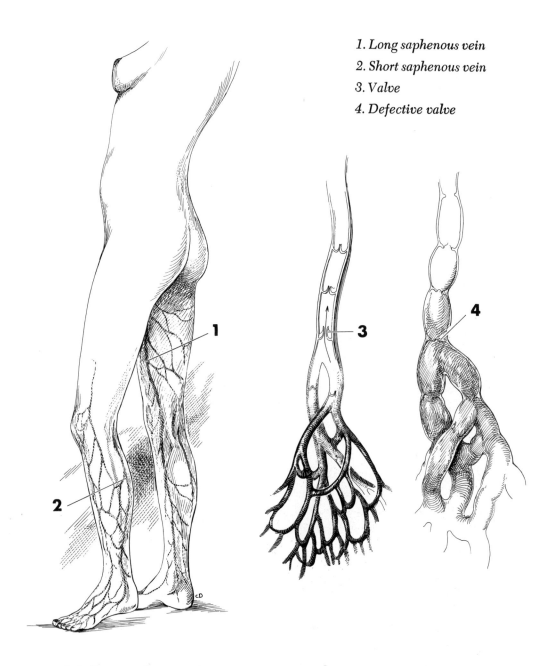

1. *Long saphenous vein*
2. *Short saphenous vein*
3. *Valve*
4. *Defective valve*

Left: Drawing of a woman's legs showing the course of the two veins that are mostly affected by varices: the long saphenous, which runs from the groin to the foot, and the short saphenous, which runs from below the knee to the outside of the ankle.

Center: A normal vein, with its functioning one-way valves, which help to evenly distribute the blood pressure along the vein's course.

Right: A varicose vein, whose valves are either malformed or weakened by illness, causing the blood to flow backward, pool in the veins, and exert pressure on the vessel walls. The veins then dilate, and the typical blue varices appear on the leg.

354

VARICOSE VEINS

Varicose veins are a common circulatory problem of the legs in which the veins become stretched and swollen because of pressure on the vein walls from the flow of blood.

Normally, the veins in the legs carry blood from the extremities back to the heart through a pumping action. In addition, leg muscles, by contracting and squeezing against the veins, help push the blood upward. Because the blood must make an uphill fight against gravity, the major veins in the legs are equipped with a series of tiny one-way valves that prevent reflux and evenly distribute the pressure along the vein's course.

Hereditary tendency to weak blood vessels and weak or malformed valves; diseases such as phlebitis; OBESITY; pregnancy; and aging can cause the blood to flow backward, which further stretches and weakens the veins and further distorts the valves below, allowing even more blood to leak back, while congested blood vessels fail to provide enough oxygen to the muscles, which may in turn become tightened. The skin itches and burns, and in severe cases breaks into ulcers that cannot heal properly because they lack healing cells normally carried in the circulating blood.

The typical blue varices appear mostly in the superficial veins located just under the skin in the fatty tissue, where the support is minimal—deeper veins, supported by muscle, do not ordinarily stretch. (The bluish color results from the lack of oxygen in the *venous* blood, as opposed to the bright, oxygen-rich *arterial* blood.)

These superficial veins are the *long saphenous*, the longest vein in the body, which runs all the way from the groin to the foot; and the *short saphenous*, which runs from behind the knee to the outside of the ankle.

For mild cases in which the valves are not involved, the following measures are sufficient to relieve most of the discomfort:

1) Wear elastic stockings or bandages; this supports the vein walls and prevents them from stretching.
2) Avoid prolonged sitting or standing; whenever possible, elevate legs to hip level.
3) Don't wear anything that constricts the upper thighs or abdomen, such as tight GIRDLES.
4) Reduce weight, as the more weight the body has to carry, the more strain on the veins of the legs.
5) Walk about one or two miles a day, provided that the legs are supported with elastic stockings or bandages.

Peripheral but unsightly varicose veins can be injected with a SCLEROSING SOLUTION, which obliterates them painlessly. For large, extended varices with defective valves, the best treatment is a surgical procedure called stripping. Despite the many complicated tests devised to recognize malfunctioning valves—"blowouts"—a competent vascular surgeon can detect them just by slowly running the index finger along the course of the long saphenous and/or the short saphenous; he will feel a sudden increase of pressure in the vein just below the damaged valve.

The stripping procedure can be performed under local ANAESTHESIA, but the patient is often more comfortable with a general anaesthesia. The varicose vein—usually the long saphenous—is marked out with surgical ink; then, through a small incision at the groin, the vein is ligated at its junction with the femoral vein. Through another incision at the ankle, a thin stainless-steel cable is inserted into the vein, slowly pushed upward until the tip surfaces at the other end. The stripper is then secured to the vein; and after the head of the operating table is lowered, the vein is slowly stripped out. An instrument widely used is the Nabatoff Intraluminal® vein stripper, devised in 1955. It is flexible, and its small tip facilitates guidance even through tortuous veins.

Elastic adhesive is wrapped over gauze from the toes to the knee, followed by an elastic bandage on the thigh, which the patient must wear for about one week. About two or three hours after surgery, the patient is already able to walk; as a result of new techniques, he can leave the hospital the same day and can return to all normal activities the following day. Both incisions, at the inguinal fold and at the ankle, heal readily. Additional small vertical incisions are made if there are large clusters of veins, but these leave very little scarring.

Varicose veins caused by pregnancy are different from other types in that they are temporary: many of them usually recede within a few days after delivery. Therefore, major vascular surgeons, among whom is Dr. Robert A. Nabatoff, associate clinical professor of vascular surgery and chief of the vascular clinic, department of obstetrics and gynecology, at the Mount Sinai School of Medicine in New York, disapprove of stripping or injecting varices during pregnancy. They prefer to recommend, in addition to leg exercises and frequent rests, rubberized elastic bandages or elastic stockings, though the latter stretch after several weeks and are not so adjustable as the bandages.

Sometimes pregnant women develop large varices at the VULVA, which result in part from the pressure exerted by the expanded uterus and which may obstruct the leg veins. For these there are specially designed supports made of foam rubber pads covered with knitted nylon tricot connected by adjustable straps.

If varicose veins persist after childbirth, surgery or injection of sclerosing solution is a much more effective treatment.

VASECTOMY

Vasectomy is a surgical operation performed on men as a form of permanent CONTRACEPTION. It consists of closing off the vas deferens, the two tiny ducts that store sperm and carry it from the bottom of the testicles up through the prostate gland and, after joining the duct from the seminal glands, into a single ejaculatory duct, down to the urethra—a long, twisting path to connect two organs only a few inches apart.

When the vas deferens are closed, the mature sperm—which is stored in a pocket (ampulla) just below the prostate—is prevented from reaching the semen. Lacking sperm, the semen ejaculated during intercourse cannot fertilize the egg.

The operation, which takes about twenty minutes, is performed under local ANAESTHESIA and is a simple, reasonably safe and effective procedure. Because there may be millions of sperm already present along the male reproductive tract, a man's semen can still fertilize an OVUM six weeks after vasectomy.

When it is performed high in the scrotum (the sack containing the testicles), vasectomy does not make a man sterile: it only prevents the newly manufactured sperm from getting into circulation. More important, it makes it sometimes possible to reverse vasectomy with a recanalization procedure called vasovasotomy.

Neither the penis nor the testicles are affected by vasectomy: semen and male hormones are produced as usual, which means that it does not interfere with potency or sexual pleasure. However, to undergo vasectomy is a serious decision to make. For one thing, it is in most cases irreversible. And for some men, the thought of voluntary sterilization is unbearable, a symbolic humiliation of their masculinity. But there are many men who are proud of and completely satisfied with their decision, which is often a gesture toward their wives, who may already have had many children and for various reasons may not be able to accept any form of contraception.

VEGETARIANISM

"Vegetarian" is a general term applied to people who live solely on vegetables, grains, fruits and nuts and who do not use foods of animal origin in their diet (though some vegetarians will eat fish).

People follow vegetarianism for several reasons. Some do it because of scarcity of meat or because of extreme poverty, or because they belong to certain religious sects that forbid eating foods obtained by killing animals. Some believe that food from animal sources, as well as all processed and refined foods, is harmful to human beings. Others believe that using meat as a primary PROTEIN source is an exploitation of the earth's limited resources. Still others believe that the slaughter of animals is wrong.

There are several different kinds of vegetarians:

Lacto-vegetarians—Vegetarians who use dairy products such as milk, butter and cheese.

Lacto-ovo-vegetarians—Vegetarians who include eggs in their diet.

Mono-vegetarians—Those who eat only one food, such as SOYBEANS or brown rice.

Natural vegetarians—Those who avoid refined or processed foods, such as white sugar or bleached flour.

Pure vegetarians—Those who eat only fruits, grains, legumes and vegetables. Some do not eat honey.

Vegans—Vegetarians who, for ethical reasons, do not use *any* animal product, including leather. Some vegans even refuse VACCINES because they are prepared from animal cultures.

VERRUCAE (WARTS)

Verrucae, better known as warts, are small nipplelike growths that vary in color and size. They are most often seen on hands, especially children's.

Warts are benign—they do not become cancerous—and result from a virus that grows in the outer layer of the skin and stimulates overgrowth.

Warts are autoinoculable, i.e., they tend to be inoculated by their own virus and tend to spread to other areas of the body, especially when they are cut open. Warts on women's legs (or on men's faces), for instance, tend to spread when cut by a razor. Women who overmanicure their nails may have the same problem, as may people who twist metal-link watchbands as a nervous habit and nick the skin of their wrists; the warts may appear in the exact pattern of the links.

Practically everything has been used in the past to destroy warts, from gunpowder to black magic. Today, warts are either briefly frozen with liquid nitrogen, electrodesiccated, or excised with a curette. But the extraordinary truth is that, in many instances, warts have actually disappeared as a result of suggestion or hypnosis. At least one dermatologist gives patients shiny bracelets to wear, with the instruction to mail them back as soon as the warts are gone. Many warts, this dermatologist is certain, have disappeared this way in a few weeks. It is also true that, if left alone, many warts tend to disappear spontaneously.

Warts are a nuisance, but generally they do not hurt, with the exception of plantar warts, which occur on the soles of the feet and are painful because they are subjected to continuous pressure from walking. They are white, are flatter than other warts and have a granular texture.

Plantar warts are also different from calluses, with which people sometimes confuse them. In a callus, the skin's surface is essentially unchanged, only thickened; whereas in a wart the normal lines of skin stop at the margins of the lesion.

Plantar warts rarely disappear spontaneously; excision is not recommended, because of the possibility of painful scarring and recurrence. Electrodesiccation is also inadvisable because KELOIDS may result, which are more painful than the wart itself. At present the best treatment for plantar warts is a daily application of linseed oil mixed with other ingredients, then covered with adhesive. Within a few weeks the wart softens and separates from the underlying normal tissue. It can then be removed painlessly with a curette, and the area heals without scarring.

VITAMINS

Vitamins are a mixed group of accessory food factors, small amounts of which are essential for health and vital body functions. Vitamins differ in both chemical structure and specification. Each vitamin performs one or more exclusive functions in the body.

With rare exceptions (VITAMIN K; also C in many animals), vitamins cannot be synthetized by the body and have to be provided in food or in synthetic form. (However, certain substances such as choline that could be considered vitamins are snythetized by intestinal bacteria.)

The vitamins that have definitely been identified so far may be classified in two groups: *water-soluble* and *fat-soluble*. Water-soluble vitamins, such as the B VITAMINS and VITAMIN C, are not stored in the body, and any excess over the body's immediate need is eliminated in the urine. Fat-soluble vitamins tend to accumulate in the body; if taken in too-large doses, some of them can cause hypervitaminosis, an excessive level of vitamins in the body that, if present for a long time, can itself cause disease.

The presence of vitamins was originally recognized when it was discovered that some unknown chemicals were needed in the diet to prevent such deficiency states as beriberi, scurvy and rickets, and that administration of certain foods would reverse most (but not all) of the symptoms of these deficiencies, though it was not yet understood that these symptoms are the end result of a long chain of reactions. First there is a depletion, then a metabolic change in the cells, and only after these changes have reached the danger level—a process that could last months—do the deficiency symptoms appear. However, even moderate depletion can cause impairment of health, lowered resistance to infections and impaired healing of wounds.

The synthesis and large-scale production of vitamins began mainly in the 1930s and 1940s, and it was then that proof became available that all vitamins, whether synthetic or natural, have the same molecular structure, and that both synthetic vitamins and natural vitamins carry on the same biological activity.

After the early period of study of the vitamins in classic deficiency states, the use of vitamins became fashionable, and dramatic cures were claimed. Subsequently, careful observations refuted some of the exaggerated claims, and over a number of years government publications methodically denied that the vitamins had any miraculous value. Another reason for loss of interest in vitamins was the general improvement in the nutrition of most people in the developed countries. A generation of physicians emerged who were not inclined to examine patients for signs of vitamin deficiency.

This negative approach began to disappear in the 1960s as modern techniques demonstrated the astonishing importance of and intricate functions performed by vitamins. By now, the biochemical function of many vitamins is known: generally, a vitamin is the main—or sole—component of a CO-ENZYME, the nonprotein substance needed by some ENZYMES to control chemical reactions in the body. Because of these co-enzyme functions, vitamins are indispensable as catalysts in the metabolism of CARBOHYDRATES, FATS and PROTEINS—that is, the provision of energy within the body.

Enzymes are developed as a result of genetic factors within the cell's nucleus, and it is now known that many examples of faulty enzyme activity are due to abnormalities in the genetic code within the nucleus, such as a faulty binding between the enzyme and the co-enzyme. In such conditions, abnormal metabolism occurs of the type seen in vitamin deficiency, even though the co-enzyme is present in normal quantities. Genetic abnormalities of the enzyme activity may explain why certain illnesses improve only with doses of vitamins that are much greater than those required for normal nutrition.

At the time when the chemical composition of vitamins was not yet known, they were identified by letters. Later, what was thought to be one vitamin turned out to be many, and the designation by groups appeared, such as the B vitamins. And when it was discovered that different chemical structures occurred within compounds having the same vitamin activity, numbers were added—B_1, B_2, etc. Popular names and synonyms were eventually applied to the chemicals and, a few years ago, internationally codified. Nevertheless, while it is now more logical to use these accepted popular names, such as ascorbic acid, riboflavin and pyridoxin, certain vitamins are still known best by their old letter designations.

Vitamins are measured in extremely small amounts, because it takes very little of them to be effective in generating the needed chemical reactions. Some vitamins are designated in IUs (International Units); others are expressed by weight only, in milligrams or in micrograms.

360

Despite biochemistry's impressive progress, scientists have not yet succeeded in correlating exactly the physiological functions of all vitamins with their respective deficiencies. But many feel that the 1970s might be the decade in which the remaining secrets of the extraordinary micronutrients will be solved.

VITAMIN A

The history of vitamin A is interwoven with the discovery of vitamins and nutrition research. At the turn of the century, biochemists were beginning to realize that certain fat-soluble fractions found in butter, egg yolk and cod-liver oil were essential for the growth of laboratory animals. Eventually, they concluded that the unknown substance was organic in nature. The word "vitamine" seemed at first appropriate to describe this growth factor. Subsequently, the phrase "growth-promoting fat-soluble A" was suggested; and finally the term vitamin A—with the final "e" omitted—was adopted.

In the early 1930s the structure of the vitamin A molecule was determined, and pure vitamin A was extracted from halibut liver oil. Although vitamin A can still be extracted from natural sources, such as fish or liver, the synthetic compound has been found equally satisfactory for human use. The synthetic vitamin A is manufactured either in liquid form or in dry granular form, in which droplets of the liquid vitamin are encased in a dry, edible substance. Other natural sources of vitamin A are vegetables rich in carotene, a so-called provitamin which is converted into vitamin A by the body through the action of an ENZYME called carotenase.

Pure vitamin A crystals are pale yellow and are soluble in fat and fat solvents. Essentially stable to light and heat, vitamin A is destroyed by oxidation and ultraviolet light. Unlike water-soluble vitamins, which are readily excreted in the urine, vitamin A can be stored in the body—90 percent of it stored in the liver and released as needed. Sometimes the liver contains enough vitamin A to last from three months to almost a year. The rest is stored in the kidneys, lungs, adrenal glands and body fat.

Vitamin A is needed to promote growth and in general to maintain good nutrition for the human body. It contributes to the health of skin, bones, teeth, hair, and the urinary and gastrointestinal tracts.

Unlike lack of VITAMIN C, which is swiftly and dramatically apparent, it takes time before a vitamin A deficiency develops. However, infection, poisoning or high temperature may use up the stored vitamin quickly. Lack of vitamin A shows itself in several ways; the so-called dark adaptation of the eyes, for instance, is diminished—the eye cannot readily adjust when moving from bright light to dim light or to darkness. Also, the skin becomes dry and the mucous membranes harden; the lining of the hair FOLLICLES becomes plugged, thus interfering with the secretion of the skin's oil glands.

Vitamin A deficiency is treated with therapeutic doses; supplementary doses are prescribed to prevent its recurrence. However, excessive doses of it over a long period of time can become harmful, causing hypervitaminosis, whose symptoms—cracked lips, hair loss, dry skin, FATIGUE, INSOMNIA, thickening of bones—become evident from six to fifteen months from the start of excessive intake. The symptoms disappear gradually after vitamin A is removed from the diet.

Because of the potential risk of hypervitaminosis, the Food and Drug Administration has recently issued regulations that it hopes will prevent people from getting too much vitamin A (as well as VITAMIN D): all vitamin A preparations above 10,000 international units must be labeled "for prescription use only."

VITAMIN B COMPLEX

B$_1$ (Thiamine)	B$_{12}$ (Cobalamin)
B$_2$ (Riboflavin)	Biotin
B$_3$ (Niacin or Nicotinamide)	Folic Acid
B$_6$ (Pyridoxine)	Pantothenic Acid

These vitamins are regarded as a "complex" because they are often found together.

Vitamin B$_1$ was isolated in 1926, fourteen years after it was discovered that beriberi—a serious, often fatal disease marked by changes in the heart and in the nervous and digestive systems—was caused by a deficiency in the diet of a mysterious substance absent in polished rice, which later turned out to be vitamin B$_1$. Early, often unnoticed signs of vitamin B$_1$ deficiency are FATIGUE, loss of appetite and weight, HEADACHE, poor sleep.

Vitamin B$_1$, a white powder soluble in water, with a yeastlike odor and a nutlike taste, is absorbed into the system through the small intestine. It is needed daily because the body does not store it in quantity; only enough for a few days is present at any time. Vitamin B$_1$, which acts as a CO-ENZYME, works within the living cells as an essential part of CARBOHYDRATE metabolism.

Unmilled cereals are excellent sources of vitamin B$_1$, though few people would like to eat raw wheat berries or rice kernels. Since during the processing of white flour and white bread natural vitamin B$_1$ disappears with parts of the grain that are milled out, flour and breads are now routinely enriched with vitamins B$_1$ and B$_2$ and niacinamide. Good sources of the vitamin are legumes, lean pork, yeast and cow's milk. More vitamin B$_1$ is needed by the human body during periods of

Crystals of vitamin A.

Crystals of nicotinic acid (vitamin B₃).

Crystals of beta carotene.

Riboflavin (vitamin B₂).

Vitamin B₆.

Biotin (vitamin B complex).

Crystals of vitamin B₁.

Crystals of vitamin C.

Crystals of vitamin E.

increased metabolism, such as fever, muscular activity, and also pregnancy and LACTATION. Cases of vitamin B_1 overdoses have not been reported, though some people may have allergic reactions to injections of the vitamin.

Vitamin B_2 was isolated in 1933, and it eventually turned out to be the essential part of a "yellow enzyme" that independent researchers had obtained from yeast. Vitamin B_2 is yellow and slightly water-soluble, and has a bitter taste.

Vitamin B_2 is widely distributed in all leafy vegetables, in the flesh of warm-blooded animals, in fish, in eggs and in milk products. In humans it is stored in the liver, spleen, kidneys and the cardiac muscle, and it is eliminated in the urine—about 12 percent of an average daily intake. Small losses occur when the body perspires. Vitamin B_2 deficiency is seen as soreness and burning of the lips, mouth and tongue; itching of the eyes, and visual fatigue.

Vitamin B_3 (niacin or nicotinic acid) is present in most body tissues and is involved in energy-producing reactions in cells. Vitamin B_3 is one of the vitamins used in ORTHOMOLECULAR MEDICINE for the treatment of schizophrenia and alcoholism. However, this use is experimental and its value is controversial.

Vitamin B_6 is produced by microorganisms of the intestinal tract of animals and men. It seems likely that little of it is absorbed and utilized (70 percent of the vitamin is excreted in the urine), though it is known that vitamin B_6 is rapidly absorbed.

In late 1973, nutritional and medical researchers published new data about the importance of vitamin B_6 in normal diets as well as in the treatment of certain diseases. Vitamin B_6 has a variety of functions: it helps the body to use PROTEINS, FATS and carbohydrates and is essential in maintaining and repairing body tissues. Some physicians believe that vitamin B_6 is also linked to the prevention of diabetes, rheumatic pains and heart disease, but this is still a matter of conjecture.

Vitamin B_6 is found in liver, whole grains, wheat germ, nuts and bananas. High temperature destroys natural vitamin B_6, sometimes as much as 90 percent.

Vitamin B_{12} is necessary in the building of the nucleic acids (vital acids found in all living cells) and in the formation of red blood cells. It is also active in the functioning of the nervous system. The absorption of vitamin B_{12} in the intestinal tract depends on a constituent of the gastric juice called "intrinsic factor."

The amount of vitamin B_{12} in food is very small. The main sources are foods of animal origin, especially liver, and, to a lesser extent, beef, herrings, cheese and eggs. Vitamin B_{12} is almost entirely absent from plants.

Vitamin B_{12} deficiency may occur as a result of inadequate diet, deficiency of the "intrinsic factor," or defects in the absorption capacity of the intestinal walls. Pernicious ANEMIA is the typical reaction of deficiency in the "intrinsic factor" and is sometimes found in VEGETARIANS.

Biotin, which was for a while called vitamin H, is widely distributed in small concentration in all animal and plant tissues. Higher quantities are found in yeast, liver and kidney. In concentrated form, it consists of fine colorless crystals that are slightly soluble in cold water and stable in heat.

Biotin is absorbed from the small intestine. It has an important co-enzyme role in the metabolism of carbohydrates, proteins and fats. Except in infants, a deficiency of biotin is extremely rare.

Folic Acid, which was once called vitamin M, is a yellowish-orange crystalline powder that is tasteless and odorless and slightly soluble in hot water. It is stable in heat but sensitive to light.

Folic acid is present in green-leaved vegetables, potatoes, calf liver, and kidney. Cooking, however, may reduce its content considerably. Folic acid deficiency can occur as a result of unbalanced diet; another cause is pregnancy, for the fetus makes demands on the mother's stores of it. The reaction of the human body to folic acid deficiency is a form of anemia.

Pantothenic Acid, which is available in meat, fish, eggs, soybeans, peanuts, cabbage and whole-grain products, is absorbed from the intestinal tract, and it helps in the metabolism of fats, carbohydrates and proteins and in the formation of certain HORMONES.

Pantothenic acid deficiency is rare, as the vitamin is widely available in ordinary food. Pantothenic acid is a pale yellow, viscous oil soluble in water, unstable in heat and acids.

VITAMIN C

Scurvy, a disease that was common among sailors on long voyages, among the Crusaders, and among entire populations during times of famine and pestilence, results from a deficiency of vitamin C in the diet. About three hundred years ago man discovered that fresh fruits and vegetables were helpful in preventing and healing scurvy. In the early 1920s an antiscorbutic substance was concentrated from lemons and isolated in cabbage; shortly after, the molecular structure of vitamin C and its ability to absorb oxygen were established.

Vitamin C, or ascorbic acid, as it is also called, not only prevents or cures scurvy (by now a rare illness) but also is a vital substance for maintaining healthy bone tissue and for forming COLLAGEN, the important PROTEIN found in skin, tendons, bones and cartilage. Vitamin C also promotes healing of wounds and fractures and helps the body to resist infection. It is believed to contribute to the formation of hemoglobin, to the maturation of red blood cells, and to the metabolism of certain amino acids, as well as to the storage of IRON in the body.

Vitamin C is found in most body tissues and fluids, but its highest concentration is in the retina, the pituitary gland, the liver, the brain, the testicles and the ovaries. However, it will rapidly exhaust its supplies if not replenished frequently, especially in pregnant and lactating women.

Ascorbic acid is a white crystalline compound with a slightly acidic taste. It is readily soluble in water and stable in dry form, though it gradually darkens when exposed to light. In the presence of oxygen, high temperature and certain FOOD ADDITIVES used as coloring, it is rapidly destroyed. Because of its ability to attach itself to oxygen, vitamin C is one of the most important ANTIOXIDANTS for certain frozen foods that have a tendency to discolor and lose their natural flavor during thawing.

Citrus fruits—oranges, lemons, grapefruits—are generally rich in vitamin C. Tomatoes and potatoes and certain green vegetables are also good sources, though there are wide differences in the amount of vitamin C found in various foods, and even in varieties of the same food.

At present, one of vitamin C's best-known functions is that of a prophylactic against the COMMON COLD. Vitamin C is believed to play a role in the tissues' defense mechanism: when the tissues are deficient in vitamin C, the defense mechanism does not work effectively. Professor Linus Pauling, the 1954 Nobel prize laureate for chemistry, made vitamin C famous with his book *Vitamin C and the Common Cold.* At first, Professor Pauling was ridiculed, and his suggestion of massive doses of the vitamin (1 to 5 gm a day to *prevent* the cold; 10 to 20 gm a day to *cure* it) was considered just another food fad, a particularly embarrassing one for the medical profession, as it was advocated by one of this century's most honored biochemists.

Then, in 1973, came the double-blind study of two Canadian doctors that, rather than disproving Professor Pauling's claim, provided a measure of support for a limited effect of vitamin C in the prevention and treatment of the common cold. By the end of 1973, reluctantly or triumphantly, some medical investigators stated that indeed Professor Pauling was partly right: some people who take vitamin C supplements are, at the very least, less disabled by illness than those who don't. However, supplements are not the same as gigantic, indiscriminate doses of vitamin C, which could definitely be hazardous to certain individuals. Moreover, some careful studies have failed to show a definite effect of vitamin C on the common cold, while others have produced ambiguous results.

VITAMIN D

Vitamin D is sometimes called the "sunshine vitamin" because sunlight is able to convert a substance present in the human skin—ergosterol—into some of the vitamin D needed by the body. The rest of the necessary vitamin D is obtained from food; however, vitamin D is not widely distributed in nature. The only rich sources are fish liver oils and fish eggs, in caviar, seal and salmon. Small amounts are found in butter, liver and egg yolk, and milk is often fortified with vitamin D.

Vitamin D is absorbed by the small intestine, then carried to the liver, where it is transformed into 25-hydroxyvitamin D_3, a metabolically active compound that is carried by a special PROTEIN through the blood into the kidneys. There it is converted into a form that carries out the main function associated with vitamin D: helping the body utilize calcium and phosphorus in the building of healthy bones and teeth in children. For women, vitamin D is important during pregnancy and lactation.

Deficiency of vitamin D during childhood leads to the development of rickets, a nutritive disturbance involving defective utilization of calcium and phosphorus in the bones, owing to inadequate diet or insufficient exposure to sunshine. Rickets from poor diet or lack of sun is practically nonexistent in the United States today, but osteomalacia—the adult version of rickets—is more common and can be caused, for example, by certain medications that alter the metabolism of vitamin D so as to lower its level in the blood and lead to defective bone mineralization.

Excessive doses of vitamin D—hypervitaminosis D—may result in hypercalcemia (an excessive amount of calcium in the blood) or in calcification of soft tissue. Because of the danger connected with excessive amounts of vitamin D in the diet, its sale has been restricted by the FDA to 400 International Units. Any preparation above 400 IU, must be labeled "for prescription use only."

Skin pigment, it was discovered, has a role in regulating vitamin D synthesis. Dark skin is an adaptive mechanism that both ensures protection against rickets and minimizes hypervitaminosis D in tropical regions. Although much is already known about vitamin D, it continues to be the subject of considerable investigation. In a current study, developed from the mid-1960s discovery that it is a metabolite, not vitamin D itself, that is active in the body, 25-hydroxyvitamin D_3 is being tested as a drug for certain serious bone diseases that are resistant to conventional vitamin D therapy. Another fascinating discovery is that, since it is made in and secreted from the skin and carried by the blood to specific organs far from its point of synthesis, vitamin D is not a simple nutrient but actually behaves like a HORMONE.

VITAMINS

Vitamin E will probably be remembered as the most popular vitamin of the 1970s: tons of it have been manufactured in the last few years and have been swallowed (or smeared on the body) in large doses by millions of Americans who attribute to it almost miraculous qualities. Vitamin manufacturers themselves are careful not to claim that vitamin E or other products containing it are necessary to treat or prevent any nutritional deficiency, and the Food and Drug Administration is even more cautious. Still, there are nutritionists, natural-food enthusiasts and many ordinary people who seem convinced that vitamin E aids in hair growth; cures ACNE, sterility and impotence; eases arthritic pain; prevents ulcers, heart disease and BODY ODOR; flattens scars; erases wrinkles; rejuvenates skin, and so on, but there is no proof for these claims.

The medical profession has been somewhat startled by this sudden popularity of a vitamin whose presence in food has been known for decades. Partly because of this "discovery" of vitamin E, many reputable researchers have become reluctant to involve themselves in studies of its possible therapeutic benefits. Some physicians have suggested that the popularity may stem from misinterpretation of experiments with laboratory animals. In other words, thousands of people seem to have substituted the word "humans" for "mice" and "rats," without waiting for the biochemist's confirmation. Vitamin E deficiency in laboratory animals does indeed cause abnormalities in gestation and in the central nervous system; it also causes eye defects and muscular dystrophy. Conversely, vitamin E supplements in rats can prevent or cure most of these conditions.

Vitamin E is a fat-soluble chemical in the alcohol family; it is stable in the presence of ordinary light, but prolonged ultraviolet light slowly inactivates it. For the moment, one of vitamin E's proven functions is that of an ANTIOXIDANT, which means that it is capable of protecting substances against damage from oxidation—their chemical breakdown by oxygen—which makes vitamin E an excellent food and cosmetic preservative. More important, vitamin E is a *physiological* antioxidant, i.e., it slows down oxidation of the polyunsaturated FATS in the body cells. The body stores excess CALORIES in the adipose tissue primarily in the form of saturated fats, but with diets low in CHOLESTEROL, for instance, the adipose tissue tends to accumulate unsaturated fats, which may form harmful peroxides and raise the body's need for vitamin E.

Moreover, certain air pollutants apparently speed up the oxidation of polyunsaturated fatty acids in the body, and supplements of vitamin E are already capable of protecting mice, at least, against this accelerated oxidation. Yet, A. L. Tappel of the University of California, one of the most active researchers on vitamin E and the man who formulated the antioxidant theory, believes that this could be true for humans, too.

However, dietary supplements of vitamin E are, as of 1975, considered superfluous, because the wide distribution of the vitamin in vegetable oils, cereal grains and animal fats (even though some vitamin E is lost in food processing) makes a human deficiency unlikely, except for premature babies or people with impaired absorption of fat. On the other hand, there is at present no evidence that excessive amounts of vitamin E are harmful, as any excess is soon excreted in the urine.

VITAMIN K

Vitamin K was discovered by Professor Henrik Dam of Copenhagen, who received the Nobel prize for the discovery. He called it *Koagulationsvitamin*, or vitamin K, because of its utilization by the body in the synthesis of prothrombin, an important blood-clotting factor needed for normal blood coagulation.

Clinically, the most important use of vitamin K is the prevention and treatment of hemorrhagic diseases in newborn babies, caused by several factors, including low vitamin K reserves in the fetus and low intake of the vitamin in the mother's diet. However, routine prophylactic doses of vitamin K for the mother during labor or to the newborn at birth usually reduces this risk.

Vitamin K compounds are present in various living organisms; they play an important role in such biochemical processes as photosynthesis in green plants, namely, the formation of CARBOHYDRATES from carbon dioxide and water in chlorophyll-containing cells of green plants exposed to light, involving release of oxygen through decomposition of water, followed by various enzyme reactions.

Natural vitamin K occurs in two forms: K_1 (phylloquinone) and K_2 (farnoquinone). Both are fat-soluble and insoluble in water. At one time, the most widely used source of vitamin K was alfalfa, but now it is being manufactured in several synthetic forms, some of whose derivatives are water-soluble. Vitamin K is found in lean meat, pork liver, cow's milk, cabbage, potatoes, carrots, spinach and tomatoes. It is also found in bacteria that normally occur in the human intestine; they serve as a source of vitamin K, provided enough bile is present.

How the body synthetizes vitamin K from food is still not well understood, but it is known that the vitamin can be properly absorbed only in the upper part of the intestine, in the presence of bile. Deficiency of vitamin K in adults is usually caused either by inadequate absorption (resulting from reduced production of bile) or utilization of the vitamin, or by disturbances in the microorganisms of the gastrointestinal tract.

As of 1974, no Recommended Daily Allowance or Minimum Daily Requirement for vitamin K has been worked out.

VULVA

The vulva refers to the external parts of a woman's genital organs. It includes:

1) the clitoris, a small, elongated, erectile body situated at the vulva's anterior angle which is homologous (corresponding in position and origin) to the penis in the man;

2) the hymen, also called the virginal membrane, the membranous fold which partially or completely occludes the external opening of the vagina;

3) the opening of the urethra, a canal 1½ inches long running above the anterior vaginal wall and conveying urine from the bladder to the surface;

4) mons veneris (literally, "mount of Venus"), also called mons pubis, a rounded prominence of fatty tissue on the pubic bone;

5) labia, two sets of lip-shaped folds of skin—the labia majora, which are on the surface, and the labia minora, which lie beneath them—surrounding the external opening of the vagina.

VULVITIS

Vulvitis is an inflammation of the VULVA that may result from many different conditions, such as trichomoniasis, moniliasis, postmenopausal VAGINITIS, viral infections and VENEREAL DISEASES. Irritation may also be caused, or worsened, by sensitivity to tight pants, close-fitting synthetic underwear that gives inadequate ventilation, colored and perfumed toilet paper, medicated SOAPS, rubber condoms, nickel-plated zippers and improperly diluted DOUCHES and vaginal sprays. More rarely, vulvitis may be caused by VITAMIN deficiency.

Sometimes vulvitis is only a symptom of a vaginal infection. Since the vagina has few nerve endings—which are responsible for the sensation of itching and PAIN—these may be mistakenly felt as originating from the vulva.

Whatever treatment follows, a woman suffering from vulvitis should first discontinue using DETERGENTS, sprays and DEODORANTS, and use cotton underwear and neutral soaps.

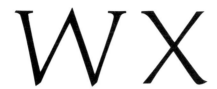

WASSERMAN TESTS

Wasserman test (or more appropriately, Wasserman reaction) refers to a number of laboratory procedures developed from the original test devised in 1906 by August von Wasserman, a German bacteriologist, and used to diagnose SYPHILIS (both active and latent) and to assess the progress of its treatment.

The Wasserman reaction is based on the identification in a patient's blood of the antibodies that are formed during an infection by the syphilis organism *Treponema pallidum.*

There are several Wasserman-type tests available, and more are being studied. Among the basic methods currently in use are: 1) fixation of complement; and 2) flocculation.

1) In the *fixation of complement,* a small amount of complement—an *active* substance of normal blood that fights bacteria—is added to a sample of a patient's blood. If the patient has syphilis, his blood will form specific ANTIBODIES when an antigen (in this case, an injection of a solution containing live or dead syphilis organisms) invades the body. Antibodies then combine with the antigen and quickly absorb the added complement, which becomes fixed, or *inactive.* Conversely, if the patient does *not* have syphilis, the complement remains *active.*

2) *Flocculation* is a chemical reaction that occurs in the presence of syphilis antibodies and which causes the blood sample to separate and settle down visibly in lumpy particles.

The result of a Wasserman reaction is called *positive* when the patient has syphilis, *negative* when he does not, and *doubtful* when more tests are needed. The tests are not always accurate: one may show a false-negative result if, for instance, the test is performed immediately after exposure to infection, because it takes about five weeks for the body's immune system to respond to syphilis. There are cases, too, in which a test performed too early may show a false-positive reaction.

Therefore, physicians prefer to repeat the Wasserman and other tests at monthly intervals for about one year until they are absolutely sure that the syphilis has been cured.

WATER

Water, the major constituent of all living matter, without which no creature could live for long, is a mysterious and unique substance, the only one that can exist as a solid, a liquid and a gas in the earth's normal temperature range—often at the same time and in the same place.

Water can be either soft, medium hard, hard, very hard or extremely hard, depending on the percentage of calcium and magnesium salts and other MINERALS it contains. Hardness is measured in grains—3 gr to a gallon is considered the limit between soft and hard water; at 20 gr, water is extremely hard.

Because of its extraordinary property of holding or dissolving so many substances, water is often called the universal solvent. As rainwater, it gathers a little bit of almost everything it touches in its long journey from the clouds to the faucet: smog, fumes, dust, microorganisms. And once it seeps into the ground, it gathers rust, acid, unpleasant tastes and odors, as well as the calcium and magnesium salts responsible for its hardness. The degree of impurities in the water depends mainly on the type of soil the rain falls on. If it were collected from an unpolluted atmosphere, rain would indeed be the softest natural water.

Hard water reacts with SOAPS to form an insoluble curd and deposits that adhere to skin, hair, fabrics, glassware and porcelain; the ring around a bathtub is a common household illustration of hard-water deposits. Hair washed with a soap SHAMPOO in hard water tends to look dull and sticky; the soap curd entraps and holds bacteria on the hair strands and the scalp, causing a dry and itchy skin and sometimes even infections. When soft water is not available, a detergent shampoo is more efficient, as synthetic DETERGENTS do not combine with the calcium and magnesium salts.

Water is the only substance the outer layer of human skin requires to retain its smoothness. No amount of expensive OIL can soften dry skin, but a few drops of water sealed into the skin by a moisturizing lotion are sufficient to restore or maintain a degree of softness. Water, says Dr. Bedford Shelmire, Jr., the well-known professor of dermatology at the Southwestern Medical School, University of Texas, is "the ultimate moisturizer."

Water in itself is never harmful to skin; in practice, however, too frequent contact with water causes dry and chapped skin, because as water flows away it literally washes off most of the skin's natural oils. A

MOISTURIZER should always be applied to the skin after each contact with soap and water.

Though not an active ingredient, water is used in the manufacture of most cosmetics and toiletries—SHAMPOOS, creams, lotions, FRAGRANCES. Here, too, soft water is preferred to obtain stable, consistent products. HAIR COLORING compounds, for instance, yield more even and long-lasting shades; permanent wave products, too, are more satisfactory when soft water is used.

Water containing excessive amounts of fluorine, chlorine or iodine may cause ACNE-like eruptions on the skin. However, public water supplies, which are currently treated with small amounts of these substances for reasons of health, are perfectly safe.

Among the various methods to improve the quality of water are:

Water softening—Water softeners are chemical substances that are added to the water to remove the elements that cause hardness.

Water-hardness map of the United States, designed by the Culligan International Company of New Jersey. Water hardness is caused by the presence of calcium and magnesium, two minerals which fresh water, in its long journey from the clouds to the faucet, collects as it seeps through soil and rocks. The degree of hardness, which is calculated in grains per gallon, depends on the geographical location. New York City water, for instance, is considered slightly hard—under three grains per gallon—while parts of New Mexico have as many as forty grains.

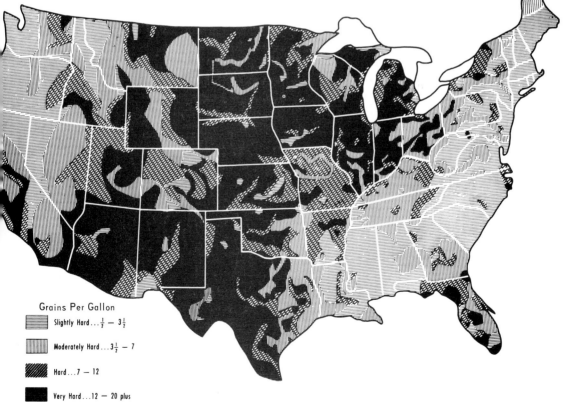

Grains Per Gallon

Slightly Hard... $\frac{1}{2}$ — $3\frac{1}{2}$

Moderately Hard... $3\frac{1}{2}$ — 7

Hard... 7 — 12

Very Hard... 12 — 20 plus

Water filtering—Water-filtering equipment removes dirt, mud, sand, iron, tastes and odors from the water supply in the house. A water filter can be either a unit installed near the main water pipe, or a smaller version attached directly to the faucet. All types of filters are equipped with cartridges that need to be replaced occasionally.

Water demineralization (or deionization)—A process, similar to distillation, that removes from the water all dissolved minerals (ions).

Water-purification tablets—When water purification units or bottled water are not available, and boiling water is not feasible—especially on a trip to the tropics—hazalone or other equivalent iodine water-purification tablets can be used.

WATER PIC®

Water Pic® is a brand name, often used as a generic term, for one of the better-known oral irrigating devices. These consist of small hydraulic appliances that force tiny jets of water (or washing solution) through a fine hand-held nozzle.

Dentists use these devices to irrigate orthodontic braces, for instance, or the crevices between gums and teeth and underneath dental bridges, in order to wash off decaying food residues and bacteria which normally penetrate those hard-to-reach areas.

The warm stream of water under pressure is excellent for removing loose debris, though care should be taken in adjusting the water pressure, since excess pressure may damage the gums. People should be reminded, too, that Water Pic® is not a substitute for a TOOTHBRUSH or DENTAL FLOSS. It does not remove the tenacious microorganisms that adhere to the surface of the teeth and form a substance called PLAQUE.

There are two basic types of irrigators. One is attached directly to the water faucet; the other uses a motor-driven pump to generate intermittent jets of water.

WATERPROOF COSMETICS

"Waterproof" ordinarily refers to cosmetics such as eyeliners, which are resistant to PERSPIRATION, tears, and moisture in the air. Some are also resistant to SOAP and WATER and require a solvent such as mineral oil, which is usually one of the basic ingredients of cleansing creams and lotions.

Many waterproof eyeliners are composed of resin solutions or a waxy base mixed with pigment and dissolved in a volatile solvent.

No makeup is *entirely* waterproof; however, those labeled as being waterproof generally stay in place longer than other products.

WEIGHT WATCHERS INTERNATIONAL

Weight Watchers International is a chain of one hundred five franchised and eight company-owned DIET clubs founded in the early 1960s by Jean Nidetch, "a Formerly Fat Baby, Formerly Fat Child, and Formerly Fat Girl," in her words during a famous interview in 1961.

The Weight Watchers diet was developed by the late Norman Jolliffe when he headed the Bureau of Nutrition of the New York City Board of Health—the same diet Jean Nidetch was handed when she went there seeking help. It is a basic, high-PROTEIN, three-meals-a-day diet relying on fish and vegetables. It emphasizes that portions must be exactly measured, and encourages dieters to weigh all foods.

Weight Watchers members meet every week. During the meetings each member is weighed, and individual losses and gains are discussed in a group-therapy kind of atmosphere.

Weight Watchers is one of the world's largest diet clubs. As of 1974, about five million people were enrolled, some for the second time. There are other clubs, such as OVEREATERS ANONYMOUS (OA), Take Off Pounds Sensibly (TOPS), and a number of small local groups. They differ in detail and in psychological approach. For instance, at TOPS, those who gain weight usually meet with ridicule, while for OA members dieting is considered almost a religious experience. However, members of these diet clubs share the belief that talking about their compulsive overeating makes the drudgery of persevering in a diet a little easier. It is an idea that has worked for alcoholics, drug addicts and compulsive gamblers. In fact, the exact method doesn't really seem to matter—it is the personal decision to lose weight added to the sense of camaraderie and support inspired by the other members that are responsible for success.

WIGS

In the past, the only wigs an elegant woman would consider wearing were human-hair wigs. Those made of synthetic fiber were usually too shiny and too stiff, with harsh, uniform colors that hardly approximated the many tones of natural hair.

Human-hair wigs can be beautiful, and the modern ones are no longer heavy or ill-fitting, as many of them used to be. The only drawback is that they are almost always very expensive. One of the reasons, apparently, is that there are fewer and fewer European country girls who still have tresses to sell to wig manufacturers. Tresses of Far Eastern women are still collected, but the texture of Oriental hair is so different from that of Caucasian hair that it makes a wig look almost as artificial as the old-fashioned synthetic kind.

In the last ten years, scientists have perfected so-called modacrylic fibers, some of which can be woven into wigs with extraordinary results. These synthetic fibers have most of the good qualities of human hair—natural luster and color, lightweight, texture—and none of the drawbacks, such as drooping in damp weather, becoming frizzy in humidity, drying out in the wind and cold weather, absorbing dirt and unpleasant odors, fading in the sun, losing curls after a rain, getting squashed by hats and scarves, requiring expensive professional grooming, and growing out of a favorite hairdo.

Not all synthetic wigs are made the same way, but the simplest and most comfortable wigs have the synthetic fibers attached to an elasticized netlike cap that fits almost all heads. Certain wigs have separate strips of elastic sewn in front, at the sides, or at the nape of the neck, where some also have hooks and eyes to allow for adjustment, in case a woman's head is slightly larger or smaller than the average. Other wigs have fibers that are woven into the elastic cap itself. All are designed to remain in the desired position despite wind or movements of the head.

Wigs of better quality have a hand-finished hairline, i.e., one with several hairs knitted together in such a way as to stand away from a woman's hairline as real hairs do and without revealing the underlying net. The base is usually skin-colored so that the wig's strands can be parted anywhere and still look natural.

Modacrylic wigs, such as Kane, Elura®, Kalon® and Venicelon®, are made in dozens of different styles, but a good hairdresser can adjust them further by thinning them at the crown or trimming the ends or the bangs. Synthetic wigs can also be restyled with curlers (ELECTRIC CURLERS can be used only when so specified on the label) but all return to the original styling after a shampoo, unless combed while still wet.

In order for a wig to look natural and avoid unsightly lumps, a woman's own hair should be arranged first. If it is short, it can just be combed back and held in place with a few pins. If it is long, it should be neatly wrapped around the head or divided and pinned into wide, flat curls, or rolled into a flat, tight chignon. *Vogue* magazine once suggested that, for extra crown height, women could knot on top of the head an old nylon stocking with the foot snipped off; the hair could then be tucked inside. The wig is put on front to back, like a bathing cap, then pulled down on both sides at the ears—without covering them—and adjusted to the right position. Sometimes a lock of front hair can be left out, set in a curler, and later combed over the wig for a more natural hairline.

Traditionally, black women have been particularly interested in wigs, mostly as a fashion accessory but often as a necessity—between hair-straightening sessions, for instance, or instead of straightening, in cases when hair is weakened by the excessive or unprofessional use of harsh straightening products. However, for years wigs have offered to

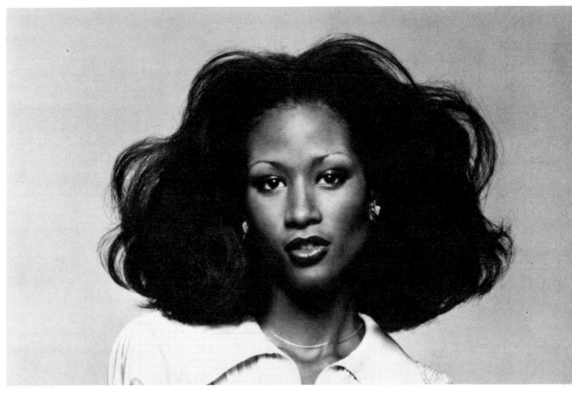

A young model wearing a wig from the Naomi Sims collection. The wig is made of a synthetic fiber called Kanekalon Presselle that looks and feels like the black woman's straightened hair. *Courtesy of Kaneka America Corporation.*

Left: Sheila Anderson, a twenty-one-year-old New York model and actress, with her own straightened hair, waiting to be fitted with a new wig.

Right: Sheila Anderson wearing the wig she has chosen from the collection of Joseph Plaskett, the owner of Hair Styling by Joseph, one of the best known interracial beauty salons in New York.

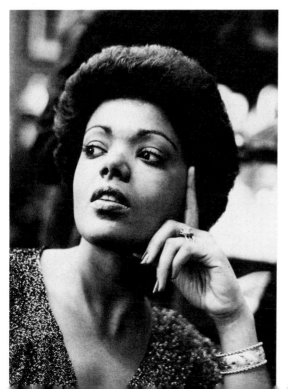
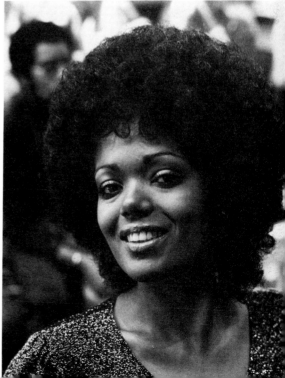

black women only simulated Caucasian hair that hardly resembled the texture and shade of either curly or straightened hair. For a short while in the 1960s, when the "natural" style became popular, many young black women dispensed with both wigs and hair-straightening. Soon, however, they found out that keeping real hair fluffy and symmetrically curled, as the "natural" style required, was just as time-consuming as, and called for even more care than, the periodic straightening. For them, as well as for women with hair that was not thick enough or curly enough for a natural "natural," the alternative became, once more, the wig.

In 1973 the first wigs for black women ever to reproduce successfully *straightened* hair finally appeared. They were created by Naomi Sims, who not only has been one of the most famous fashion models in the United States but has always been keenly aware of black women's special hair problems. Together with the research staff of Metropa Company, Ltd., Naomi Sims developed Kanekalon Presselle®, a special modacrylic fiber that duplicates the texture, body and sheen of the black woman's hair—both straightened and curly.

Kanekalon's raw material is provided by the Kanegafuchi Chemical Industry Co., Ltd., of Japan. The wigs themselves are manufactured in Korea by the Metropa Company and distributed in the United States and abroad.

Modacrylic wigs should be brushed once in a while with a wire-bristle brush and combed with a wide-toothed comb. They can all be shampooed—once a month is more than sufficient. They should be soaked in cold water and a mild SOAP (or wig cleanser) for five minutes, then squeezed gently and rinsed repeatedly. Then they should be shaken and hung to dry; an ELECTRIC HAIR-STYLER should never be used. Once they are dry, they should be shaken and gently brushed.

Unless so specified on the label, modacrylic wigs should never be dyed or color-rinsed. Neither should they be brushed while wet, which may cause them to become permanently straightened. There is no need for a wig block: most of them can be stored or packed in their own boxes or rolled inside plastic bags without ever losing their shape.

WITCH HAZEL

Witch hazel is distilled from the leaves and/or the bark of a common shrub of eastern North America, *Hamamelis virginiana*. It may be used as a skin freshener, a local ANAESTHETIC and an astringent.

Witch hazel contains about 75 percent ethanol, an antibacterial used in many cosmetic products, and about 5 percent tannin, an astringent. Commercially available witch hazel is a diluted solution containing only 15 percent ethanol.

XEROGRAPHY

Xerography is one of the most recently developed methods for early detection of BREAST CANCER. It resembles MAMMOGRAPHY, except that the X-ray image of the breast is recorded on a selenium-coated plate rather than on photographic film. In other words, xerography is a *photoelectric* process, whereas mammography is a *photochemical* one.

The accuracy of xerography is higher than that of mammography—95 percent. It results in a picture in which all the tissues of the breast, including the skin, are better defined in a single exposure. Also, there is less X-ray exposure; no darkroom is needed, the image has the same size of the object, and its interpretation is extremely easy and rapid.

Incidentally, the principal aim of xerography is not accuracy, but the discovery of very small tumors that escape detection by other means. Xerography is also useful for patients who are about to undergo BIOPSY, or patients with a family history of cancer.

Since physical examination, THERMOGRAPHY and xerography (or mammography) seem to detect different types of cancers, their combined use in screening for breast cancer is most important.

RELIABLE SOURCES OF
INFORMATION FOR LAYMEN

Allergy Foundation
80 Second Avenue
New York, N.Y. 10017

American Cancer Society
19 West 56th Street
New York, N.Y. 10019

American Dental Association
211 East Chicago Avenue
Chicago, Ill. 60611

American Dietetic Association
629 North Michigan
Chicago, Ill. 60611

American Lung Association
1740 Broadway
New York, N.Y. 10019

American Medical Association
535 North Dearborn Street
Chicago, Ill. 60610

American Society of Clinical Hypnosis
800 Washington Avenue
Minneapolis, Minn. 55414

Better Business Bureau
115 Fifth Avenue
New York, N.Y. 10003

Consumer Product Safety Commission
7315 Wisconsin Avenue
Bethesda, Md. 20016

Consumers' Research, Inc.
Bowerstown Road
Washington, N.J. 07882

Department of Health, Education and Welfare
330 Independence Avenue S.W.
Washington, D.C. 20201

La Leche League, International
9616 Minneapolis Avenue
Franklin Park, Ill. 60131

Maternity Center Association
48 East 92nd Street
New York, N.Y. 10028

National Hearing Aid Society
24261 Grand River
Detroit, Mich. 48219

National Migraine Foundation
2422 West Foster Avenue
Chicago, Ill. 60625

New York Academy of Medicine
2 East 103rd Street
New York, N.Y. 10029

RELIABLE SOURCES OF INFORMATION FOR LAYMEN

New York Academy of Science
2 East 63rd Street
New York, N.Y. 10021

New York City Department of Health
Bureau of Nutrition
93 Worth Street, Room 714
New York, N.Y. 10013

New York State Chiropractic Association
45 John Street
New York, N.Y. 10038

Planned Parenthood World Population
Information and Education Department
810 Seventh Avenue
New York, N.Y. 10019

Scientists' Institute for Public Information
30 East 68th Street
New York, N.Y. 10021

Society of Cosmetic Chemists
52 East 41st Street
New York, N.Y. 10017

Superintendent of Documents
U.S. Government Printing Office
Washington, D.C. 20402

The Contact Lens Association
of Ophthalmologists
40 West 77th Street
New York, N.Y. 10024

U.S. Department of Agriculture
Office of Information
Washington, D.C. 20250

READING LIST

ALLEN, LINDA, editor, *The Look You Like; Answers to Your Questions About Skin Care & Cosmetics*, Chicago, Ill., American Medical Association, 1971.

ANDELMAN, SAMUEL L., *The New Home Medical Encyclopedia*, New York, Quadrangle Books, 1973.

BING, ELISABETH, *Six Practical Lessons for an Easier Childbirth*, New York, Bantam Books, 1969.

DEUTSCH, RONALD M., *The Family Guide to Better Food and Better Health*, Des Moines, Ia., Creative Home Library, 1971.

DORFMAN, Wilfred, *Closing the Gap Between Medicine and Psychiatry*, Springfield, Ill., Charles C Thomas, 1966.

EIGER, MARVIN S. and SALLY WENDKOS OLDS, *The Complete Book of Breastfeeding*, New York, Bantam Books, 1973.

EWY, DONNA and RODGER, *Preparation for Childbirth, a Lamaze Guide*, Boulder, Colorado, Pruett Publishing Company, 1970.

FREESE, ARTHUR S., *Headaches: The Kinds and the Cures*, New York, Doubleday, 1973.

FRIEDMAN, AROLD P. and SHERVERT H. FRAZIER, *The Headache Book*, New York, Dodd, Mead, 1973.

GALLWEY, W. TIMOTHY, *The Inner Game of Tennis*, New York, Random House, 1974.

GERRARD, JOHN W., *Understanding Allergies*, Springfield, Ill., Charles C. Thomas, 1973.

GUTCHEON, BETH, *Abortion: A Woman's Guide*, for Planned Parenthood of NYC, Inc., New York, Abelard-Schuman, 1973.

LUCE, GAY GAER, *Body Time: Physiological Rhythms and Social Stress*, New York, Pantheon Books, 1971.

LUCE, GAY GAER and JULIUS SEGAL, *Sleep*, New York, Coward, McCann, 1966.

MARGOLIUS, SIDNEY, *Health Foods: Facts and Fakes*, New York, Walker, 1973.

——, *The Consumer's Guide to Better Buying*, New York, Simon & Schuster, 1972.

MARX, INA, *Yoga and Common Sense*, New York, Bobbs-Merrill, 1970.

MAYER, JEAN, *Overweight: Causes, Cost and Control*, Englewood Cliffs, N.J., Prentice-Hall, 1968.

MORINI, SIMONA, *Body Sculpture*, New York, Delacorte Press, 1972.

READING LIST

NETZER, CORINNE, *The Brand Name Calorie Counter*, New York, Dell, 1971.

NEWBOLD, H. L., *Mega-Nutrients for Your Nerves*, New York, Peter H. Wyden, 1975.

RANDOLPH, THERON G., *Human Ecology & Susceptibility to the Chemical Environment*, Springfield, Ill., Charles C Thomas, 1972.

SAGARIN, EDWARD, *The Science and Art of Perfumery*, New York, Greenberg, 1955.

SAGARIN, EDWARD and M. S. BALSAM, editors, *Cosmetics: Science and Technology*, New York, Wiley-Interscience, 1972.

SHELMIRE, BEDFORD, JR., *The Art of Looking Younger*, New York, St. Martin's Press, 1973.

SIMS, NAOMI, *Naomi Sims' All About Health and Beauty for the Black Woman*, New York, Doubleday, 1976.

SOLOMON, NEIL and SALLY SHEPPARD, *The Truth About Weight Control: How to Lose Excess Pounds Permanently*, New York, Stein & Day, 1972.

TODD, MABEL L., *The Thinking Body: A Study of the Balancing Forces of Dynamic Man*, New York, Dance Horizon, 1968.

Vogue magazine, "Health and Beauty," New York, The Condé Nast Publications.

Vogue Beauty & Health Guide, New York, The Condé Nast Publications, 1973–74 and 1974–75.

VOLIN, MICHAEL and NANCY PHELAN, *Yoga for Women*, New York, Harper & Row, 1973.

ZIMMERMAN, DAVID R., *Rh: The Intimate History of a Disease and Its Conquest*, New York, Macmillan, 1973.

SOURCES AND ACKNOWLEDGMENTS

ADAMSON, DR. JAMES, chief of department of plastic surgery, Norfolk General Hospital, Norfolk, Virginia   (HAND LIFT)

AITKEN, DR. GERALD J., internist, New Jersey   (DRUG INTERACTION)

ALTCHEK, DR. ALBERT, associate professor of obstetrics and gynecology, Mount Sinai School of Medicine, New York City   (ABORTION)

ANDERSON, SHEILA, fashion model and actress, New York City   (BLACK HAIR)

ARTINIAN, GARO, director, Kree Institute of Electrolysis, Inc., New York City   (ELECTROLYSIS)

ASHLEY, DR. FRANKLIN L., chief of division of plastic surgery, UCLA, Los Angeles, California   (SILICONES)

ASLAN, PROFESSOR ANA, director, Institute of Geriatrics, Bucharest, Rumania   (AGE RETARDATION)

BAUM, DR. GILBERT, director, ultrasound laboratory, Albert Einstein College of Medicine, New York City   (MAMMOGRAPHY)

BAUM, DR. JULES L., associate professor of ophthalmology, Tufts University School of Medicine, Medford, Massachusetts   (SOFT CONTACT LENSES)

BEHRMAN, DR. STANLEY J., oral surgeon in charge, oral surgeon and dentistry department, New York Hospital–Cornell Medical Center, New York City   (ORAL SURGERY)

BLACKMON, ROSEMARY, editor, *Vogue* Magazine, New York City   (FATIGUE)

BRALEY, SILAS, director, Dow Corning Center for Aid to Medical Research, Midland, Michigan   (SILICONES)

BRUCH, DR. HILDE, professor of psychiatry, Baylor College of Medicine, Houston, Texas   (ANOREXIA NERVOSA)

BUONOCORE, DR. MICHAEL, dentist, Rochester, New York   (DENTAL SEALANT)

CAMMER, DR. LEONARD, author, *Up From Depression*   (NERVOUS BREAKDOWN)

CANNON, DR. WALTER B., physiologist, Harvard University Medical School, Boston, Massachusetts   (HOMEOSTASIS)

CODDON, DR. DAVID R., associate professor of neurology; founder, Headache Clinic, Mount Sinai Medical Center, New York City   (HEADACHES)

COX, DR. CHARLES D., University of Massachusetts Medical School, Worcester, Massachusetts   (SYPHILIS)

SOURCES AND ACKNOWLEDGMENTS

CRILE, DR. GEORGE, JR., emeritus consultant, department of general surgery, Cleveland Clinic Foundation, Cleveland, Ohio   (MASTECTOMY)

CRONIN, DR. THOMAS D., clinical professor of plastic surgery, Baylor University, Houston, Texas   (PLASTIC SURGERY)

DAM, PROFESSOR HENRIK, Copenhagen, Denmark   (VITAMIN K)

DEBEVOISE, CHARLES R., inventor, France   (BRASSIERES)

DUFOURMENTEL, DR. CLAUDE, plastic surgeon, Paris, France   (MAMMAPLASTY)

DUKAN, DR. PIERRE, author, *La Cellulite en Question*, France   (CELLULITE)

DURHAM, OREN C., American Academy of Allergy   (RAGWEED POLLEN INDEX)

FIEVE, DR. RONALD R., chief of psychiatric research, New York State Psychiatric Institute, Columbia Presbyterian Medical Center, New York City (LITHIUM CARBONATE)

FISCHER, DR. JACK C., associate professor of plastic surgery, University of Virginia School of Medicine, Charlottesville, Virginia   (PLASTIC SURGERY)

FLEMING, SIR ALEXANDER, chemist, England   (ANTIBIOTICS)

FREESE, DR. ARTHUR S., author, *Headaches: The Kinds and the Cures* (HEADACHES)

FUTORAN, DR. JACK M., gynecologist, University of California, San Francisco, California   (INTRAUTERINE DEVICES)

GARCIA, DR. RAYMOND L., dermatologist, Lackland Air Force Base, Texas (EARLOBE PIERCING)

GERRARD, DR. JOHN W., professor of pediatrics, University of Saskatchewan, Canada   (ALLERGY)

GILLIES, SIR HAROLD, plastic surgeon, England   (PLASTIC SURGERY)

GWALTNEY, DR. JACK, head of division of epidemiology and virology, University of Virginia School of Medicine, Charlottesville, Virginia   (COMMON COLD)

HAWKINS, DR. DAVID, director of psychiatric research, Brunswick Hospital, Long Island, New York   (ORTHOMOLECULAR MEDICINE)

HIRSCH, DR. JULES, head of department of human behavior and metabolism, Rockefeller University, New York City   (OBESITY)

HODGE, DR. JAMES R., head of psychiatric section, Akron City Hospital, Akron, Ohio   (HYPNOTHERAPY)

HOFFER, DR. ABRAHAM, biochemist, Huxley Institute for Biosocial Research, New York City   (ORTHOMOLECULAR MEDICINE)

JACOB, DR. STANLEY W., professor of surgery, University of Oregon, Portland, Oregon   (DIMETHYL SULFOXIDE)

JOLLIFFE, NORMAN, one-time head of Bureau of Nutrition, New York City Board of Health   (WEIGHT WATCHERS INTERNATIONAL)

KALSØ, ANNE, costume designer, Denmark   (EARTH SHOES)

KARMAN, HARVEY, psychologist, Los Angeles, California   (MENSTRUAL EXTRACTION)

KIPPING, FREDERICK STANLEY, chemist, England   (SILICONES)

KLIEFF, DR. GILBERT, oral surgeon, Michigan   (DIETS)

KLIGMAN, DR. ALBERT M., professor of dermatology, University of Pennsylvania School of Medicine, Philadelphia, Pennsylvania   (ACNE)

KNUDSEN, DR. VERN O., pioneer in acoustics   (NOISE POLLUTION)

KRAKOWSKI, DR. ADAM J., chief of division of psychiatric liaison and research, Champlain Valley-Physician's Hospital Medical Center, Plattsburgh, New York   (PSYCHOSOMATIC DISEASES)

KREE, PAUL M., inventor   (ELECTROLYSIS)

LAMAZE, DR. FERNAND, gynecologist, France   (PREPARED CHILDBIRTH)

LEIS, DR. HENRY P., JR., clinical professor of surgery; chief of breast surgery service, New York Medical School, New York City   (MAMMOGRAPHY)

LEWIS, DR. HENRY M., dermatologist, Denver, Colorado   (HERPES SIMPLEX)

LING, PER HENRIK, medical-gymnastic practitioner, Sweden   (MASSAGE)

LUBIC, RUTH, general director, Maternity Center Association, New York City   (MIDWIFERY)

LUCE, GAY GAER, author, *Body Time*, et al.   (BODY CYCLES; HYPERSOMNIA)

MAIBACH, DR. HOWARD I., department of dermatology, University of California School of Medicine, San Francisco, California   (PATCH TESTING)

MAYER, DR. JEAN, professor of nutrition, Harvard University Medical School, Boston, Massachusetts   (DIETS)

MC GRATH, MARIE, hair colorist, New York City   (HAIR FROSTING)

MC INDOE, SIR ARCHIBALD, plastic surgeon, England   (PLASTIC SURGERY)

MELZACK, DR. RONALD, professor of psychology, McGill University, Montreal, Canada   (PAIN)

MELNICK, DR. JOSEPH L., professor of virology and epidemiology, Baylor College of Medicine, Houston, Texas   (HERPES SIMPLEX)

MICHAEL, DR. RICHARD P., department of psychiatry, Emory University School of Medicine, Atlanta, Georgia   (PHEROMONES)

MILLER, DR. CHARLES CONRAD, general practitioner and surgeon, Chicago, Illinois   (RHYTIDECTOMY)

MOULY, DR. ROGER, plastic surgeon, Paris, France   (MAMMAPLASTY)

MONROE, MARILYN, Hollywood film star   (BRASSIERES)

NABATOFF, DR. ROBERT A., associate clinical professor of vascular surgery, chief of vascular clinic, Mount Sinai School of Medicine, New York City   (VARICOSE VEINS)

NIDETCH, JEAN, founder, Weight Watchers International, Inc.   (WEIGHT WATCHERS INTERNATIONAL)

NIEHANS, DR. PAUL, founder, Clinic La Prairie, Clarence-Montreux, Switzerland   (AGE RETARDATION)

NOËL, DR. SUZANNE, plastic surgeon, Paris, France   (RHYTIDECTOMY)

NOLEN, DR. WILLIAM A., author, *The Making of a Surgeon*   (MASTECTOMY)

OLDS, SALLY WENDKOS, author, *The Complete Book of Breastfeeding* (LACTATION)

OSMOND, DR. HUMPHREY, biochemist, Huxley Institute for Biosocial Research, New York City   (ORTHOMOLECULAR MEDICINE)

PAPANICOLAOU, DR. GEORGE, Greek anatomist and physician   (PAP SMEAR TEST)

PARÉ, AMBROISE (1510–90), personal surgeon of Charles IX of France (PLASTIC SURGERY)

PATERSON, JOYA, vice-president, S & S Industries, Inc., New York City (BRASSIERES)

PAULING, PROFESSOR LINUS, biochemist, New York City   (ORGANIC FOOD; ORTHOMOLECULAR MEDICINE)

PAULSEN, DR. C. ALVIN, University of Washington, Seattle   (MALE CONTRACEPTIVE PILL)

PAVLOV, IVAN, Russian physiologist   (PREPARED CHILDBIRTH)

PEEL, ROBERT, senior research consultant, Hanes Corporation, New York City   (PANTYHOSE)

PHILLIPS, DR. DAVID M., scientist, Population Council, Rockefeller University, New York City   (CONCEPTION)

PILATES, JOSEPH H., German gymnast   (EXERCISE)

PITANGUY, DR. IVO, plastic surgeon, Rio de Janeiro, Brazil   (MAMMAPLASTY)

PLASKETT, JOSEPH, hairstylist, New York City   (HAIR STRAIGHTENERS)

POPOV, DR. IVAN, director, Renaissance Revitalization Center, Nassau, Bahamas   (BEAUTY SPAS)

RAITEN, ALLEN, certified hearing-aid dealer, New York City   (HEARING AIDS)

RANDOLPH, DR. THERON G., internist, Lutheran General Hospital Park Ridge, Illinois   (FOOD ALLERGY)

RAPP, DR. FRED, virologist, Milton S. Hershey Medical Center, Pennsylvania State University, Hershey, Pennsylvania   (HERPES SIMPLEX)

RIEGER, DR. MARTIN M., chemist, associate director of chemistry, consumer products division, Warner-Lambert Company, Morris Plains, New Jersey   (HAIR WAVING)

RODIN, LINDA, photographer, New York City   (MAKEUP)

RONSARD, NICOLE, beautician, New York City   (CELLULITE)

RUSSELL, JANE, Hollywood film star   (BRASSIERES)

SAXENA, DR. BRIJ B., professor of endocrinology and biochemistry, New York Hospital–Cornell Medical Center, New York City   (PREGNANCY TESTS)

SCOMMEGNA, DR. ANTONIO, gynecologist, department of obstetrics and gynecology, Michael Reese Medical Center, Chicago, Illinois   (INTRAUTERINE DEVICES)

SCHAEFER, DR. GEORGE, obstetrician, New York City   (NAUSEA)

SCRIBONIUS LARGUS, court physician to Emperor Claudius   (PAIN)

SEGAL, DR. JULIUS, co-author, *Sleep*   (HYPERSOMNIA)

SELYE, DR. HANS, director, Institute of Experimental Medicine and Surgery, University of Montreal, Canada   (FATIGUE)

SHEALY, DR. CLYDE NORMAN, director, Pain Rehabilitation Center, St. Francis Hospital, La Crosse, Wisconsin   (PAIN)

SHELDON, DR. WILLIAM H., physical anthropologist, Massachusetts   (SOMATOTYPE)

SHELMIRE, DR. BEDFORD, JR., professor of dermatology, Southwestern Medical School, University of Texas   (CHEMICAL PEEL)

SIMS, NAOMI, former fashion model, author, *Naomi Sims' All About Health and Beauty for the Black Woman*   (WIGS)

SNYDERMAN, DR. REUVEN K., plastic surgeon, Princeton, New Jersey   (BREAST RECONSTRUCTION)

SOICHET, DR. SAMUEL, professor of obstetrics and gynecology, Cornell Medical College, New York City   (INTRAUTERINE DEVICES)

SORENSEN, DR. JOHN R. J., University of Cincinnati Medical School, Cincinnati, Ohio   (ASPIRIN)

STRÖMBECK, DR. OLOF, plastic surgeon, Stockholm, Sweden   (MAMMAPLASTY)

STRONG, DR. DANIEL, dentist, New York City   (ELECTROSURGERY)

SWANSON, DR. ALFRED B., chief of department of orthopedic surgery, Blodgett Memorial Hospital, Grand Rapids, Michigan   (ARTHRITIS)

TAGLIACOZZI, GASPARO (1546–99), surgeon from Bologna; author, *The Surgery of Deformities by Transplantation*   (PLASTIC SURGERY)

TAMBURINO, ELBA, manicurist/pedicurist, New York City   (MANICURE)

TAPPEL, A. L., researcher, University of California, San Francisco, California   (VITAMIN E)

TATUM, DR. HOWARD J., associate director, biomedical division, Rockefeller University, New York City   (intrauterine devices)

TRIER, CAROLA, instructor, body conditioning and rehabilitation, New York City   (EXERCISE)

TURNER, SHIRLEY, housewife, England   (DIETS)

VON BAEYER, ADOLF, German chemist   (BARBITURATES)

VON WASSERMAN, DR. AUGUST, German bacteriologist   (WASSERMAN TESTS)

WATSON, DR. JOHN E., chief of audiology-speech pathology service, Veterans Administration Hospital, Palo Alto, California   (NOISE POLLUTION)

WITTIG, DR. HEINZ J., professor, division of allergy and clinical immunology, University of Florida College of Medicine, Gainesville, Florida   (FOOD ALLERGY)

ZUCKERMAN, DR. HERMAN C., radiologist, New York City   (MAMMOGRAPHY)

INDEX

Following each entry is a list of the main headings under which that subject is discussed. **Boldface** *indicates that the entry is itself a main heading.*

ABORTION
  Contraception; Intrauterine Device;
    Pregnancy Tests; Prostaglandins
ABRASION
  Acne; Dermabrasion
ABRASIVE CLEANSERS
  Thinners
ACEROLA
  Organic Food; Vitamin C
ACETAMINOPHEN
  Aspirin; Headaches
ACIDITY
  Cosmetics; pH
ACNE
  Actinotherapy; Antibiotics; Chemical Peel;
    Contraceptive Pill; Cysts; Dermabrasion;
    Detergents; Silicones; Thinners;
    Vitamin E
ACRYLIC
  Contact Lenses
ACTINIC KERATOSES (SOLAR
    KERATOSES)
  Skin Cancer
ACTINOTHERAPY
  Acne

ACUPUNCTURE
  Backache; Headaches; Pain
ADDICTION
  Anorectics; Barbiturates; Food Allergy
ADDITIVES
  Food Additives; Shampoos
ADIPOCYTES
  Obesity
ADIPOSE TISSUE
  Cellulite; Fats; Glucose; Obesity; Silicones
ADRENAL GLANDS
  Asthma; Cholesterol; Hirsutism; Insect
    Stings; Vitamin A
AEROSOL
  Antiperspirants; Hair Sprays; Mouthwashes
AFTERBIRTH
  Placenta
AFTERPAINS
AGE RETARDATION
AGING
  Age Retardation; Bath Oils; Brassieres;
    Hypertension; Immunology; Varicose
    Veins
AIR POLLUTION
  Allergy; Noise Pollution

393

INDEX

INDEX

INDEX

INDEX

INDEX

INDEX

404

INDEX

INDEX

INDEX

INDEX

INDEX

INDEX

416

INDEX

INDEX

INDEX

INDEX

INDEX